The
30-Day
Diabetes
Miracle

Lifestyle Center of America's Complete Program for Overcoming Diabetes, Restoring Health, and Rebuilding Natural Vitality

Franklin House, M.D.
Stuart A. Seale, M.D.
Ian Blake Newman

A PERIGEE BOOK

A PERIGEE BOOK
Published by the Penguin Group
Penguin Group (USA) Inc.
375 Hudson Street, New York, New York 10014, USA
Penguin Group (Canada), 90 Eglinton Avenue East, Suite 700, Toronto, Ontario M4P 2Y3, Canada (a division of Pearson Penguin Canada Inc.) • Penguin Books Ltd., 80 Strand, London WC2R 0RL, England • Penguin Group Ireland, 25 St. Stephen's Green, Dublin 2, Ireland (a division of Penguin Books Ltd.) • Penguin Group (Australia), 250 Camberwell Road, Camberwell, Victoria 3124, Australia (a division of Pearson Australia Group Pty. Ltd.) • Penguin Books India Pvt. Ltd., 11 Community Centre, Panchsheel Park, New Delhi—110 017, India • Penguin Group (NZ), 67 Apollo Drive, Rosedale, North Shore 0632, New Zealand (a division of Pearson New Zealand Ltd.) • Penguin Books (South Africa) (Pty.) Ltd., 24 Sturdee Avenue, Rosebank, Johannesburg 2196, South Africa

Penguin Books Ltd., Registered Offices: 80 Strand, London WC2R 0RL, England

While the author has made every effort to provide accurate telephone numbers and Internet addresses at the time of publication, neither the publisher nor the author assumes any responsibility for errors, or for changes that occur after publication. Further, the publisher does not have any control over and does not assume any responsibility for author or third-party websites or their content.

Copyright © 2008 by Ardmore Institutes of Health
Interior photos by Davidography
Interior illustrations by David S. Hemmer
Text design by Pauline Neuwirth, Neuwirth & Associates, Inc.
Cover design by Elizabeth Sheehan
Cover photos by JupiterImages

PRINTING HISTORY
Perigee hardcover edition / January 2008
Perigee trade paperback edition / January 2009

Perigee trade paperback ISBN: 978-0-399-53476-8

The Library of Congress has cataloged the Perigee hardcover edition as follows:

House, Franklin.
The 30-day diabetes miracle : Lifestyle Center of America's complete program to stop diabetes, restore health, and build natural vitality / Franklin House, Stuart A. Seale, Ian Blake Newman.
p. cm.
"A Perigee book."
Includes bibliographical references and index.
ISBN-13: 978-0-399-53386-0
1. Diabetes—Diet therapy—Popular works. 2. Diabetes—Nutritional aspects—Popular works. I. Seale, Stuart A. II. Newman, Ian Blake. III. Title.
RC662.H68 2008
616.4'620654—dc22   2007034901

PRINTED IN THE UNITED STATES OF AMERICA
10 9 8 7 6

PUBLISHER'S NOTE: Neither the publisher nor the author is engaged in rendering professional advice or services to the individual reader. The ideas, procedures, and suggestions contained in this book are not intended as a substitute for consulting with your physician. All matters regarding your health require medical supervision. Neither the author not the publisher shall be liable or responsible for any loss or damage allegedly arising from any information or suggestion in this book.

The recipes contained in this book are to be followed exactly as written. The publisher is not responsible for your specific health or allergy needs that may require medical supervision. The publisher is not responsible for any adverse reactions to the recipes contained in this book.

Most Perigee books are available at special quantity discounts for bulk purchases for sales promotions, premiums, fund-raising, or educational use. Special books, or book excerpts, can also be created to fit specific needs. For details, write: Special Markets, Penguin Group (USA) Inc., 375 Hudson Street, New York, New York 10014.

WE INVITE READERS of *The 30-Day Diabetes Miracle* to access extensive supplementary materials on our website. You can download articles, view success stories, get recipes, connect with other readers, and find many other exclusive resources.

www.diabetesmiracle.org
(password: miracle)

WE GRATEFULLY DEDICATE this book to two of Lifestyle Center of America's legends: Layton Sutton, MD, and Ruth (Selby) Brown Martin.

Layton was a member of our board from its inception in 1963 until his death in 2007 after a valiant battle against cancer. He served as its chairman from 1998 to 2004, and president thereafter. His leadership and quiet, thoughtful diplomacy were prized by all of us.

"Ruthie" grew up with Lifestyle Center of America's founder, Otey Johnson, and was his childhood chum and lifelong confidant. She is an inspiration to us, and an indefatigable ambassador of our mission.

•

Contents

Stop Diabetes
Before It Stops You

COULD YOU CALL IT A CURE?

CONGRATULATIONS! BY PICKING up this book you've taken the first step toward a lifestyle that is a big leap in beating your diabetes—even vanquishing its nasty ravages, and soon.

We're going to assume that you or someone you care about has diabetes or is worried about it. You might be suffering right now from the devastating complications of uncontrolled diabetes—bad eyes, beat-up kidneys, a weak heart, and numb or painful feet. Maybe you've been told you have "prediabetes." Or maybe you still *feel* okay, but you're aware that your extra pounds, your high cholesterol, and your up-and-down blood sugar levels are going to get you in the end.

There are more than 21 million people with diabetes in the United States—7 percent of the population. More than 41 million more people have prediabetes.[1] In some places, like New York City, more than *1 in 8* people already have diabetes.[2] And soon even those numbers will seem small: The Centers for Disease Control and Prevention (CDC) estimates that *1 in 3* children born in the United States in 2000 are expected to get diabetes in their lifetimes.[3] We're not talking about a minor inconvenience here or even just a run-of-the-mill epidemic. Diabetes is a serious, chronic, pervasive disease that has rapidly grown into a crisis and will soon become a bona fide catastrophe. We probably don't have to tell you that. After all, your own life is on the line.

Sound pretty grim? Well, we have great news. There's an excellent chance that if you follow our counsel you can stop the progress of diabetes in its tracks and even *reverse* some of the damage that diabetes might have already done to your body. We know this is a radical claim, but we've seen it time and again with thousands of our own patients. In the 1990s, when Dean Ornish, John McDougal, and Caldwell Esselstyn, our colleagues in lifestyle medicine, proved that coronary artery disease could be reversed with a healthy, low cholesterol diet—and in most cases with *no* cholesterol-lowering drugs—many mainstream doctors scoffed. Now the evidence is overwhelming.[4] Ornish, McDougal, and Esselstyn pioneered the lifestyle medicine approach to the treatment of coronary artery disease, and we've done the same with diabetes.

HEALING VS. CURING

●

HEALING and curing are related but not equivalent concepts, and they should not be confused.

Curing is the province of the physician in an acute medical care setting. Doctors are trained to try to cure disease and alleviate pain. Within the existing system, a good patient *is* patient; he or she is a passive recipient of the physician's art and skill.

Healing is something quite different. Healing is something a physician *can't* do for a patient, no matter how hard he or she might want to. Healing can come only from within each individual. Healing is the physical, mental, emotional, social, and spiritual process of becoming whole again.[5] At Lifestyle Center of America, and in this book, we're interested in both healing and curing.

For the past 11 years at Lifestyle Center of America (LCA), our not-for-profit intensive health resort in southern Oklahoma, we've proven that if you follow the 30-Day Diabetes Miracle program of eating *the right kinds of foods, getting active in the right way,* and *thinking the right way,* you can conquer diabetes just as dramatically and very likely with much less medication—even much less insulin. For years, our patients have been asking us to put our intensive 18-day program into a book so millions of diabetes patients could learn at home. Well, here it is. We're going to focus on people with type-2 diabetes, but the information can be very relevant for those with type-1 diabetes as well, for reasons we will explain later. Whether you've been diagnosed with type-1 diabetes, type-2 diabetes, prediabetes, insulin resistance, syndrome X, or metabolic syndrome, the 30-Day Diabetes Miracle program will help you feel better; worry less; live a fuller, more meaningful life; and assume responsibility for your health and future. We call that *quality of life*. And we'll show you how to get it now and how to hold onto it forever.

How much can we promise? Most doctors and patients still think of diabetes as incurable. We don't exactly agree. What would you call it if your doctor were eventually unable to detect *any evidence of diabetes*, or see *any sign of the disease process* at work? Could you call it a genuine cure? That would be your call.

DIABETES:
Good News, for Once

MUCH OF WHAT you hear or read about diabetes is riddled with myths, ignorance, and misconceptions. Here are a few encouraging truths about diabetes, right up front.

- **Diabetes is *not* a death sentence.** A diagnosis of type-1 or type-2 diabetes does not mean you will have to die earlier than your peers who do not have diabetes. While it's true that the risk for death among people with diabetes is about twice that of people without diabetes of similar age,[6] your *lifestyle choices* about diet and physical activity can have a tremendous influence on your health, well-being, and longevity. And the lifestyle option is often much better than the drug option. If you make well-informed choices, diabetes doesn't have to affect how healthy you are, how good you feel, and how long you live. In fact, as a consequence of following the 30-Day Diabetes Miracle program, there's a good chance you'll be able to live even longer than your peers who don't have diabetes, despite your diabetes!
- **Having diabetes does *not* mean you will have awful complications.** Your diabetes diagnosis does not mean you will eventually go blind, require dialysis, and suffer the trauma of amputations. The commonsense lifestyle changes in diet and

activity outlined in *The 30-Day Diabetes Miracle* can drastically reduce and often eliminate such complications.

- **Diabetes is *not* primarily a genetic disease.** Because your parents had diabetes does not mean you will, too. The only certainty is that if you *live your life the way your parents did,* you'll increase your chances of getting diabetes yourself and of suffering the way they did.

- **Type-2 diabetes is *not* something you catch like the flu.** While it's true that 1.5 million new cases of adult diabetes will be diagnosed this year,[7] almost all of these people developed their chronic disease through the foods they ate and other lifestyle choices, all of which were *totally within their control.* We're going to help you make the best choices.

- **A diagnosis of type-2 diabetes does *not* mean you will have to take large doses of medicine for the rest of your life.** Medications, including large doses of insulin, should not be the basis for diabetes care. Although some diabetes medicines can be effective and helpful, they are usually overprescribed, and often unnecessary, provided the patient is willing to make important lifestyle changes. A majority of our patients on the 30-Day Diabetes Miracle program significantly reduce or eliminate at least some of their diabetes medicines—including their insulin—after just a short time. This is true even for people with type-1 diabetes: They must take some insulin in order to live, but we find that, for most of these patients, less insulin leads to better health. We also find that our patients are able to reduce or eliminate many of their other medicines (such as for cholesterol and high blood pressure). There is no magic pill or secret cure for diabetes; the power comes from the *choices* you make each day.

- **It is *not* best for you to place your diabetes management solely in the hands of your doctor.** Unfortunately, even many well-meaning healthcare providers mismanage diabetes, with dire consequences for their patients and, ultimately, for our economy and our society. Of course we believe in the role of a properly trained physician with expertise in lifestyle management of diabetes. But it is also important for patients to take responsibility for their disease. An *educated, proactive patient* will work cooperatively with an encouraging doctor, jointly making key decisions for conquering the disease. You can generate your own 30-day diabetes miracle.

■ **Many healthcare experts are *not* recommending target goals that are optimal for diabetes care.** Some guidelines for diabetes control—for example, recommended blood sugar range and diet and physical activity guidelines—are *significantly suboptimal*. Although the big national diabetes organizations are respected, noble, and valuable institutions offering vital research and many fine services for people with diabetes, we believe a number of their guidelines are *not on target* for optimal health for people with diabetes. Same goes for many doctors and federal health institutions. Despite remarkable advances in research and technology, the whole diabetes industry—including the medical profession and the pharmaceutical companies—is not necessarily giving you the whole truth all the time.

■ **Diabetes is *not* uncontrollable.** We believe that *90 to 95 percent* of patients' health outcomes are attributable to lifestyle factors. Even type-1 diabetes, though it's not yet curable, can be made much easier to live with through wise lifestyle choices.

THE DIABETES HAMSTER WHEEL

WE'VE HEARD THIS tale a thousand times (literally!) from patients and their loved ones, and we're afraid we'll keep hearing it until doctors and patients recognize a major paradigm shift in the way to think about and treat diabetes.

The typical session with a certified diabetes educator begins with the pronouncement that there's "good news and bad news for people with diabetes." The good news, they'll say, is that there's tons of information available, and if you apply this newfound knowledge, you will be able to manage the progression of your disease. The bad news, they'll continue, is that everyone with diabetes will eventually die of some complication of the disease.

You might be told to eat right, watch your sugar, test your blood regularly, take your medicine, and check your feet regularly. And you might find yourself on a "spinning hamster wheel," as one of our patients put it. If you have type-2 diabetes, you probably already know this routine: You're constantly hungry, but you have no energy. For a while, your blood sugar levels might be pretty good, but soon, they creep up again. That means more and more medicine over time, but less and less understanding of what's happening to you—and what you can do about it. Even as your doctor tells you to lose weight, your oral diabetes medicine will likely lead to more and more weight gain. You feel more sluggish, so you become even less inclined to get active. Soon you find you're going on high cholesterol and high blood pressure medicines, too; this is really depressing. But it isn't until you hear your doctor use the dreaded I-word—*insulin*—that a sense of utter hopelessness washes over you. Perhaps you remember a parent or someone else close to you going on insulin—not long before they died. "If you don't *change your ways*," the doctor might say, "you're going to have to start those shots." It's a horrible prospect, but you *still* don't understand exactly what you're supposed to do to change your ways.

IF YOU KEEP DOING WHAT YOU'VE BEEN DOING, YOU'LL KEEP GETTING WHAT YOU'VE GOT

WHY SHOULDN'T YOU just stick with your current plan for managing your diabetes? After all, it's probably your doctor's orders. Consider how well your doctor's advice has been working:

- Is your need for medication or insulin decreasing or increasing?
- Is it getting easier to manage your blood sugar or harder?
- Are you losing weight or gaining?
- Do you feel more lively and energetic or less so?
- Are you now in less pain or more?
- Is your health in general and diabetes in particular getting better or worse?
- Who's in charge? You or your diabetes?

Alcoholics Anonymous has shared a wonderful maxim with the world that we think applies to the usual routine of so-called diabetes self-management: "Insanity is defined as doing the same thing again and again but expecting different results." Our 30-Day Diabetes Miracle program will show you a path back to sanity, a path to health, a path to *hope*.

IF IT'S TO BE, IT'S UP TO ME

WE CALL MANY of our patients "pushees," because their spouses, friends, or coworkers pretty much insist they come see us. Maybe someone is pushing you to read this book. Many of our patients arrive at LCA in a skeptical frame of mind. And we assume that, at this point, you might be skeptical, too. We don't expect you to just accept our word as gospel. So we ask you only to lend us your trust until we earn it for keeps. We believe that you can see dramatic results in blood sugar control, in weight loss, in cholesterol levels, and blood pressure control, all in a relatively short time and with less medicine. That should come as good news, right?

But this good news comes with a serious caveat. We'll remind you throughout this book that "If it's to be, it's up to me." In other words, your doctor won't do it for you. Even this book won't do it *for* you. You have to take charge of your own body, your own disease, and your own destiny. You have to make some fundamental but doable changes in your thinking and your behavior.

The benefits and results you get from our program will be directly related to what you put into it. If you decide you don't want to change at all, then you "will keep getting what you got," and we suspect that isn't too good or you wouldn't still be reading this book. If you pick and choose only some suggestions, we really don't know what results you will obtain. You might improve or you might not. This is the danger in going only part way with your lifestyle changes: You will likely feel continuously deprived and disappointed because you stopped some of your bad habits (though you wish you were still doing them), and at the same time, you'll likely not see the results you hoped for. It will seem as if all the effort just wasn't worth it, and you'll probably give up, ending up right back where you are now—or worse. On the other hand, we know that if you follow our plan completely for 30 days (lend us your trust), you'll experience the same impressive results we see when we treat our patients at LCA. We feel confident that when those 30 days are up, you'll keep following the plan because you feel, look, and "test" better than you likely have in a long time.

For patients who attend LCA's 18-day program, the results are amazing, especially considering there's only 15 days between the "before" and "after" laboratory tests. Many of our patients use the term *miraculous*, and we don't argue with them. Before they come to LCA, many people are told there's little or no chance they'll ever see any improvement in their diabetes. Yet, after 18 days, our patients with type-2 diabetes experience[8]:

- A nearly 20 percent drop in triglyceride levels
- Total cholesterol reduction of 16 percent (patients with type-1 diabetes do even better: 19 percent)
- A decrease in serum levels of low-density lipoprotein (LDLs), the "bad" cholesterol, by 22 percent (31 percent for those with type-1 diabetes)
- A 17 percent reduction in fasting blood sugar
- Weight reduction equal to 4.6 percent of body weight (3 percent for patients with type-1 diabetes)
- A decrease of just over 3 percent in waist circumference
- A drop in serum fructosamine[9] of 8.7 percent (13 percent for patients with type-1 diabetes)
- More than a 5 percent reduction in resting heart rate (8 percent for those with type-1 diabetes)
- A 12 percent improvement in the 1-mile walk test
- A nearly 6 percent drop in systolic blood pressure (the top number)
- A 4 percent decline in diastolic blood pressure (the bottom number)
- An 18 percent increase in flexibility (patients with type-1 diabetes improved 16 percent)

Remember—that's after only 15 days. Continuing with the lifestyle changes for the long haul will breed very dramatic results.

Not to say it's easy at first. For most of you, our program will require a major departure from the way you've been brought up to think about healthcare, disease, food, and other basic tenets of our culture. For many, this is a big adjustment. Most of us are still caught up in negative, pessimistic thinking when it comes to our health. We think:

- Our chronic disease determines our fate.
- Our doctor is our healthcare boss.
- The all-you-can-eat buffet table determines our food intake.
- When we get sick, the latest wonder drug is the solution.

- Our fear of change is in control of our behavior.
- Our unhealthy habits are binding, too potent, and too ingrained to ever change.

You get the idea. And you probably know by now that we disagree wholeheartedly with such counterproductive ways of thinking. We believe, like thousands of our patients, that the sheer will to get better can triumph over current patterns of thinking and behaving, and you can experience a 30-day diabetes miracle.

Our most successful patients are *proactive*. They have what Dr. Dennis Deaton has called an "ownership spirit."[10] They take responsibility for their thinking, their behaviors, and their consequences. For most of us, though, there are major challenges to overcome first—societal, familial, even biological and neurochemical. So we'll help you throughout this book with reminders, encouragement, and lots of practical counsel on how to start incorporating the ownership spirit into your attitudes about your diabetes and the rest of your life.

We'll spend a whole chapter (Chapter 9) describing how to motivate yourself to do what you know you should but somehow haven't been able to do—getting more active, for example, or eating the right foods for optimal health. We expect that by incorporating the basics of this scientifically validated, rational, and commonsense form of therapy, called cognitive behavior therapy (CBT), you can accelerate major change that you might otherwise feel is too difficult or even impossible to achieve.

ISN'T THIS JUST MORE OF THE SAME EAT-RIGHT-AND-EXERCISE STUFF?

PRACTICALLY SPEAKING, THE 30-Day Diabetes Miracle program is fundamentally different from the diabetes information and treatment millions of Americans have been given in the past. Here are the top 10 reasons our program substantively differs from others:

- **It actually works.** Between two of us, we have 60 years of clinical experience treating diabetes, have seen thousands of patients, and have reviewed hundreds of rigorous scientific studies that back up our program. We'll introduce you to the research and to many patients who've *reversed their diabetes* and gone on to live happier and more productive lives. We also have as a co-author Ian Blake Newman, a former patient who's experienced both the "usual" diabetes treatment as well as LCA's way, outlined in this book—Ian's our proof positive.

■ **It's all-inclusive.** The 30-Day Diabetes Miracle program brings together sensible, scientifically sound information and advice about all aspects of living healthy. And it's tailored specifically for people with diabetes.

■ **It's about lifestyle choices.** These choices are made in conjunction with the latest science and medical methods. Our program is a straightforward, realistic, and sustainable one that can quickly produce striking changes.

■ **Medications—including insulin—are secondary, not primary, for managing diabetes.** By strictly following the 30-Day Diabetes Miracle program, many of our patients can significantly reduce their oral diabetes medications, their insulin, and their blood pressure and cholesterol drugs—some within months, some within weeks, and some within mere days.

■ **It's based on a diet that's very different from the standard American diet.** There are decades worth of rigorous studies that prove irrefutably that the standard American diet (SAD, isn't it?) is killing us through obesity, high blood pressure, diabetes, and other chronic diseases. And now there are many important studies that confirm undeniably the diet we recommend to all our patients works to curb the scourge of those diseases. It's true that most doctors and diabetes organizations don't prescribe our diet, but they should. We *know* it will make people with diabetes (and almost everyone else, too) much healthier, because we've seen it with so many of our own patients. The 30-Day Diabetes Miracle diet is plant based. This means it consists of fruits, vegetables, whole grains, legumes, and nuts and seeds (in moderation). The diet is filling, thanks to high fiber; it's naturally low fat; it provides plenty of good-quality protein; and it's *high in complex carbohydrates*. We know this will surprise many people with diabetes. You'll have to read on to get the details.

■ **It gives you the complete truth.** The average person is bright, motivated, and deserving of the full truth about diabetes. We believe that we must give our patients the whole truth without dumbing down the medical evidence by assuming that our patients "will never follow the plan anyway." You and all our patients deserve the opportunity to achieve far greater health than just managing your diabetes as your condition gradually deteriorates over time. We don't want you to just get by with marginal, incorrect, or incomplete information. It's *up to you* to act on the information we provide.

- **It promotes the health benefits of a physically active lifestyle without unpleasant side effects.** The 30-Day Diabetes Miracle program incorporates a unique form of physical activity, unlike the kind you're probably used to doing—or *not* doing. Intermittent training (IT) is easier to learn, easier to do, and easier to maintain than the usual exercise prescription so many of us suffer through or strive to avoid. IT works without pain, and with little specialized training. We reject the notion of "no pain, no gain" and show that you can get *more benefits for less effort* than you've probably thought possible.

- **It helps you achieve your goals by helping you train your brain.** The CBT approach gives you the rational, down-to-earth tools you need to change your attitudes and behavior to maximize the overall benefits to your health and emotions. We help you every step of the way with practical advice about how to build all the foundations of the program into your daily life—starting today.

- **It will improve nearly all facets of your health, not just your diabetes.** The 30-Day Diabetes Miracle program integrates healthy lifestyle choices that will not only help you master your diabetes but also help you lose weight, lower your blood pressure, lower your cholesterol, escape depression, and appreciably reduce your chances of many other chronic diseases—from stroke and heart attack to arthritis and cancer.

- **It helps you address the key question of, "Good health—for what?"** Most popular health programs and most doctors overlook this question. You might say this is the spiritual side of the equation, an important pillar of the program. We ask you to consider *why* you want to overcome your diabetes, why you want to live better and longer. Is it just to get a few more years of languishing in a nursing home? We suspect there's more to it, and we want to help you articulate your answers to this important question.

CHOICES 101

ANOTHER CRITICAL POINT to the 30-Day Diabetes Miracle program is that it will allow you to make *basic choices*, tailored to your needs and abilities, about how strictly or liberally you choose to follow each part of the program. Think of it as a "choice adventure" in which you can tackle your most pressing concerns first, then move on to secondary problems. If you want maximum gains and dramatic impact in a short time—if you want miraculous results in 1 month—we recommend you follow the program to a tee, taking advantage of all our advice. If your blood sugar levels are way out of control, you're obese, have had a heart attack or stroke, smoke, and/or can't control your eating, we recommend you do this, starting ASAP.

WHO ARE WE, WHAT IS LIFESTYLE MEDICINE, AND HOW CAN WE HELP YOU STOP DIABETES?

AT LCA, INSTEAD of simply fixing the symptoms of various conditions, we help individuals get to the root of their problems—*their lifestyle*. We use the enormous power of diet, physical activity, and stress management as well as intensive, personal medical supervision to overcome disease, restore health, and build lasting vitality. We empower our patients by leading each of them through a life-changing experience to restore and maintain health. While we were designed to live in good health, misguided choices have caused many of today's chronic diseases, and diabetes tops that list. More than 2,000 people have come through our program in the past 11 years, and those who've stuck to their new lifestyle have shown remarkable results, which they frequently call "miraculous." We're setting up now for a large, comprehensive, peer-reviewed study, but we believe it's critical to get this information to you right now. Because we're asking you to lend us your trust, we want to introduce ourselves, and tell you a little about how we came to embrace the 30-Day Diabetes Miracle program.

Dr. Franklin House

I was born in Mexico City, into poverty, and came to America when I was 15, feeling culturally challenged. Education was in my blood and

DNA. So medical school seemed natural for me—the perfect synthesis of altruism from my family's missionary past and an emergent capitalism I found in the American land of opportunity. I went to Loma Linda University, got my M.D. in 1962, and did a rotating internship at the Loma Linda University Hospital. The following 2 years were devoted to military service at Fort Hood, Texas, in the U.S. Army as surgeon of the 1st Battalion of the 13th Armor.

I stayed on in Texas, and founded a multispecialty clinic, a community hospital, and a long-term-care company. Throughout medical school and in the years afterward, my altruistic and acquisitive tendencies did battle, as I suspect they do for most doctors. Things started to change for me during my time working in obstetrics. I became keenly aware of the need for basic nutritional knowledge among my young maternity patients. It comes as a shock to people that most medical school students get very limited education in nutrition, at least not in the way that nutrition education can be really useful. I could see the consequences of this omission in the prevalence of chronic disease among so many of my patients. You might come to the same conclusion just strolling though your average shopping mall.

Around this time my attention became focused on my family. My dear wife, Bonnie, had suffered with pain for years. She had what appeared to be a familial arthritic predisposition. Since the time we courted, this miserable nuisance had interfered with our lives. I started out resenting this intruder when she reacted with an "ouch" the first time I hugged her. As time passed, her pain progressed, and more joints became involved in spite of my best diagnostic and therapeutic efforts.

After my graduation from medical school, we eventually settled on a small Texas ranch. One Sunday after feeding the cows, I heard some stirring in the bedroom. What I discovered next changed my plans for that week and every one since then. Bonnie was crawling to the bathroom. "The pain is so severe I can't walk," she said, groaning. "I do this almost every day, Franklin; it's just that you leave so early you never see me do it."

That incident motivated a systematic search for an answer that we had failed to find in the many prescription drugs we had used through the years. We began exploring lifestyle treatments, mainly dietary changes. When we implemented a plant-based diet and altered our lifestyle, Bonnie found total and enduring relief. When I could squeeze her again, I began to embrace lifestyle medicine.

With this experience, I reorganized my practice to include thorough wellness evaluations, physical activity assessments and prescriptions, and lifestyle lectures. For the next dozen years Bonnie held healthy-cooking classes in our home. As I saw my patients get better, I was hooked.

When I was chairman of the board of a nonprofit organization that provides medical care to the people of Micronesia, I made some 15 medical trips between 1985 and 1996. There I saw on a large scale how lifestyle medicine can begin the process of radically altering the course of a culture's health and well-being. Currently, there are Micronesians in their early 20s who are already suffering long-term complications related to diabetes, such as amputations, blindness, and kidney failure. In my experience, North America is not more than a decade or so behind Micronesia in the demographics of diabetes.

Since I came to LCA in 2000, first as its president and now as chairman of the board, I've been encouraged that we've planted this same seed in rural Oklahoma, a place no less in need of a change in thinking and in treatment of diabetes. By now we've cared for patients from nearly every state in the union and from many different countries.

My great motivation as I enter my 70s has been to use my own vitality and health to promote lifestyle medicine to a world in need— a world very close to home now. I want to tell all the indelible individual stories of so many of our patients whose diabetes has been *stopped* and whose lives have been *restored* by following our program. The fact that you're reading this book gives me as much hope as we want to give you.

Dr. Stuart Seale

By the age of 15, I knew I wanted to become a doctor. It was the late 1960s, and everyone was watching *Marcus Welby, M.D.* on TV. In 1976, I was accepted into Loma Linda University School of Medicine, and I graduated in 1979. The pull of Dr. Welby won me over to family medicine, and after I completed residency in 1983, I entered the private medical world on top of my game. I had received excellent medical education and residency training, and felt I was competent to handle whatever came my way. The American medical system is one of the best in the world when it comes to intervening and treating the acute crises our patients face in their battles with disease, but we fall far short of other Westernized countries in terms of overall healthcare measurements. Despite spending nearly twice as much per capita on healthcare as other Western countries, the United States is ranked 37th in the world by the World Health Organization based on healthcare performance.[11]

Even though I managed the health of several thousand patients in my practice, I let my own health deteriorate. In the early 1990s, on a muggy July day in Missouri, I had an epiphany. I was only in my 30s, but I was exhausted from mowing the lawn. I was 40 pounds overweight, and because I never did routine aerobic activities, I was breathless. As I watched my 5- and 9-year-old boys riding their bikes, I told myself it was time for a change. I wanted to keep up with my sons and daughter as they grew, to be involved in their activities, and to enjoy life with them. I also felt professionally ashamed. I likened myself to those cardiologists I had seen perform coronary angiograms on patients and then go to the doctor's lounge to smoke.

The first thing I did was buy an expensive pair of running shoes. I knew if I invested heavily in the shoes, I would use them. And I did. The first few times I ran, I could go only a few blocks before slowing to a walk. But I persevered, and within 6 months I was running 25 miles per week. The craving for better physical performance fueled a desire to improve my nutrition, so I began to eat more fruits and vegetables and fewer animal products. It's a cliché, but true—the pounds started to melt away. This increased my desire even more to learn about good nutrition, a subject sorely lacking in my formal medical education, as Dr. House mentioned.

By 10 years after my transformation began, my diet was totally plant based. My nutritional beliefs changed as I studied the scientific research, which is readily and abundantly available to anyone who is interested enough to look for it—there's a lot of it among the notes and resources of this book and available at www.diabetesmiracle.org. I became convinced beyond a doubt that for virtually every common disease afflicting American society, a plant-based diet not only is the best prevention but also the best treatment.

As my knowledge of nutrition, physical activity, and health developed, it became increasingly frustrating for me to keep treating patients as I had been in my medical practice. For 20 years, I saw many patients with diseases that really weren't getting any better. The problems were just being managed, not eradicated or reversed. Usually this was because the only accepted treatment was medications, which were routinely increased to keep up with the progression of the problem. On hospital rounds, I observed patients eating the very diet that had put

them in the hospital in the first place: plates loaded with refined carbohydrates, colorless food, and fatty meat dishes drenched in gravy. I
began taking time to counsel my patients, not only on the importance
of diet and physical activity but also on how to affect change. I told
them what the research said was best. Most of the information fell on
deaf ears, and I got discouraged. From time to time someone showed a
real interest, and in my enthusiasm over having a receptive listener, I
would blow my whole schedule, creating a waiting room full of
unhappy patients. My growing desire was to educate and treat all my
patients in a manner that would motivate them to change their lifestyle
as the best means to improve or eliminate their diseases. I no longer fit
into the medical system as well as I had initially.

Determined to change my medical practice, I contacted Lifestyle
Center of America. My initial interest was to visit Oklahoma to see how
they treated and educated patients on lifestyle medicine. The call turned
into a recruitment effort on their part, and 10 months later I joined them
as a staff physician, clinic director, and educator. Now I'm medical director, program physician, and educator for LCA's Diabetes Wellness program in Sedona, Arizona. The patient improvements I have witnessed
during my time with LCA have been nothing short of miraculous. In less
than 3 weeks, patients with type-2 diabetes who eat a totally plant-based
diet and engage in a moderate physical activity program go from more
than 100 units of insulin per day to no insulin at all—and their blood
sugar levels are under better control! Along the way, blood pressure and
LDL cholesterol levels drop significantly. LCA patients have more energy,
less constipation, less joint pain and stiffness, and even less depression
than other diabetes patients. Even patients with diabetic neuropathy
(nerve pain or numbness in the feet and legs), one of the most frustrating
conditions to treat in a conventional manner, show signs of improvement
in the short time they are with us. My experience at LCA has only confirmed to me what the research predicts will indeed happen.

We have a way to go, though. It frustrates me that the traditional
medical community has largely ignored the most effective and powerful method of disease prevention and treatment we have. For most doctors, the lifestyle approach seems too extreme to recommend. Their
alternative is to put patients into a medical system that accounts for
more than 200,000 deaths per year because of medication error, physician error, or adverse events associated with medications or surgery![12]

If the information in this book could be packaged in a pill form, it would undoubtedly become the world's most prescribed drug. It would not only prevent but, research has shown, could also *reverse* type-2 diabetes, obesity, coronary artery disease, hypertension, and elevated blood lipids. It could prevent the majority of cancers from which Americans die. It would give relief to arthritis sufferers, help prevent osteoporosis, relieve constipation, and even help those with hemorrhoids. This "wonder pill" would have no adverse side effects and would cost nothing. So, take this healthy lifestyle information and devour it, digest it, and put it into practice. Let it do its magic for you, and your life will be transformed forever!

Ian Blake Newman

My worried assistant found an ad for LCA in a diabetes magazine. It showed a handsome fisherman casting a fly across a stream. Confident and vigorous, he looked like a man running for governor of Missouri. "He swears LCA saved his life," Genie told me. "You could use a little of that."

Grudgingly, I called for a packet of information. Soon I was squinting in front of the LCA video—everything was blurry lately—with a heaping bowl of ice cream and an equal measure of doubt. It was 2004. I was 36 years old. Since college, I'd gained 35 pounds, eating like a guy going to the electric chair. Food was a kind of convenient consolation prize for my hard luck in the health department. I'd been diagnosed with a rare, complicated cancer at 27 and suffered, too, from a degenerating back and joints; crippling, almost daily migraine headaches; chronic sinus infections; Lyme disease; and awful allergies to boot. I joked that it was only a matter of time until I got scurvy or beriberi. But it was no joke. I was on the brink of clinical depression, and who could blame me?

I'd had more than a dozen surgeries by age 30, one more traumatic than the last (imagine how much fun a "radical neck dissection" can be). For years I was either locked for days on end in a lead room for massive radioactive iodine ablation treatments or hooked up to intravenous antibiotics for 6-week stints, or connected to an electric stimulator literally wired into my spine to jolt my limbs and help me walk (which I did like Frankenstein's monster). Whenever I could work, I overworked and stayed stressed most of the time. Several times over those years, I'd drive straight to the hospital after toiling my usual 15-

hour days as professor and journalist, and pull down my pants for a shot of narcotic painkillers.

Then one day in 2004, I experienced a wonderful turning point: My insurance company informed me that, based on my latest clean blood work, I was officially cured of cancer. Then 6 months later, my pancreas quit its day job, and I had type-1 diabetes.

I was prescribed a big dose of insulin, offered a (literally) 20-second demonstration on how to use a syringe, and given to understand that I could expect serious complications like blindness, stroke, and amputations—if not now, then later. Meantime, five shots a day, in the stomach. At least it was a big target.

At first my blood sugar was 565 one hour and 64 the next. I couldn't see. I couldn't drive. I couldn't control my mood swings. In short, I couldn't cope.

I read books, went to doctors on both coasts. They bandied medical jargon: *supercalifragilistic ketoacidosis*. One doctor in New York informed me of another threat: My triglycerides were so high they were unmeasurable. One doctor in California told me I was a ticking time bomb. I was boggled and desperately forlorn.

I tried to commit to various radical diabetes diets. The theme seemed to be, "Protein is good; carbs are bad." I'd never been big on meat, but suddenly I was eating sausages and pork chops on a daily basis. I tried to stay as active as possible, but I wasn't losing weight, I was gaining.

I certainly had no confidence that some place in the middle of Oklahoma would offer me anything useful, new, or inspiring. What could "them Okies" possibly teach a savvy New Yorker like me?

And what if they tried to convert me into some kooky lifestyle cult? They all seemed so nice on the phone, but that's how they get you. They invite you over for tofu and smile a lot. But next thing you know you need to be rescued and deprogrammed.

Another problem—how could I spend that kind of money on myself? But I looked at that scary number in my blood test meter and decided that a stint at LCA would be cheaper than a funeral.

Of course it was the wisest, most gainful decision I ever made. At LCA, I found my Oklahoma antidote. It was worth 10 times what I paid. I didn't wind up in a cult. Instead, I met the best-informed and most compassionate doctors and nurses I'd ever known. I learned more in 18 days than I would have in 25 years of following my routine and my usual assumptions.

But, literally and figuratively, it was not a piece of cake. I realized after a few days there it was a radical lifestyle intervention. It was boot camp—my fellow guest Bill called it "Sugarless Farm," and it was exactly what I needed. It knocked me out of my poor-eating, not-moving groove and taught me the difference between that groove and a grave is only a matter of depth.

I saw the spread of gorgeous food laid out on the first morning and thought it was some kind of cruel joke. But no, it was breakfast. And it was delicious, wholesome, and filling. Lunch was even better. I was eating fruit and bread and rice and even some gourmet desserts. Despite that, within a few days, I cut my insulin intake by nearly half. "It's a miracle," I thought. They even taught me how to make the food, so I could keep eating as well at home.

I dropped 35 pounds, meaning I'm back at my high school weight and waist size (it's weird to even write that!); I cut my insulin intake by *more than half*—which is why I was able to lose the weight; I came off my triglyceride drug and two other medicines; I lowered my resting heart rate to an athletic level, according to my doctor; and I adopted a whole new way of thinking about food, stress, and physical activity. I've got my blood sugars under super tight control—better than most people who don't have diabetes. My doctor back home now asks me to print out my blood sugar patterns using the software that came with my insulin pump. He makes copies and shows his other patients what's possible with good education and motivation—with good *choices*. I got my life back, and my hope.

And I can see again! Maybe I'll go fishing and consider a bid for Missouri governor.

I'm convinced now that there's no reason I should suffer the usual complications of diabetes. As you'll see in Chapter 3, those complications are a function of high blood sugar *and high insulin levels*, both of which I have under tight control by following the LCA prescription.

Meantime, I want to spread the word about what LCA's 30-Day Diabetes Miracle program has done for me—and can do for you. I'd met one of the guests at the airport when we both arrived; I pushed her wheelchair. She wept the whole time. She said she expected to die by the following Christmas. Just 2 weeks later, she was walking (albeit slowly!) around the track and crying for a different reason—because she knew she'd get to see her grandkids grow up.

I saw enormous changes in just a few weeks, too. I noticed something interesting after a while. By eating on the LCA food plan, moving on the LCA activity plan, and thinking on the LCA behavior therapy plan, a whole lot more than just my blood sugars improved. I no longer needed painkillers, my headaches were gone, my sleep was better, I was much less depressed and stressed, and even my allergies were abating. One day I was in an elevator with Dr. House in New York, marveling at this weird new high I felt, which was surprising because I'd given up caffeine the year before. I told him I had more energy, more zest for life, more optimism. "That new feeling you have," Dr. House informed me, "is called 'health.'" I could get used to it.

When I realized that every 18 days, dozens of lives are transformed at LCA that same way—thousands have already been restored to health—I just had to get involved, spreading the LCA program to a wider audience. The idea for this book was born out of many conversations I had with the LCA staff and administration during that first stay and several subsequent trips. On one visit, in the winter of 2005, we sat around the board room talking about two articles on diabetes that had come out in the same week in major newspapers, the *Boston Globe* and the *New York Times*. This is from the *Globe*:

> Type-2 diabetes is sweeping so rapidly through America we need not waste time giving children bicycles. Just roll them a wheelchair. Forget the basketballs and baseballs. Give them Braille flash cards. The next thing you know, iPods, Game Boys and Xboxes will come with glucose meters.[13]

This is from the *Times*:

> Within a generation or so, doctors fear, a huge wave of new cases could overwhelm the public health system and engulf growing numbers of the young, creating a city where hospitals are swamped by the disease's handiwork, schools scramble for resources as they accommodate diabetic children, and the work force abounds with the blind. . . .[14]

Scary stuff. But it doesn't have to be that way. Type-2 diabetes is *preventable*. The LCA doctors and their colleagues in lifestyle medicine had proven it. Diabetes, like most chronic diseases, is a disease of our *culture*, a disease about *choices*. That means that it's also a disease that's reversible. Different inputs, different outputs. Different choices, different outcomes. So we had the brash idea that winter to try to get America to start making different choices. To offer a diabetes miracle, to one person at a time, through an easy-to-understand book that translates what LCA does in its residential program into one you can do at home. We're confident that if you follow LCA's no-nonsense, scientifically sound plan, your health will improve dramatically in as little as 30 days. It's our singular wish to someday see headlines in the *New York Times* and the *Boston Globe* tell the story of a global miracle: millions of people conquering the negative forces of our culture and living in renewed health and optimism. We hope for you to be there in that picture standing with us, beaming, proud, and healthy again. Doesn't that sound good?

Could you use a little miracle in your life? We encourage you to read on.

1

Nature vs. Nurture in the Development of Diabetes

I N THIS CHAPTER, we highlight the main anthropological, psychological, and cultural bases for the counterproductive lifestyle choices we make and discuss their serious consequences. We explain how diabetes, obesity, and other chronic diseases are, in fact, the body's natural adaptations to the choices we make in our rapidly evolving society. You'll learn how to begin to overcome the enormous forces—cultural, physiological, and psychological—compelling so many of us to continue down this doomed, diabetic path.

AMERICA THE BEAUTIFUL?

SURE, AMERICA'S BEAUTIFUL. But consider also: America the obese. America the critically, chronically ill. This is a classic paradox if ever there was one. Despite inestimable advances in medicine, pharmacology, and health education over the past few generations, a greater percentage of our population suffers now and suffers earlier from diseases and conditions that in the past had been reserved only for a few— namely the elite and extremely wealthy. Diabetes and the other "diseases of kings," as cultural anthropologists have called them, were far rarer in the past than they are now. They emerged only as culture and diets changed through a benign-sounding but ultimately hazardous process called *Westernization*.

That is to say, diseases of kings, such as diabetes and heart disease, go hand in hand with the culture of the West. In most of the developing world, the common chronic diseases we suffer in America are nowhere near as prevalent. Although rural East Africans, South Americans, and Asians might still fall victim to infectious and parasitic ailments— diseases associated with poverty and lack of proper nutrition—these people are not suffering a crisis of heart disease and diabetes . . . yet. Compare this to New York City, the epitome of Western culture, and you'll find that 1 in 8 people suffers from diabetes.[1] Even a society's cancer rates appear to be directly proportional to their proximity, either geographically or culturally, to the Western world: to *us*. Why? Well, to paraphrase a quip by Walt Kelly, creator of the classic *Pogo* comic strip, "We've created an enemy, and it is edible."

CASTLE CREEP

WHAT ACCOUNTS FOR this historical sea change and this geographical paradox? What do we regularly consume now that only kings could access in the past, and that only the very rich exploit in the still non-Westernized corners of the world? The answer is in what we call our *culture of abundance*. During the age when humankind lived a nomadic life, moving from place to place in search of food, starvation was an ever-present threat. When early humans got their hands on some chow—let's say a meaty bison they felled after an exhausting 3-day hunt—they were lucky. They would survive a little longer, whereas many of their weaker, slower, and sicker fellow humans might starve. Our forebears' bodies were hardwired to convert the high concentration of fat and calories from meat into body fat, which they stored for those inevitable long periods of hunger when the hunts were not so productive. In between times, they gathered berries and other plant-based foods; they were omnivorous, but plant foods were not always abundant in the wild, and of course they (like their animal counterparts) depended on unstable variables like the weather and competition from other species.

In many places, humankind began congregating into communities and abandoning their nomadic existence in favor of the comforts of group protection. Agriculture and the domestication of animals made possible this dramatic change in lifestyle. Civilizations—including stable villages, economies, and trade; new technology; and sophisticated cultural hierarchies and distinct social classes—arose around food-production areas. And quite suddenly, there was a relative abundance of food. That was a good thing for the short-term survival of our species, of course. But our bodies back then were just not used to getting so much food. Remember, for countless generations we had been used to going hungry—and our bodies did what they were designed to do: happily pack on the pounds anticipating the usual famine. This time, though, famine never came. That is, at least not for the wealthy: The serfs were still skin and bones, but the rich got fatter (it's been called "castle creep" and "palace paunch" by anthropologists[2]).

As we humans got better and better at producing and later *processing* food (grinding wheat into flour to make bread, for example) our culture of abundance escalated. It was all feast, on concentrated calories from meat and processed food, and no famine. On top of that, we were suddenly burning far fewer calories in the pursuit of our food. It no longer required a 10-mile hike just to collect our lunch—now food was a 5-minute trip to the village garden or quick visit to one's personal larder. As a result, we started to develop all the major chronic diseases we know and fear so much today: heart disease, diabetes, and even cancer. It's an ironic result of the momentous advances of agriculture and food processing, but one that makes sense in light of the way we're biologically programmed. The average person's body is wired in such a way that it feels good to eat calorie-dense food like meat and cupcakes because our bodies and our brains think we need it to survive the coming famine and to reproduce, sending our genes into the next generation. We'll go into more detail about why such hardwiring exists in Chapter 9.

MCDEATH WITH BACON AND CHEESE, PLEASE

FAST-FORWARD A FEW thousand years, and humans have now mastered all facets of agriculture and food processing. We in the Western world need never go hungry again. Forget the 5-minute trip to the village garden. Mechanized and industrialized agriculture and modern food processing mean our food arrives on the plate after 30 seconds in the microwave (they even have portable microwaves for your car now!). In fact, in the modern West, the vast majority of us live in an age of *all* feast and *no* famine—and this includes most poor people, too, in an ugly little paradox. Highly processed and calorie-laden foods are cheap, abundant, and very well marketed: think doughnuts, soda, chips, and candy. To reiterate, this "advance" has come at tremendous cost. All our major chronic diseases have resulted from this abundance. Not only that, virtually every major infectious threat to human survival—microorganisms and viruses such as smallpox, influenza, tuberculosis, malaria, plague, measles, and cholera—has mutated from diseases of domesticated animals and has adapted to affect humans in dire ways. The fear of avian flu is not new.[3]

We eat too many calories in the form of meat, dairy, processed foods, and sugar. On the flip side, we eat too little when it comes to healthful foods like whole grains, fruits, vegetables, and legumes. But, of course, you've known that ever since your mother told you, "Eat your veggies!"

For the real key to our culture of abundance, you need look no farther than a universal symbol for excess, a symbol that, incredibly, is much more recognizable across the planet than the Christian cross: the Golden Arches.[4] No, we don't blame the Big Mac per se for single-handedly dispersing and contributing to chronic disease throughout the world, from west to east. But some people do lay significant blame quite squarely at Ronald McDonald's feet, and they make a decent argument.[5]

We weren't surprised that in the 2004 documentary *Super Size Me*, filmmaker/guinea pig Morgan Spurlock, who set out to eat only McDonald's food for 30 days, soon began to see signs of many serious ailments. His doctors warned him to call off his experiment. Spurlock gained nearly 25 pounds by the end of the month; his cholesterol skyrocketed, he had heart palpitations, he lost his energy—as well as his libido. One alarmed doctor, worried Spurlock had seriously damaged his liver with all the fat and toxins in his fast-food diet, told Spurlock he was "pickling" his liver and turning it into "pâté." If only doctors everywhere insisted we "call off our experiment" with the standard American diet.

Extend that dangerous fast-food diet for a year, and the body will be overwhelmed trying to regulate itself under adverse conditions. Now extend that diet over decades (and this will approximate the *real* diets of millions of people in the West), and you'll begin to understand why obesity, diabetes, and heart disease rates have escalated into pandemic proportions.

As we said before, McDonald's is a very appropriate *symbol* for why we're less healthy than our grandparents were. Fast food represents, both literally and figuratively, a half-century-old trend in our daily diets of easy access to and indulgence in high-calorie, high-animal-fat, high-animal-protein, high-sugar, highly processed carbohydrate "food" in super-size portions. Simply put: It's excess. Surplus. Overload. Overindulgence.

And excess, as much simple folk wisdom and religious dogma preach, comes at a grave price. Over*kill*. Remember, the body likes this kind of food because it *thinks* it needs it to survive—the body stores it for a future famine that never comes. The body never burns off excess calories through increased activity because we have developed into a sedentary society. Our weight increases, and with it comes the deadly process of insulin resistance and the metabolic syndrome we discuss in detail in Chapter 3.

T. Colin Campbell, who conducted the single largest study of human nutrition ever undertaken, shared the results of his landmark research in a remarkable book titled *The China Study*.[6] Campbell proves that, in addition to diabetes and coronary artery disease, even cancer (leukemia, breast, colon, lung, stomach, liver, childhood brain) is directly related to what he calls the West's "nutritional extravagance."[7] The prevalence of type-2 diabetes among adults in rural, traditional communities in the developing world is less than 3 percent, but among their counterparts who live in more Westernized cities, there's a 5 to 10 times higher prevalence.[8] In the United States, the rates are increasing every year.

In other words, in impoverished places and places that haven't been infiltrated by fast-food companies, people don't get these diseases at nearly the same rate. A small part of it might be genetics. But the overwhelming cause has to do with dietary habits. As former Arkansas Governor Mike Huckabee says, we're digging our graves with a knife and fork.[9] This is happening as a worldwide pandemic. As the non-Western world Westernizes, the process escalates for them, too. Obesity, diabetes, heart disease, cancer, and autoimmune diseases that were nearly unheard of a few generations ago in some corners of the world, such as Micronesia and rural India and China, are on a steep rise, consistent with the decline in traditional plant-based diets and the influx of Western dietary habits.[10]

In China, only 7 percent of the protein in an average diet comes from animals. That's 10 times less than in the average American diet. "While most Chinese suffer very little from the major chronic killer diseases of the West, those affluent Chinese who consume similar amounts of animal protein to Westerners also have the highest rates of heart disease, cancer, and diabetes."[11] Recently, a contingent of 20 Chinese doctors and government health ministers from Hong Kong, Taiwan, and mainland China visited Lifestyle Center of America (LCA) for the express purpose of developing a plan for addressing emerging obesity and diabetes in their cultures. We hope that some experts from Micronesia will come to LCA, too.

The same thing happens when Chinese and Japanese people move to Hawaii and then farther to Washington State or California, which are even more entrenched in the West. With every mile, the chance of Asian immigrants getting diabetes goes up. Is it in the air? The water? Nope—it's on their plate.[12] As their diet becomes closer to the standard American diet, chronic disease rates increase proportionally.

DON'T PULL THAT TRIGGER!

SO WHAT WE have here is an interesting, and not at all balanced, combination of nature and nurture. These diseases of the West are the result of our bodies' natural adaptive responses to their environment. In Chapter 3, we'll go into more detail about the body's process for dealing with what we eat. For now, though, it's important to understand that disease processes like diabetes make a lot of sense physiologically when we consider what we do to our bodies and, more specifically, what we put into them. In a weird way, these diseases prove that the body is *working*. But only for so long. We're adaptable, but we're not indestructible.

We're also not simple slaves to our genes. Just look at the Pima Indians of Arizona. The prevalence of type-2 diabetes among the Pima is pretty remarkable. About half of them have the disease. This is the highest prevalence of obesity and type-2 diabetes in the country.[13] While we'll argue strongly in this book that diabetes is a lifestyle disease largely under your control, it's clear that there is a genetic factor at play as well. Innumerable generations of adaptation have made it harder for the Pima to lose weight. As the adage goes, though, "Genetics only loads the gun— lifestyle pulls the trigger." That means a lot of it is up to you. Here's a good example of how that works: The Pima are genetically very similar to several native populations in what is today Mexico. The Pima's Mexican counterparts live a more traditional (less American) life and eat a more traditional (more rural Mexican) diet. As a result, the incidence of type-

2 diabetes among them is far lower, almost nonexistent.[14] The adoption of an Anglo diet and lifestyle plays a major role in the development of diabetes among the Pima and in other peoples across the globe.[15]

Native Americans, including tribal officials, from many tribes have visited LCA or gone through our residential program: We've welcomed Mohawk, Shoshonee, Seminole, Oneida, Shawnee, and Mashantucket Pequots. We've also lectured on several reservations. And through dialogue with our Native American patients and tribal elders, we've learned that modern Native American life in America is now a far cry from that of past generations, when, among the Iroquois of upstate New York, for example, the "three sisters" (corn, beans, and squash) reigned supreme as the principal crops, and everyday life included much more vigorous physical activity.

It's clear to us that Westernization is pulling the trigger of our genetic guns very hard. "A low-fat, high-fiber diet can do more to help most diabetics than insulin pumps and medication," writes Howard Lyman,[16] a former cattle rancher who became the president of the International Vegetarian Union. Vegetarian author and health expert John Robbins writes that diabetes "worldwide is rare or nonexistent among peoples whose diets are primarily grains, vegetables, and fruits. If these same people switch to rich meat-based diets, however, their incidence of diabetes balloons."[17]

To help you make that switch and start reclaiming your life, we need to say a few words first about what you can do to overcome the seemingly gargantuan forces that stand in the way of you overcoming your diabetes. We're going to deal with the body's reaction to the standard American diet (SAD) in the next few chapters. But here we want to start with some cultural forces that work to sabotage our health and well-being, and then we want to dip into what's going on in your brain to thwart this mission.

One insidious force supporting the SAD is modern advertising—it's a big reason it seems so difficult to break the cycle of Western habits. You'll notice that you don't see many TV commercials for scallions and beans, but you do see a lot of ads for soft drinks, candy, sugary cereal, and other junk food. Writer and human development expert Dr. Dennis Deaton describes an experience many of us have had:

One time I was driving down the street with my toddler in the car seat. The child did not yet have a vocabulary that exceeded 12 words. But as we drove past the "golden arches," he lit up like he'd seen an angel descend from heaven, and he said, "Donald's!" He knew "mama," "dada," and "Donald's"?![18]

In the next chapter, we'll take a closer look at "Donald's" and some other stars in the SAD to see if we can isolate the problems and determine how they contribute to diabetes.

STRESS SUCCESS

THE LIES OF advertising, in addition to the other troubles of modern living, can be very stressful on our systems. Stress is a holdover from our old fight-or-flight days. It's still helpful if you're called to lift an I-beam off a small child or to fight off an enemy armed to the teeth. But nowadays, when most stressors are rather less dire (a boss in a bad mood, a traffic jam), stress really does more harm than good. In addition to increasing our risk of heart attacks, stomach cramps, headaches, injuries, mental impairment, and other common ailments, stress can also exacerbate—and in some cases possibly even cause diabetes—a fact we'll detail in Chapter 9. Major stress increases blood sugar levels, whether you have diabetes or not. Extreme stress on the body, such as occurs during serious illness or trauma, causes the body to release hormones to keep enough sugar in your system as energy to weather the intense situation.[19] That's why we react to stress the way we do—to survive immediate threats while remaining more or less in equilibrium.

But even moderate stress, largely because of its association with increased glucose in the bloodstream, can prevent you from keeping your diabetes in check. Over the long haul, this can seriously damage your body. For one thing, while you're stressed, some of the short-term body processes that are less essential than survival, such as sleep and digestion, are inhibited. And, of course, stress can also cause you to eat more, decrease your physical activity, feel exhausted and depressed, and fall off your health program altogether. It is alarming that extreme stress seems to be one possible culprit in the onset of type-1 diabetes, in which the part of the pancreas that makes insulin essentially dies. Some of our type-1 acute-onset diabetes patients report having gone through traumatic events in their lives—the death of a spouse or the loss of a job—usually just a few months before their diagnosis. There's controversy on this subject: Some reports back the claim,[20] but at least one recent large systematic review of past studies reveals that stress and the diabetes process are *related* but refutes the idea that type-1 diabetes is *caused* by stressful life events.[21]

The other scary problem with stress happens within our brains. As stress increases, the pituitary gland in the brain sends out an "I'm stressed" message to the adrenal glands, which then release a hormone called cortisol. When enough cortisol builds up in the brain, it can cause brain damage in the form of shrinking cells and blocked nerve connections. Meantime, excessive cortisol in the body is also responsible for increasing abdominal fat as well as suppressing the immune system, both of which are unwelcome side effects, especially if you have diabetes.

When the brain recognizes that you're experiencing a lot of stress, it has a defense mechanism built in—but, unfortunately, not a benign one. Somehow we become convinced that if we do something self-destructive (getting stoned, drinking until we pass out, or engaging in some kind of other risky behavior), our stress will go away. Such actions might work in the short term (there's no stress in unconsciousness), but they don't resolve the cause of the stress, inhibit future stress, or teach us to deal better with the inevitable stresses that recur in our lives. In fact, next time we undergo stress, we'll be less likely to wait for it to get as bad as the last time before we seek detrimental coping behaviors. The good news is that the right kind of physical activity, such as we describe in Chapter 8, can protect you from the damaging artery inflammation that flares up during times of mental stress.[22] In Chapter 9, we detail a plan for easing stress and negotiating your way toward good health amid the mess of modern life.

YOU'RE ON YOUR OWN

THERE'S A CRITICAL concept you need to accept to triumph over the obstacles you'll face in reclaiming your health: The world is not necessarily going to rush to support you. You will certainly encounter great ignorance. For example, most people will immediately balk at the idea of the plant-based diet and the type of physical activity we advocate. You and others will ask: Why are you eating rabbit food? Where will you get your protein? How do you expect to lose weight if you're not working out to the point of pain? No pain, no weight loss, right? We're certain that when you're through reading this book, you'll be armed with solid answers to these questions. And we're certain that if you follow our precepts, the results will speak vividly for themselves. But in the meantime, this is going to take some trust on your part. Remember, this program has provided miracles for many hundreds of our patients. We want you to be among them.

You will definitely face temptation along the way. Those Golden Arches will yet gleam and beckon you inside for just one helping of burger, fries, and a shake. Those poker friends will urge you to "just live a little." Those doughnuts will still arrive on the conference table at work. And that chocolate cream pie will still be placed in front of you at a dinner party. "I made this just for you. One bite won't kill you!" Your emotions will vie to control your food intake. Bad days will beg you to dive headfirst into a pint of Häagen-Dazs.

You might even slip a little one day and be tempted to forget the whole thing. *Don't let a lapse turn into a relapse.* The research we've done among our own patients has shown the difference between the consequences of "cheating" occasionally and those of cheating most days a week is enormous.

Another big challenge is that your close friends, spouse, and family will probably not understand right away what you're trying to do. Sometimes deliberately, often unknowingly, they will work hard to sabotage your strategy.

In the end, though, this is about you, and only you can make it happen. Please don't be discouraged by this notion. You ought to feel quite the opposite: Your health and well-being, including your attitude, are all under *your* influence.

We're going to help you navigate through all the obstacles—internal and external—to train your brain so that positive changes stick, even during the really tough times. In Chapter 9, we outline sustainable steps you can take to adhere to the program for life. But we'll give you the gist of the secret right now: *You're in charge of your brain.* You're in charge of the way you think about things, the way you react to things, and the way you talk to yourself and others about things. We know this sounds deceptively simple, but it's worked for hundreds of our patients and millions of people who've embraced cognitive behavior therapy. And it certainly can work for you, if you understand it, practice it, and sharpen your expertise in it regularly. Don't give up.

2

Good Health—For What?

KEY CONCEPTS FOR LASTING HEALTH

YOU NO DOUBT recognize that becoming healthy requires more than simply obtaining reliable health information. How many times have you heard, "Be sure to eat your veggies"? We are aware that knowing is never enough. *Decisions* and *commitments* to better health spring from the interaction of multiple stimuli—not just mere knowledge. Consider the key concepts presented in the following sections as you embark on your own journey toward health and mastery over counterproductive ideas and emotions.

The first question you might ask yourself is a big one, which may seem obvious until you really think about it. Dr. House defines this questions as, "Good health—for what?" In other words, we can tell you *how* to get better through the right foods, the right form of physical activity, and the right mind-set, but *why* you want to feel better, to be healthier, and to live longer is entirely up to you. Honestly and earnestly searching your mind and soul for answers to this profound question could be the *key determinant* to your level of success in changing your life for the better. Here are a few things to think about as you embark on your new lifestyle.

Goals

The absolute best thing you can do to defeat your diabetes and achieve optimal health is to follow all our dietary and physical activity recommendations to the letter. But we recognize that for many people this means a lot of sweeping changes that might feel like too much to swallow all at once. So focus on your priorities first and plan to tackle them head-on. One wise and simple proverb says it all: "He who fails to plan, plans to fail." Setting clear and reasonable personal goals is the first step in their attainment. Make sure your goals and expectations are realistic. They should be achievable in the near to intermediate future. As you achieve success, go ahead and set another batch of goals. It's good also to have a long-range objective and work toward it incrementally. For example, you might consider tackling the challenge of your after-breakfast blood sugars first. You can do this by cutting out the junk, increasing your fiber intake, and strolling after the meal. When you're satisfied with that success, move on the next goal, which might be substituting cow's milk with soy milk.

Change

Change takes place at such a fast pace in our culture that we become dizzied by it, and desensitized to its potential benefits. Some of us find respite from change in our habitual, predictable lifestyle. We are comfortable with our routines and resist change for fear of some perceived or imagined discomfort or displeasure. But we all know that diabetes won't cease its relentless progression of degeneration and disability unless *you* make a change. Consider the genius Albert Einstein's words: "We can't solve today's problems by using the same thinking we used in creating them."[1] In other words, some change is good and even necessary; sometimes things *need* to change. Sooner than you might expect, you'll find you've incorporated the positive changes into your life, and they've become part of your comfortable routine. If you wake up at 7:00 every morning and eat a big bowl of oatmeal with berries, you'll find after only 3 weeks that it's exceedingly difficult *not* to do this. Your new routine will now be leading you toward better health.

Courage

Maya Angelou says, "Courage is the most important of all the virtues."[2] Courage is *a character trait expressed in action*. Courage is a key concept in health success because it's usually required to make changes. Courage drives the engine of choice, which is the fountainhead of hope. You need simply to believe (which takes courage) that you are the master of your fate, then that belief will carry you home—not circumstances, not culture, not heredity. Go ahead and decide to get better, to refuse to allow yourself to be dominated by your diabetes.

Hope

Happy people look to the future and expect it to be good. Hope allows us to look outward, away from what we perceive to be our limitations, and into a new reality. Hope catalyzes our effort to find meaning in life and to experience fulfillment. Einstein understood something fundamental about life besides quantum physics. He said, "Learn from yesterday, live for today, and hope for tomorrow."[3]

Very often at Lifestyle Center of America (LCA), we hear our patients proclaim our residential treatment program to be their last hope. By the end of the program, their hope is nearly universally rewarded. Of course, this is hugely rewarding for us, too. We recognize during every tearful graduation ceremony that there are very few jobs in the world in which you get to see the fruits of your mission so obviously (and gratefully) manifest. Recently an LCA patient actually said, "I came here 18 days ago as an overweight atheist, and I'm leaving 26 pounds lighter, and *God bless you* all for that." Many of our patients credit God, and many credit good medicine and a healthful lifestyle; but hope, in the end, must reside inside you. We've all been through awful times, and it's tempting during those midnight hours to just let go. Hope doesn't always spring eternal. You have to search for it amid the dirt and weeds.

Just 10 years ago, Ian was a very young man and very sick. There came a dark time when his physical and spiritual agony was so severe, he nearly gave up. Chronic disease can be cruel and disheartening. At one point, Ian did not believe that he would walk again without intense, debilitating pain. All he wanted was some glimmer of hope, some shred of evidence that there might be a future ahead without pain, without disability. For Ian that evidence had to come from within. He had to *decide* to go on, to overcome the problems he could and live with those he couldn't, without complaint. Hope starts out one day at a time and builds, incrementally and even exponentially. Now Ian's in the best shape of his life.

Hope and optimism actually boost our immune systems,[4] helping us live better and longer. A University of Pennsylvania study showed that optimistic adults had the strongest immune response, whereas pessimistic people had the weakest.[5] One study at the Mayo Clinic in Rochester, Minnesota, showed that optimistic patients had a lower mortality rate over 30 years than patients who were pessimistic.[6]

Optimism

Optimism is an attitude worth cultivating. If you have had diabetes for some time, it might feel like a stretch to consider being optimistic. You might already be experiencing the major complications of diabetes, or maybe you've attended diabetes education classes and learned what might be ahead for you. You might assume that optimism would be foolish and unrealistic for you.

Viktor Frankl, an Austrian psychiatrist who outlived one of Hitler's most appalling death camps, was convinced that his attitude was the key to his survival. He said of his experience, "[E]verything can be taken from a man but one thing: the last of human freedoms—*to choose one's attitude in any given set of circumstances*, to choose one's own way."[7] Frankl believed that every conceivable circumstance of life, no matter how terrible, could be experienced positively by maintaining an optimistic "search for meaning."

Our highest function, the capacity that distinguishes us from all other life forms, is our capacity to choose. In the very act of choosing, we are exercising the highest quality of which a human is capable. *Choice is optimism in action.*

Having trouble cultivating optimism? Start by trying a little humor. Dr. Sven Svebak of the medical school at the Norwegian University of Science and Technology recently reported a study of 54,000 people conducted over 7 years. Those participants who appreciated humor the most were 35 percent more likely to be alive at the end of the study than those in the bottom quartile of humor appreciation—and the survival edge was particularly large for people with cancer. "Humor works like a shock absorber in a car. You appreciate a good shock absorber when you go over bumps, and cancer [like diabetes] is a big bump in life."[8]

Endurance

Once you are clear about your personal goals and how to attain them, once you've summoned the courage to change to reach those goals (really believing all the while that you *can* do it), and once you've learned to have a sense of humor about the whole thing, the next characteristic you need is endurance. Some call it stick-to-itiveness. As we learned from Aesop's fable "The Tortoise and the Hare," it's not how you begin the race, it's how you end: *Slow and steady wins the race.* Good health, for the long term, requires a lifestyle change, not just a diet. A diet is something we tolerate until we achieve a short-term goal, and then we go back to doing what we really want to do, which is pig out in front of the TV. For long-term success, it's important that we go with what works and make it *stick.* We'd say strive to endure until the end (that is, until the achievement of your goals becomes second nature), but we want you to do more than simply endure. We want you to stick to it so that you can have a more fulfilling life, day in and day out.

Endurance requires discipline. The word *discipline* might conjure unpleasant memories of mean gym teachers or drill sergeants, but the word really means that you're a *disciple* of your own beliefs, values, and mission. Every time you make a promise to yourself and break it through lack of discipline, you erode the trust you have in yourself. Your own word loses value, which can really harm your self-esteem. So think seriously about what you value (health, for example), what matters to you, and what you'd sacrifice for. Then set achievable goals that are aligned with those values and stick to them.

ASKING WHY

THE SUPREMELY EVOCATIVE question of why should occupy some of your time as you digest the counsel of this book and define your own course of action.

Our experience as doctors and patient tells us that if your answer fails to promise a good return on your investment of time and effort, your commitment won't last. Restoration from diabetes requires a lifestyle change, and that's not a weekend's trivial activity. Street wisdom tells us, "Life's a bummer—and then you die." Toiling to merely escape the ultimate reach of the Grim Reaper is not an activity that promises big dividends; it's also a losing battle for all of us, isn't it? So why the fuss about diabetes anyway? Or any other condition for that matter?

The answer to the question of why usually flows easily in a moment of personal crisis, such as after a heart attack. "I'm willing to 'suffer' without this hamburger, because I'd like to live a little longer." But it's in the intervals between crises that we have a tendency to give freedom to the remnants of the whiny kid inside each of us. In childlike ways, we rationalize our inaction with excuses like, "It's too hard," "I don't like it," "It takes too much time," and "It's no fun."

So before such crises come—and come they will, for all of us—we recommend you formulate your very personal answers to the why question. Why do you want to live? Why do you want good health and vigor? Why do you want to be out of pain and misery and hopelessness? Why—*specifically* why? The following ideas might spark possible answers for you as you ponder this important question.

For Happiness

Consider happiness in the sense of fulfillment, the joy of life, and satisfaction as distinguished from pleasure, amusement, glee, or fulfilled sensual desire. If experiencing good health brought you happiness, what would you do that you are not now doing? Throw your grandkids into the air? Hike up the pyramids in Mexico? Walk hand in hand with the love of your life around your favorite pond? Run with your dog? Ride horses? Write a book to help others? This answer will be intensely personal to you.

For Service

A life lived in service to others is one that pays in ways that monetary compensation can never reach. This is a good thing for lifestyle medicine doctors and writers who don't choose their specialties for the money!

- Jesus said, "Greater love hath no man than this, that a man lay down his life for his friends."[9]

- Before Jesus, there were Damon and Pythias of Greek mythology. Damon stood for his comrade Pythias at his execution, while Pythias scrambled to keep his word on promises to others he'd tendered. They were both rewarded for their service to each other and set free.
- Albert Schweitzer, the beloved Alsatian missionary to Africa—who literally gave his life for the people of Gabon—mused, "I don't know what your destiny will be, but one thing I do know: the only ones among you who will be really happy are those who have sought and found how to serve."[10]

These are pretty high marks, of course. This kind of service might seem unattainable for us mortals, so what can it mean to you? Find your own way to serve. Volunteer somewhere. Create art or poetry or music. Serve your family, your community, your country, or your religious organization. In doing so you might discover your life's meaning and receive happiness and longevity as a pleasant coincidence. "Nobody made a greater mistake than he who did nothing because he could do only a little," said Edmund Burke.[11]

For Legacy

Here's a big one. Most of us don't spend much time thinking along the lines of legacy until later in life, and often when it's nearly too late. Regardless of your age and current health condition, you might find it valuable to ask yourself, "How do I want to be remembered?" Your answer might include how you would want your family, your religious group, your children, your significant other, or your workmates to remember you. Then start living that way, *today*. Maybe there's important unfinished business in your life. Perhaps there are some emotional fences to mend. Those are good places to start answering the why question.

"Too old to plant trees for my own gratification, I shall do it for my posterity," said Thomas Jefferson.[12] We want you to live, to be healthy, happy, fruitful, and free from the shackles of hopelessness and unnecessary pain. We want you to trust that we did not casually choose to use the word *miracle* for our program: We believe with all our hearts (and scientific minds) that the plan offered in this book can yield results that are nothing short of miraculous.

For Commitment

You get back from life what you put into it. Make a commitment, starting today, to gain the sort of mastery you want over your diabetes and the rest of your life. It's redundant to word it this way, but we mean *really* commit. Make a promise to yourself, one small promise at a time, and keep it. It helps as well to share the promise with someone you care about and trust. In *The Book of Mind Management,* Dr. Dennis R. Deaton writes, "Without question, your words can become forceful vectors of creation when you establish an impeccable state of integrity. When (you and) others can trust what you say, your word creates rippling spheres of influence."[13]

If you choose, your commitment might be with God or your house of worship: 95 percent of Americans believe in God, more than half of us pray daily, and more than 40 percent attend a religious service weekly.[14] That might not surprise you, but this might: Those whose approach to life is grounded in their religious faith are probably doing their health a favor.[15] Did you know that more than 350 studies have looked into religious beliefs, faith, spirituality, and health? A majority of those (up to 80 percent) have found that those who believe in something are physically healthier, lead healthier lifestyles, and require fewer health services than those who do not believe.[16] This can be as beneficial to your survival as giving up cigarette smoking, adding 7 to 14 years to your life![17]

3

Insulin Resistance
The Real Culprit in Diabetes

TO GET TO the bottom of what a diabetes diagnosis means—what's *wrong* with you when you have diabetes—we need to start by understanding the way things are supposed to work. The body is an awesomely complex and brilliant machine. A constellation of intricate systems, machines within the machine all working together, keeps us alive and healthy. At least these systems are supposed to. It's clear that when one process isn't operating at its best, it's likely to adversely affect others; and if you don't do something to correct the problem, sooner or later you've got a major health crisis—a chronic disease.

Sometimes problems happen from the inside out, and sometimes from the outside in. In other words, sometimes processes within the body itself cause harm. We call these *endogenous,* or internal, processes. For example, one of the body's organs might secrete too much or too little of a given substance to maintain optimal health. Other times, factors from outside the body do damage. These are called *exogenous,* or external, processes. Accidents, pollution, and diet are external factors that can affect our health. When it comes to diabetes, both internal and external processes are at work.

NORMAL BY DESIGN

PICTURE A NORMAL, busy cell, anywhere in the body. It has some job to do; and whatever the job, it requires energy. Each cell's demand for energy is unique and depends on its function. Some cells require much, and others not so much. This energy comes in the form of fuel from digested food. Specifically, most of the energy that fuels the cells comes from the carbohydrate portion of foods—the portion that ultimately breaks down into simple forms of sugar. The important thing to know is the process by which your soup or your oatmeal becomes fuel energy for cells.

Even before you take your first bite, your body begins the digestion process when your brain signals your salivary glands to start producing saliva. This process you probably remember from grammar-school biology: Food goes through the mouth, down the esophagus, into the stomach, and then into the intestines. Various enzymes and acids help digest, or break down, nutrients into smaller components. As the digested nutrients snake along through the intestines, they are absorbed into the bloodstream, where they're used for various purposes. Most of the nutrients will supply energy to the body's cells, in the form of blood sugar (glucose).

But here we want to introduce another player: the banana-shaped organ that sits behind the stomach—the pancreas. It has two main jobs: It makes digestive enzymes and it makes a few very important hormones that help the body use the onslaught of energy from food you eat. The most well-known hormone produced in the pancreas is insulin. Its immediate job is to let the cells of the body know how much glucose energy is available so they can prepare to use that energy for fuel.

Insulin can be described as a key that unlocks the cell to let the needed energy in. The insulin locks onto a specific receptor on the cell's surface, which then allows the transfer of the energy from the blood, through the cell membrane, and into the cell. Our favorite analogy for insulin is one we've been using at Lifestyle Center of America (LCA) since Dr. George Guthrie, our former medical director, first introduced it. We call insulin "the Paul Revere Hormone." Paul Revere navigated the dark roads between Boston and Lexington, rousing patriots in every village with his alarm, "The Redcoats are coming! The Redcoats are coming!" In a similar way, insulin travels through the bloodstream, shouting, "The energy's coming! The energy's coming!" It tells the cells that there's energy in the blood, in the form of simple sugars, which have been broken down from carbohydrate foods, and asks the cells to open up and let it in.

Insulin can shout its vital message at different volumes: If there's only a little energy in the blood, if you haven't eaten much carbohydrate, it might barely whisper, "The energy's coming." But if it knows there's a lot of energy on its way because you've consumed a large portion of carbohydrate, it will shout, "The Energy's Coming!" Either way, when things are working properly, healthy, busy cells in need of energy will listen to the Paul Revere Hormone and open up accordingly, based on the amount of energy they need to do their jobs and the amount of energy on its way through the bloodstream.

The pancreas is pretty smart. It sends out only the amount of insulin it thinks is necessary to get the energy into the cells, and it makes this decision by sensing how much energy there is in the blood passing through it. So if there's a lot of sugar energy on its way to the cells, it shouts (secretes a lot of insulin into the blood), but if there's not so much energy on its way, it whispers (secretes a small amount of insulin into the blood). Cells will let in only the amount of energy they need, and they determine this by how busy they are, how much you're asking them to do, or how much the body's natural processes require them to do.

Let's look at this process in action. Pretend for a moment that you're a long-distance runner. You've been training for months, and you're in peak form. It's 6:00 a.m. You've drunk water. You've stretched. You've loaded up on carbs—great fuel for your cells, which are about to become very busy. There's the gun! In the first mile, your body uses fuel that it's been storing, mainly in the muscles and in the liver, for just such a quick fix. This kind of short-term fuel is called glycogen. Glycogen's a kind of blood sugar in stored form, useful for short bursts. But there's only so much of it—just enough for a fast burst. Supplies dwindle rather quickly with such intense physical activity.

By the second mile, the cells that are really busy on your run—such as the muscle cells in the legs—are looking for more fuel, more energy, to accomplish their arduous task. By the third and fourth mile, those cells are really hungry for that energy. You can almost feel that hunger in every cell of your legs, can't you?

Coming around a bend, you spot one of the race staff holding out a bottle, and you snatch it as you pass. It's one of those sweet, iridescent sports drinks. You chug it. Within a few hundred yards you start to feel better. Why? Well, the sports drink has that all-important H_2O (water) to replenish your fluids. When dehydrated, none of your systems can function very well. You've also been losing electrolytes through sweating, and they're in the drink, too; these are minerals like sodium, potassium, and chloride, which your cells need to regulate their electric charges as well as the flow of water molecules across their membranes.

But another key ingredient in the sports drink is glucose. That's a form of simple sugar, a kind of sugar that occurs naturally in plants and animals. It's also the main kind of sugar that circulates in our blood. This is why you might have heard blood sugar referred to as *blood glucose,* and why you might be familiar with glucose tablets, which people with diabetes can take as a quick fix for low blood sugar. Glucose is the main kind of sugar used by our cells for energy. In fact, for the purposes of discussing food metabolism and diabetes, the terms *sugar, glucose,* and *energy* are synonymous.

So, imagine the effect of a whole sports drink worth of glucose as it's absorbed through the blood vessels of the small intestine and sent through the pancreas. Do you suppose the pancreas is going to interpret that glucose as a lot of energy on its way to the cells—or a little? The answer, of course, is *a lot.* So the pancreas is going to shout: "*The Energy's Coming!*" In other words, it's going to send out a lot of insulin, enough to match all that sugar and get it all into all those cells. The formula's simple in the healthy pancreas: The more sugar you put into the system, the more insulin the pancreas will produce.

Keep in mind here the all-important fact that *sugar* means the carbohydrate portion of foods, which breaks down into glucose through digestion. There are differences in the time it takes to digest and metabolize different kinds of carbs—you'll learn a lot about this in Chapter 6—but, ultimately, a slice of white bread is not much different from a candy bar or a bowl of spaghetti with marinara sauce or a quantity of plain table sugar.

All those cells in your thigh and calf muscles that are working overtime on your run open up wide to heed that call of the Paul Revere Hormone. All that insulin helps the free-floating sugar in the bloodstream become useful energy to be burned by busy cells. This is an example of what we call *homeostasis,* a stable, healthy state. Lots of sugar's okay in your system right now; after all, you're on a long-distance run, and the cells are so busy, they need lots of energy. And lots of insulin in the system is okay, too, because the pancreas needs to shout loud for all the cells to hear about all that sugar. Your body is working as it should.

TROUBLE IN PANCREATIC PARADISE:
The Seeds of Type-1 and Type-2 Diabetes

IN DIABETES, THOUGH, we have fundamental problems with this process. There are two main types of diabetes—type 1 and type 2. Type 2 is far more common, accounting for 90 to 95 percent of all diabetes. Both types are tied up in metabolic malfunctions, both can be characterized by roller-coaster blood sugars, and both can have devastating long-term consequences if left unchecked. But having said that, they're actually almost opposite diseases, tending to even affect different types of people.

The basic difference might be presented in this way: In type-1 diabetes, Paul Revere doesn't ride and shout at all, and in type-2 diabetes, he rides and shouts, but no one along the way seems to listen. In type-1 diabetes, the pancreas is not producing sufficient insulin to usher needed energy into cells. In early type-2 diabetes, the pancreas is making more than enough insulin, but the cells are *resisting* its efforts to let energy pass through their membranes.

THE SECRET'S IN THE CELLS:
Insulin Resistance

IF YOU THINK about the management of energy in normal physiologic circumstances, it makes sense. The body doesn't manage energy intake very well at the mouth. We eat for lots of reasons—not just because we need energy. We might be eating for emotional reasons, for example, because we're depressed or because we're celebrating. We might eat out of boredom or habit, because we think something smells good or because our mamas told us we had to finish everything on our plate. The esophagus doesn't manage energy intake either. Everything that falls into it goes down for processing. The stomach mixes and stores food temporarily during digestion, but it doesn't control energy distribution or consumption either—whatever's there is going into the small intestine. The stomach doesn't withhold some energy or disperse energy directly to various parts of the body according to need. Even the pancreas doesn't control the energy delivery.

Instead, *each cell of the body decides how much energy it needs* at any given time and adjusts its intake accordingly, by either accepting it or rejecting it. Each cell has a relative insulin *sensitivity* or *resistance*. This is an extremely important lesson about normal physiology, worthy of repetition, especially for people with diabetes: The body disseminates energy it takes in from food. Each cell decides how much it needs and adjusts its response accordingly. Cells that are bathed in *excess* energy become resistant to the insulin's message. Thus a big secret to managing diabetes is to manage energy metabolism, meaning to manage not just the intake (what you're eating) but also the processing (how sensitive your cells are). Increasing your physical activity level, lowering your weight, and consuming the right kinds of energy—the right amount of the right kind of carbs at the right time—can all contribute substantially to increasing your insulin sensitivity and lowering your insulin resistance. Both of these weaken the diabetes process and move you toward greater health. If all you do is keep your eye on your blood sugar, it's likely your diabetes will eventually get worse.

LAZY CELLS:
Too Much Energy In, Not Enough Energy Out

THE MODEL OF healthy energy metabolism occurring in the long-distance runner, described earlier, is not the way it works in the average person. Most of us don't have cells as busy as a runner's. Yet we don't reduce our consumption of energy (carbs that break down into sugar) in proportion with our low physical activity level. In fact, the way it usually works is just the opposite. People with low physical activity levels tend to be even more likely to consume the kinds of foods that contain excess energy. This paradox will eventually knock a normal, healthy person's metabolism out of homeostasis. You're going to have too much energy (sugar) going into your body and not enough energy (physical activity) going out. This condition is the seed of both obesity and type-2 diabetes.

You can think of the first part of this problem as *lazy cells*. Imagine you're not on the running track but on your recliner in front of the TV.

There's an empty bowl of ice cream on the coffee table, two empty sleeves of cookies, and a couple of empty soda cans on the floor. After all that energy goes down your hatch, into the small intestine, and then into the bloodstream to the pancreas, the latter is going to boom out to all your cells, *"The Energy's Coming!"* But your thigh muscles will say, "No, thank you." You see, they don't need all that energy. Or think of it this way: If your car is full of gas, but you don't drive it anywhere, you don't have to fill it up again.

So, after you eat, your bloodstream's got a lot of energy (sugar) floating around with no place to go, and it's also got a lot of insulin floating around, shouting vainly, hoping for a taker. This process is more likely to occur if you develop a *habit* of too much energy in, not enough energy out. If you usually run every day, but don't run for a few days, your cells will probably still welcome much of that cookie and cheese puff energy even though you're in your recliner today. You might have heard this erroneously referred to as a "good metabolism." But note it's a person's good *habits* that will have led to this condition—not some lucky gene or other mysterious internal cause.

It might also be the case that, depending on your physical activity level, only some of your cells resist Paul Revere's call and reject the energy in the bloodstream. Not such a big deal. But many of us subject our bodies to a consistent pattern of too much energy in (too many calories broken down into sugar) and not enough energy out (too little physical activity). So our pancreas keeps shouting louder and louder, releasing insulin to match all that energy, and our cells have gotten into the habit of shouting back, "No, thank you!" to the high levels of energy consumed. Eventually, all or most all of our cells begin to say, "No thank you," and now the whole body's got a problem that we call insulin resistance.

Insulin resistance is the lazy cells' rejection of the insulin's call to usher in energy. Insulin resistance causes many serious problems that are the foundation of the type-2 diabetes process as well as the origin of other serious, chronic diseases (it can be present in type-1 diabetes, too).

HIGH INSULIN AND HIGH BLOOD SUGAR:
A Recipe for Diabetic Disaster

THERE ARE TWO principal components of the type-2 diabetes process. The first is high insulin levels, and the second is high blood sugar. That's a paradox, isn't it? Under normal circumstances, you'd expect that with high insulin levels, blood sugar would be low. Why isn't that the case?

First, if the pattern of too much energy in, not enough energy out continues long enough, and the cells keep saying no to the energy coming in, the insulin levels eventually start going up. Remember, the pancreas is smart. It's reading (sensing) the amount of energy in the blood and secreting insulin proportionally. So if the blood recirculating back through the pancreas on the next round is still full of sugar (because the resistant cells of the body rejected some or most of it), the pancreas is going to secrete even more insulin. It's going to shout louder. It's going to yell, *"Hey! Maybe You Didn't Hear Me the First Time, but . . . The Energy's Coming!"* Meantime, the owner of those cells is likely consuming even more energy (the blood sugar's still high from the previous meal, but the next meal or snack is on the way). Over a 24-hour period, a lot of insulin accumulates in the bloodstream.

The pancreas is a workhorse. It's okay on overtime—for a while. It can produce only so much insulin anyway, so the insulin levels in the blood will eventually reach a maximum. Should this pattern continue for a long time, though, the pancreas is going to start to suffer. Too much shouting for too long—too much insulin secretion, too often—and it can start to burn out. Technically, the pancreas doesn't fatigue from overproducing insulin for a long period. It's actually destroyed through a complex set of chemical processes. But the effect is the same as if the pancreas was getting tired, and this is a simpler way to think about the condition. In the worst-case scenario, a person with type-2 diabetes could begin to act like a patient with type 1, by exhausting and eventually shutting down the part of the pancreas responsible for insulin production.

The second step in the type-2 diabetes process is also pretty logical. The average blood sugar levels will start to sneak up. Blood sugar is a measurement of how much sugar (energy) is free floating in your blood at any given time. In other words, how much energy is still in your bloodstream because it hasn't gotten into busy cells. Again, if you're not putting your cells to work through physical activity, then they're going to ignore the insulin's call, they're going to *resist*, or reject, the energy.

If the sugar energy can't get into the cells, it will continue to float around in the blood, and a lot of it will filter out through the kidneys into the urine. Some years ago, a patient told us at the end of providing a lengthy medical history, "Oh, by the way, when I forget to flush, the ants come to drink out of my toilet!" That was an easy one: What's an ant's favorite snack? Sugar! We tested her, and sure enough, she had diabetes. In fact, the official name of the disorder is *diabetes mellitus,* which means, more or less, "sweet urine" in a combination of Greek and Latin. In the old days, before more sophisticated blood testing, people with diabetes tested their urine for sugar. And in even older days, it was a "taste" test.

It's important to remember that in the type-2 diabetes disease process, *high insulin levels come first.* When cells become resistant to insulin, high blood sugar follows. Most doctors seem to ignore this fact—to their patients' peril. The body doesn't want the blood sugar so high; it recognizes that this will cause damage. So the pancreas keeps producing insulin, pours it out to match all that sugar, and get it into the cells. As we've said, the pancreas is smart at detecting the *amount* of sugar in the blood, but it's not clever enough to know whether the cells of the body are busy and *need* that energy, or lazy and don't.

You might already be familiar with the ramifications of high blood sugar. The main one has to do with small blood vessel diseases. When there's too much sugar circulating in the blood, it can clog up small blood vessels by several different methods. The lining of the blood vessels don't have the ability to say no to the sugar like the other cells in the body. This leads to a clogging of the cells' energy-management process; the result is increased free radicals, sugar attached to proteins and other damaging compounds. Injured blood vessels in the eyes can cause blindness. Small blood vessels damaged in the kidneys can cause kidney failure. If it happens in the nerves, it can lead to neuropathy— each nerve contains a tiny blood vessel that supplies it with energy, and when the supply chain is broken, the nerve will begin to complain, by burning, itching, or going numb. Small blood vessel disease caused by chronic high blood sugar can affect the circulation in the extremities. If, for example, a person with diabetes injures his or her foot, proper energy, nutrition, oxygen, and infection-fighting substances can't get to the site in adequate amounts and serious consequences, like gangrene and eventual amputation, can ensue.

But did you also know that there are serious problems associated with high insulin levels? High insulin tends to cause another kind of circulation problem, called large blood vessel disease. Now we're beyond the eyes, the kidneys, and the feet, and we're dealing with the coronary arteries—with the heart itself. Strokes and heart attacks are much more common in diabetes patients than in the general population. In fact, 65 percent of people with diabetes die from a heart attack or stroke.[1] A male with diabetes has twice the risk of coronary artery disease as does a male without diabetes. For women, it is even worse— a 5 fold increase in risk![2] But don't panic: We're going to explain why this doesn't have to be the case for you.

How's high insulin related to heart disease? At the core of the relationship is the fact that insulin is a *growth hormone*. In simplified terms, the more you have of it in your system, the more likely you are to gain weight. This is one of the main reasons people with type-2 diabetes are often overweight (another reason is that the standard American diet [SAD] is high in fat, calories, and processed foods). And, with overweight comes lazier cells, more resistance, and worsening diabetes. Remember, we said that insulin's *primary* job is glucose transport? Well, like many hormones, insulin has a few side jobs, too. One of them is to hinder the breakdown of fat, protein, and glycogen (the complex carbohydrate stored in the liver as an emergency energy source for muscles). What this means is that insulin is responsible for *storing energy for future use*, and, as a result, for *building up tissue*. In short: growth. That's the last thing someone with type-2 diabetes needs. If you gain weight, you're probably going to become even less physically active, and your cells are going to become even more resistant to insulin. Eventually, you're going to have to take more diabetes medicine, which can contribute to even more weight gain.

High insulin levels also correspond with high blood pressure. This seems to have to do with insulin's effect on the pliability of blood vessels (the less pliable, the harder to dilate, and the less dilated, the higher the pressure). It may also have something to do with the fact that insulin tends to make the kidneys hang on to sodium. Water follows the sodium and this means more water in the pipes of the body. A combination of rigid pipes (blood vessels) and more fluid in the pipes leads to higher pressure.

High insulin levels also cause total cholesterol and low-density lipoprotein (LDL), the bad, cholesterol to go up, and the high-density lipoprotein (HDL), the good, cholesterol to go down. We discuss cholesterol in more detail in Chapter 5. For now, it's important to understand that this collection of events increases our risk of heart attack and stroke very dramatically.

High insulin levels can have other insidious consequences, too. Studies show quite conclusively the negative effects of high insulin on sex hormones like testosterone and estrogen.[3] Insulin resistance can, therefore, cause problems related to the prostate, the gonads (the testes in males and ovaries in females), and other systems affected by sex hormones, such as skin and hair. In women, high insulin levels are a likely contributor to polycystic ovarian syndrome (PCOS), ovarian cysts, and irregular menstruation (especially in overweight women).[4] A fundamental mistake that many doctors make in treating diabetes is *ignoring the negative effects of high insulin levels and associated insulin resistance while focusing only on treating the blood sugar.*

THREE CHANCES TO DETECT IMPENDING DIABETES

IF YOU'VE BEEN diagnosed with diabetes, it's likely that diagnosis was made using a fasting blood sugar test. It might have been the first you heard of having diabetes, but did you know that by the time your fasting blood sugars became elevated, your disease process was already very well under way?

It makes us lifestyle medicine advocates wonder why more physicians don't use high insulin levels to diagnose type-2 diabetes. It's this test that marks the earliest stage a doctor can clinically diagnose impending diabetes. Unfortunately, serum insulin levels are rarely checked by anyone but lifestyle medicine doctors. Most doctors depend on the clinically associated findings, such as high cholesterol, increasing abdominal girth, and elevated blood pressure—and often they don't even make those associations.

At the next stage of the disease process, you can detect the problem at home, using a blood test meter. This way of identifying prediabetes is to measure your blood sugar 2 hours after a regular-size meal. If the blood sugar is over 140 milligrams per deciliter (mg/dL) 2 hours after beginning the meal, there's a good chance that you will develop diabetes within the next 5 years or so unless you make some lifestyle changes. You should see your doctor and have a fasting serum insulin test done to confirm there is a high level present, which is defined as greater than 6 micro International Units per milliliter [μIU/mL]). High postprandial (after meal) blood sugar means the pancreas has maxed out its production of insulin and can keep up during the fasting state but can't keep up when more energy is added after a meal (so the blood sugar rises abnormally). At this stage, you've already got higher levels of both sugar and insulin in the body—the hallmark of insulin resistance.

Dr. Seale often tells his patients that the best thing they can do for their friends, neighbors, or family members who have a waist size of 40 inches or more in men, or 35 inches or more in women, is to tell them to check their blood sugar 2 hours after a meal. The earlier insulin resistance is discovered, the easier it is to reverse the process, avoid the eventual complications of diabetes, and prevent the damage done by high insulin and high after-meal blood sugar levels.

It isn't until *still later* that the fasting blood sugar goes up. This happens when the pancreas can't even keep up with energy input when *no food (no extra energy) is consumed*. So by the time your doctor determines your fasting blood sugar is elevated, the diabetes process is in full swing. It's been estimated that by the time the clinical diagnosis of type-2 diabetes is made, many patients have had the disease for 5 to 8 years—enough time to develop complications.[5] By this time, it's common to see 50 percent or so of beta-cell function in the pancreas already gone (beta cells are discussed later in this chapter).

LADIES ONLY:
Gestational Diabetes

GESTATIONAL DIABETES IS a temporary form of diabetes that can occur in the late stages of pregnancy among some women. Insulin levels increase during pregnancy to provide enough energy for the growing fetus. There's also a kind of competition between mother and fetus for this energy. Resistance in the mother can increase as sensitivity in the baby increases. Meantime, the mother's pancreas is working overtime and getting stressed. Gestational diabetes will reverse itself once the baby is born. All pregnant women—not just older ones—should be screened somewhere between weeks 24 and 28.[6] Treatment for gestational diabetes is usually with lifestyle (diet and physical activity), but some women will need to take insulin to bring down very high blood sugars, which can be harmful to both mother and baby.

OTHER TYPES OF DIABETES

●

THERE are at least two more types of diabetes—type 1.5 and type 3—which you can read about in the endnotes and in the resource section at www.diabetesmiracle.org.[7]

HUNGRY CELLS:
The Dynamics of Type-1 Diabetes

REMEMBER THAT IN type-2 diabetes a working pancreas produces insulin that the body's cells resist. A diagnosis of type-1 diabetes, on the other hand, means that the pancreas has stopped functioning properly in terms of insulin production. Specifically, certain cells called beta cells, responsible for the production of insulin and other hormones, have stopped working properly. There are several chief causes of this failure, though there's still debate about the details. What seems clear at present is that the problem starts with an autoimmune response gone haywire: The body's own immune system attacks the beta cells responsible for insulin production. It's likely this response is based in the body's natural reaction to infection. In other words, a viral infection, probably unrelated to the pancreas itself (a virus in the coxsackievirus family is a usual suspect[8]), might somehow establish itself within the pancreas. When the immune system goes in to do its job, to fight the bug trespassing in the pancreas, it either mistakes the beta cells for the virus (the protein portions of each are similar) or the cells just somehow get swept up in the housecleaning process. Either way, once the beta cells have been diminished, insulin production will be reduced or halted entirely. By now you know what that means: Sugar energy cannot get into the cells for use as fuel because the Paul Revere Hormone is not there to let the cells know they should prepare to accept the energy arriving via the blood.

Other sources of beta-cell damage include pancreatic trauma, such as automobile accidents; tumors, whether benign or malignant; and pancreatitis, severe inflammation or infection of the pancreas. These can all result in reduction of insulin production. Certain drugs and chemicals have also been linked to the death of beta cells in the pancreas.

Another theory about the cause of type-1 diabetes is very compelling to lifestyle medicine proponents. It posits that the destructive autoimmune response is likely rendered by antibodies against the proteins contained in cow's milk. A large retrospective study published in 2006 found that infants who were never breast-fed had twice the risk for developing type-1 diabetes than did infants who were breast-fed for at least 12 months.[9] Other studies support these findings, that children weaned too early and fed cow's milk have on average a 50 to 60 percent higher risk of developing type-1 diabetes.[10] This might mean that breast-fed babies are introduced to helpful antibodies from their mothers or that an early introduction to cow's milk protein—as opposed to human milk protein—is harmful to the pancreatic beta cells.

There's also a lot of evidence now that a vitamin D deficiency is linked to type-1 diabetes.[11] For example, a study in northern Finland, where individuals do not produce a lot of vitamin D because of the lack of sunshine, showed that giving children a high dose (2,000 IU daily) of vitamin D in their first year of life reduced the risk of type-1 diabetes by 80 percent.[12] (See Chapter 5 for information about vitamin D and type-2 diabetes and Chapter 9 for information on sunshine and vitamin D.)

As with most medical conditions, one can't escape the nature vs. nurture debate when seeking a cause of type-1 diabetes. It would seem that people with type-1 diabetes have a genetic predisposition to the disorder that's somehow triggered by one or more exogenous (external) causes. But whatever the cause, the results are the same: very little or no natural insulin production. And because insulin is necessary for shepherding sugar energy into cells, people with type-1 diabetes will die in a matter of days or weeks if they don't take insulin (in some combination of injection, pump, or inhalation). This is why type-1 diabetes is also known as insulin-dependent diabetes; without insulin, the cells will starve for lack of energy.

We should note, however, that people with type-1 diabetes shouldn't take more insulin than the pancreas would ordinarily secrete if it were working on its own. *This means any excess injected, pumped, or inhaled insulin in the system can easily lead to insulin resistance* because of the same dynamic of too much energy in, not enough energy out as we see in most type-2 diabetes patients. This will worsen the diabetes condition. How much insulin is potentially too much to take? In a normal, healthy adult, the pancreas secretes 20 to 30 units a day.

Whereas in type-2 diabetes, we describe the body's cells as lazy and resistant to energy, it helps to imagine that in type-1 diabetes, the cells are *hungry* because the pancreas is producing no insulin. We therefore think of the cells of the type-1 diabetes patient as being insulin *sensitive*. For the usual patient with type-1 diabetes, it takes only a little injected, pumped, or inhaled insulin (at the right time, of course) to get energy into the cells. As we noted earlier, in type-1 diabetes, the cells are starving—literally dying to get some energy in. And because that can't happen unless some insulin comes along to open the receptors, the cells are listening very attentively for the faintest whisper of the Paul Revere Hormone.

At LCA we find that, contrary to what most doctors prescribe, just a little bit of insulin goes a long way for the patient with type-1 diabetes whose lifestyle is tuned to peak performance. With a little bit of insulin, the cells open up, saying, "Finally, we're getting that energy we need to survive." It is not incidental that this hungry-cell phenomenon is why people with type-1 diabetes tend to be thin. Because of the lack of natural insulin, there's very little energy or fat stored in the cells.

INSULIN RESISTANCE IN TYPE-1 DIABETES

●

THE process of insulin resistance in type-1 diabetes is so important it bears further explanation. The understanding that just a little insulin is adequate for people with type-1 diabetes is critical for treating this disease. Just as it is for patients with type-2 diabetes, a chronically high insulin level can prove a major problem for those with type 1, even though their bodies don't produce enough of their own insulin. In one type of diabetes, the insulin is secreted by the pancreas; and in the other type, it's injected (or pumped or inhaled). But either way, the relative level of resistance or sensitivity will determine how well the energy is metabolized.

If the diet of a person with type-1 diabetes is not controlled, the blood sugar rises. The way this is typically managed is by increasing the doses of administered insulin (much like the functioning pancreas does in a person with type-2 diabetes). This will allow the sugar (energy) to enter into the cells, but it can also lead to weight gain and, ultimately, insulin resistance, just as in type-2 diabetes. The patient is then left with not only a pancreas that can't make insulin but also body cells that are resistant to the insulin that is being injected, pumped, or inhaled— the worst of both worlds. Therefore, people with insulin-dependent diabetes will be much better off maintaining a balanced caloric intake of low-glycemic foods, allowing them to take as little insulin as possible to maintain good blood sugar levels (low-glycemic foods are discussed in Chapter 6). This means that if you're on insulin, you should not think of it as a magic bullet for slaying the high blood sugar dragon. It is a mistake for anyone to accept that it's okay to use high doses of insulin to make up for poor lifestyle choices in diet and activity. If you have type-1 diabetes, you *could* eat a whole wedding cake and then inject enough insulin to "cover" that amount of sugar. You could then check your blood sugar reading and find it's within range. But as you've seen, high-dose insulin only compounds the problem.

Traditionally, dieticians, nutritionists, and even many doctors have advised patients with type-1 diabetes to eat six meals a day to prevent low blood sugar. This pattern made sense when the only available treatment was 3-hour regular and 6- to 8-hour neutral protamine Hagedorn (NPH) insulin. But nowadays, subscribing to this prescription starts an unhealthy pattern familiar to many people on insulin: insulin to cover food, and food to chase insulin. If you're used to this pattern, you should remind yourself regularly that too much energy in (too much food) and not enough energy out (too little physical activity) is the chief cause of type-2 diabetes! Higher insulin levels begin to have the expected effects of increasing weight, cholesterol, and blood pressure, and the person with type-1 diabetes begins to look and act like someone with type-2 diabetes.

Eventually, a person can have both type-1 and type-2 diabetes at once. A cornerstone of the 30-Day Diabetes Miracle treatment plan is to keep both blood sugar and insulin levels as low and as stable as possible for people with either type-2 or type-1 diabetes. We do this primarily through lifestyle choices centered on nutrition and physical activity.

DIABETES BY THE NUMBERS

THERE ARE FOUR effective and informative tests you can take if you want to know whether you've got diabetes or you're likely to get it down the road.

First, you can take your blood sugar 2 hours after the *start* of a normal meal. We call this a *postprandial glucose test*, meaning "after-meal blood sugar test." If this reading is 140 mg/dL or higher, there's a good chance that in about 5 years or less, you'll have full-blown diabetes if you don't change your lifestyle. The number 140 tells us the process toward a metabolic abnormality is underway: Your pancreas either is working too hard because of insulin-resistant cells (the beginning of type-2 diabetes) or, much less likely, is starting to fail already (type-1 diabetes).

Another useful measurement is your fasting blood sugar. The technical name is a *fasting plasma glucose test*. This number, usually taken on waking because it's been about 8 hours since your last meal, should be no higher than 125 mg/dL. If it is, it is very likely you have diabetes now. If it's higher than 100, you have impaired fasting glucose and also it's likely you have insulin resistance, or "prediabetes." After 8 hours, the pancreas should be producing enough insulin, and the cells sucking up consumed energy, for the level of sugar in the blood to be relatively low, certainly less than 100 and preferably less than 90.

Both of those tests can be done at home with a blood test meter. These meters are ubiquitous at pharmacies and relatively cheap. You might even be able to get a free one from your doctor. They're also pretty easy to use without much training, and they're fairly accurate.

A more clinical test that requires medical supervision is called an *oral glucose tolerance test*. Here, you're asked to fast for 8 hours and then to consume 75 grams (g) of glucose in a very sweet syrupy drink. A medical professional will test your blood sugar periodically to see how well your body's metabolizing all that sugar. After 2 hours, your plasma glucose reading should be no more than 200, preferably quite a bit lower. If you're healthy, the pancreas should be able to deal with this temporary overdose of fast-acting sugar. People with advanced diabetes will often see readings of 400 or more.

The fourth, and probably the best, test also requires medical supervision. It is the *fasting serum insulin test*, used in combination with a fasting plasma glucose test. From these two tests, it is possible for your doctor to calculate how much insulin resistance is present in your body and also how well your pancreas's insulin-producing cells are functioning. We feel testing of this type will most accurately determine whether or not you have prediabetes and also will reveal it at its earliest stage.

With each of these tests, you must remember three important things: The first is that you're getting only a snapshot—one recorded moment, frozen in time. You don't know, for example, whether a given blood sugar reading is holding steady, going steeply up, or gradually coming down at the moment you record it.

Second, an individual test is not statistically relevant, so you should test several times to confirm patterns, especially for diagnostic purposes. There are many variables that can affect given blood sugar readings, including the time of your last meal, the type of food consumed, the mix of food consumed, your level of physical activity, the presence of infection or fever, even the amount of stress you're under.

Last, some of these numbers are merely benchmarks set by medical scientists. They're somewhat arbitrary and capricious, they tend to change with time, and they're generally not optimal. As it stands now with the medical establishment, until your fasting blood sugar reaches that magic level of 125 mg/dL, you don't have diabetes. In other words, at 126 mg/dL you *do*, and at 125 mg/dL you *don't*. When Drs. House and Seale went to medical school decades ago, they were taught to make a diagnosis of diabetes when the blood sugar level reached 145 mg/dL.[13]

We think it's a good sign that the establishment has finally lowered the diagnostic threshold. It's a step in the right direction. The addition of the prediabetes category when the fasting blood sugars fall between 100 and 124 mg/dL is a recognition that the disease takes years to develop—and *can be recognized early*, giving the patient an opportunity for effective intervention and prevention. It seems that many doctors have come to realize that type-2 diabetes is a lifestyle disease. It's not an acute, traumatic disorder, such as a broken toe that happened when you stubbed it on a curb. It's about *choices gone wrong* in a culture that promotes such wrong choices. And now that it's pandemic, many more doctors see that the sooner we diagnose the condition and set patients on the right track, the better.

BLOOD SUGAR TESTING

WHETHER YOU ARE diagnosed with type-1 or type-2 diabetes or prediabetes, you need to test your blood sugar consistently, several times a day. You simply can't make the best decisions about food, physical activity, or medicine without knowing your blood sugar levels and their patterns. We recommend using your blood test meter six to eight times a day (see Chapter 6 for more details) to better understand how foods, physical activity, and medicines affect your blood sugar. If this advice sounds like we've just recommended you pet a porcupine eight times a day, we understand. We strongly suggest that you get a newer model blood test meter that requires only a microdroplet of blood. The lancet device that comes with such monitors is as close to pain free as possible. The FreeStyle meters from Abbot (the Flash and the Freedom models) take a very small blood sample and barely cause pain. We've also found them to be the most accurate. Generally, the OneTouch monitors produced by LifeScan are accurate and relatively pain free, too. Of course, all brands of blood test meters must be cleared by the U.S. Food and Drug Administration (FDA) for accuracy before they are allowed to be sold to the public. One more piece of advice from Ian: Try testing on the backs or tops of your fingers near the nail—many people find it both easier to draw blood and less painful than using the pads of the fingertip.

THE CHICKEN AND THE EGG:
More on Prediabetes

BECAUSE WE NOW know the process of type-2 diabetes starts well before that day you wake up with a fasting blood sugar at 126 mg/dL, there's a whole new diagnostic category. Thanks in part to the influence of the lifestyle medicine approach, the medical establishment has recognized a new condition called *prediabetes*. The benchmarks for prediabetes include a fasting blood sugar of 100 to 125 mg/dL (until recently, it was 110 to 125, another step in the right direction). A blood sugar level over 140 mg/dL, taken 2 hours after starting a regular-size meal, signals that the body is having a hard time putting sugar away after a meal, indicating growing insulin resistance. The same thing is probably happening (to a lesser degree) even when the blood sugar level 2 hours after a meal are between 120 and 140 mg/dL. While this is not an official range, you could very well consider it a telltale sign of increasing insulin resistance (pre-prediabetes, if you will), especially if it happens on a regular basis.

We say that things are moving in the right direction, but traditional medicine is not there yet. If you are a male, your risk of heart attack, stroke, eye disease, neuropathy, and other chronic complications is raised when your fasting blood sugar is over *90 mg/dL!*

How long do you have between prediabetes and full-blown type-2 diabetes? Will prediabetes necessarily lead to a diagnosis of diabetes? That depends mostly on you. Specifically, it depends on your lifestyle choices, primarily on what you eat and how physically active you are. *Prediabetes and type-2 diabetes are 95 percent lifestyle and environmental diseases.* It's clear that people in our culture are coming down with both prediabetes and type-2 diabetes earlier and earlier.[14] Just a few decades ago, only the autoimmune version of diabetes, type 1, was prevalent in children. In fact, until quite recently, people used to call type-1 diabetes *juvenile diabetes.* There was no confusion in this term, because it was highly unlikely a child could have had enough time to do enough damage through poor lifestyle choices to develop type-2 diabetes. No more. The youngest patient with type-2 diabetes in the state of Oklahoma was *only 3 years old at the time of diagnosis.* It's important to note that there are no 3-year-olds with type-2 diabetes in the Congolese or the Brazilian rain forest. A major cause of type-2 diabetes (too much energy in, and not enough energy out) is living in the United States.

In the next chapters, we're going to propose an antidote to diabetes that treats the cause of insulin resistance. Its keystone is a plant-based diet that's nutrient dense—high in vitamins, minerals, and phytochemicals—and low calorie. It's also high in fiber, which aids in slowing down sugar metabolism, and high in the *right kind* of carbohydrates. The right kind of physical activity will also help increase cell hunger (insulin sensitivity) and decrease insulin resistance, for better energy absorption in people with type-2 or type-1 diabetes.

SCIENCE OF THE TIMES:
Where Medication Fits into Your New Lifestyle

As you begin to follow the principles of lifestyle change outlined in this book, you'll find that the most powerful treatment for Western disease is what you eat and how physically active you are. It's likely that most of you have not been given this powerful treatment. Instead, you've been placed on medications. We're not opposed to the use of medications when other, more effective measures have been used and are still not enough. It just makes more sense to first do the things that work the best, cost nothing, and have no adverse side effects—namely, modifications of lifestyle through proper nutrition and sensible physical activity. But what are you to do with the medication you now take?

Here's the dilemma: If you're already being treated with medication for a lifestyle-related disease such as diabetes, heart disease, high blood pressure, or elevated cholesterol and then you add the powerful effects of proper lifestyle, you'll be at risk for developing problems from *overtreatment* of your condition. Your blood sugar and blood pressure might go lower than desired—perhaps even dangerously so. On the following few pages we'll outline some of the medications commonly used, in the order they're usually prescribed to people with diabetes. We'll also discuss the adjustments usually needed when our patients embark on the lifestyle changes we recommend. It's important for you to understand that the list cannot be all-inclusive and that we are not advocating that you attempt to adjust your medication on your own. It is also essential for you to *make all medication changes only under the direct supervision of a trusted healthcare professional*. We'll give general recommendations that may assist your doctor, based on our experience with the patients who have followed our program, but you should rely on your doctor's judgment and advice. If you're concerned about your relationship with your doctor, check out Chapter 10, which gives advice on how to find a doctor who can be a good lifestyle medicine coach.

Let's take a look at the medications for which the dosages often have been adjusted or even stopped completely when patients go on the 30-Day Diabetes Miracle lifestyle plan. These include medications for diabetes, high blood pressure, and high blood lipids (cholesterol and triglycerides). Please note that new medicines are frequently introduced and older medicines are phased out, and reports of the effects and side effects of pharmaceuticals are regularly updated, so please check with your doctor for the most up-to-date information.

Diabetes Pills

There are several types of pills used to treat type-2 diabetes.

Sulfonylureas

The sulfonylureas include the first-generation medicines Tolinase (tolazamide), Orinase (tolbutamide), Diabinese (chlorpropamide), and Dymelor (acetohexamide); the second-generation medicines Glucotrol and Glucotrol XL (glipizide), DiaBeta, Micronase, and Glynase (glyburide); and the third-generation drug Amaryl (glimepiride). Whether first, second, or third generation, these drugs all lower blood sugar by stimulating the pancreas to secrete more insulin, to shout *"The Energy's Coming!"* even louder than normal. Initially, this can help force more glucose (energy) into the cells that have been resistant to allowing more energy in, but these medicines really don't address the underlying cause of the problem—the consumption of too much energy (calories) and the expenditure of too little energy (physical activity). Early in the type-2 diabetes process, there's usually not a problem with the pancreas producing enough insulin. The pancreas will produce large amounts of insulin in an attempt to force extra energy into resistant cells. The resulting high insulin levels contribute to insulin resistance, weight gain, high blood pressure, high triglycerides and cholesterol levels, and premature large artery disease.

Late in the type-2 diabetes process, the pancreas will be failing and unable to produce adequate amounts of insulin to overcome the resistance of the body's cells. This will usually be the case, even when stimulated by prescribed drugs. By this time, it doesn't seem to make much sense to use these medications because they either stimulate an already overproducing pancreas or they flog a pancreas that cannot produce adequate amounts of insulin regardless of the stimulation. We commonly stop these medications completely early in the LCA program, usually on the first or second day. We typically will have problems with *low* blood sugar if the drugs are not stopped, as the effects of nutritional and activity changes rapidly begin to reverse the disease process. We monitor all of our diabetes patients closely, using blood sugar readings taken at least six times per day—before each meal, and 2 hours after each meal (we also recommend you test when you wake up and right before you go to sleep).

Meglitinides

The meglitinides, which include Starlix (nateglinide) and Prandin (repaglinide), also stimulate the pancreas to secrete more insulin, but they do so in a more specialized way. They are very fast acting and have a short duration of action, so they are usually taken with a meal in an attempt to keep the blood sugar under control in the first few hours after consumption of food. They're probably best used for type-2 diabetes when the pancreas is beginning to burn out and can't keep up with the increased glucose (energy) load after a meal. Usually, we stop these medications early in the program, on the first or second day. If, as the program progresses, the patient consistently has difficulty with high blood sugar (greater than 140 mg/dL) 2 hours after meals that contain adequate but not excessive carbohydrate and if blood testing indicates possible pancreatic sluggishness, we may restart the meglitinide and continue to monitor. The expectation is that as the patient loses weight and increases activity, insulin resistance will decrease and the pancreas's natural response to meals will be adequate. If that occurs, the medicine is stopped again, possibly for good.

Biguanides

Glucophage (metformin) is the only biguanide; it works by increasing insulin sensitivity of the liver. The liver stores energy in the form of glycogen and continually tries to convert glycogen into glucose (blood sugar). This is a good thing under normal circumstances because it prevents low blood sugar during times of fasting. When a meal is eaten, blood sugar rises, so there is no need for the liver to also contribute blood sugar. Insulin also increases after a meal, and it's insulin that shuts off the liver's conversion of glycogen into blood sugar. In someone who has developed insulin resistance, not only are muscle and fat cells resistant to insulin letting more blood sugar (energy) inside but the liver is also resistant to insulin's attempts to keep it from converting glycogen into more blood sugar. Glucophage increases the liver's sensitivity to insulin and helps prevent the liver from producing blood sugar when it's not needed. It does little to improve insulin sensitivity of muscle or fat cells, however. Because of this, Glucophage use is not associated with episodes of low blood sugar, even when lifestyle changes are made. At LCA, we routinely continue the use of Glucophage in our patients with type-2 diabetes. After a period of time on the program (which depends on the individual patient), when the patient loses weight and becomes more active, insulin resistance drops and the drug can then be stopped.

Thiazolidinediones

The thiazolidinediones include Actos (pioglitazone) and Avandia (rosiglitazone), which increase insulin sensitivity in the muscle and fat cells of the body. This allows the pancreas's secreted insulin to do its job more effectively; the blood sugar (energy) is more easily allowed into the cells, thus lowering the blood sugar level. Unless lifestyle change is done in conjunction with taking these medications, all of the extra blood sugar let into the cells of the body will lead to more weight gain. This, in turn, leads to even more insulin resistance. A higher dose of medication is, therefore, needed, and the vicious circle continues. Because we know the 30-Day Diabetes Miracle program will lower insulin resistance, we routinely stop the thiazolidinediones in the first few days. By doing so, patients lose weight much easier, and we avoid episodes of hypoglycemia (low blood sugar) that can occur if the drugs are continued.

Dipeptidyl Peptidase 4 Inhibitors

The only dipeptidyl peptidase 4 (DPP-4) inhibitor available as a pill to treat type-2 diabetes is Januvia (sitagliptin phosphate). In the pancreas, beta cells manufacture insulin, and alpha cells produce glucagon. Glucagon's role is to counteract the blood sugar–lowering effect of insulin. It does this by stimulating the liver to produce more blood sugar. As stated earlier, this is a good thing, in certain circumstances. As type-2 diabetes develops, three things occur in regard to blood sugar control. Insulin resistance develops in the liver and in fat and muscle cells; insulin production by pancreatic beta cells eventually decreases; and the secretion of glucagon, which raises blood sugar, isn't inhibited in a normal fashion. Also, certain hormones called *incretins* are secreted by the intestinal lining in response to eating, and these hormones increase insulin and decrease glucagon release by the pancreas. In a normal setting, incretins help keep blood sugar levels under control after a meal is eaten. However, incretins do not seem to work effectively in people with type-2 diabetes and thus are a contributing cause of elevated blood sugar, especially after meals. Januvia works by increasing the efficiency of intestinal incretins. At the time this book was being written, the drug had been available for only a short time, so we are not as experienced with it as with the other diabetes pills. Because it doesn't cause low blood sugar or weight gain, we usually continue this medication after the patient starts our program. As the patient makes lifestyle changes, begins to lose weight, and becomes regularly physically active, the diabetes process starts to reverse; Januvia can then be stopped and blood sugar is monitored.

Insulin

A common reason people with type-2 diabetes come to LCA is because they want to stop insulin or they are afraid of eventually needing it. Despite the common assumption, we can reassure you that *the vast majority of type-2 diabetes patients who are not already taking insulin will never need to begin, provided they adhere to the lifestyle changes we teach.* But how do we manage patients who are already using insulin when they come to us for treatment? As in the case of patients who are taking pills that stimulate secretion of insulin from the pancreas, we have found that if we do not decrease or discontinue insulin doses early in the program, our patients will begin to have trouble with low blood sugar events.

We have had patients who were taking 150 units or more of insulin per day when they arrived at LCA. They had been placed on such large doses in an incremental fashion, as they and their physician struggled to keep their blood sugar controlled. The real problem was not the disease progressing in and of itself but a lack of adherence to a lifestyle of proper nutrition and activity. By increasing the insulin doses in an attempt to counter unhealthy habits, the problems of weight gain, insulin resistance, high blood pressure, high cholesterol, and high triglycerides are only intensified. Even worse, blood sugar levels were not typically under control in those patients, despite such large insulin doses.

Our general approach for patients with type-2 diabetes is to reduce their daily insulin total dose by 50 percent in the first 24 hours of the program while we continue to monitor blood sugar six times per day. It's usually possible to reduce the dose again, by another 50 percent, in the next 2 or 3 days. In many cases, by the end of the 1st week of the program, we can have patients off insulin entirely—something they might have thought was impossible to do! Of course, these are only general guidelines, and treatment must be tailored to the individual patient, based on close monitoring of blood sugar. Again we remind you, *don't do this without your doctor's supervision.*

There are some type-2 diabetes patients who, like their type-1 counterparts, will not be able to stop insulin because they no longer have enough pancreatic beta-cell function remaining to sustain normal blood sugar, even with lifestyle change and the use of appropriate pills. By following our program, however, the patient can be assured that the dose of insulin will be the *lowest possible*, and they can avoid the undesirable effects of high insulin levels. The same is true for people with type-1 diabetes who are not able to stop insulin entirely. For many of these patients, insulin doses have been taken from exorbitant levels down to total daily doses that approximate the amount of insulin normally secreted by people who do not have diabetes.

Some people may be using newly available inhaled insulin. Although there hasn't been enough time for us to have adequate experience with this product, there should, theoretically, be no difference in the manner in which we would manage patients who are using it and those who are injecting insulin.

Obviously, there are many nuances to managing patients who require insulin, whether they have type-1 or type-2 diabetes, and it is not a topic that can be fully addressed in this book. We recommend you discuss our general guidelines with an understanding and supportive physician who is open to working with you and monitoring you closely before you make any adjustments in your insulin dose.

Byetta

Byetta (exenatide) is an injectible medication used for the treatment of type-2 diabetes. It is a protein originally discovered in the saliva of the Gila monster; hence it is sometimes referred to as *lizard spit*. It is now made synthetically. When injected, it mimics the effects of incretins (see "Dipeptidyl Peptidase 4 Inhibitors" earlier in this chapter) in the body, which helps control blood sugar levels. Our approach is to continue Byetta at the beginning of the lifestyle program, with the anticipation it can be stopped after the patient has lowered his or her insulin resistance. Of course, frequent blood sugar monitoring is also done.

Symlin

Symlin (pramlintide acetate), which is injected like insulin, is used by people with insulin-dependent (type-1) diabetes. It's a synthetic version of the pancreatic hormone amylin, which is made by the same pancreatic cells that make insulin, the beta cells. It stands to reason, then, that patients with type-1 diabetes and people with type-2 diabetes who have pancreatic burn-out have diminished amylin levels. Amylin helps inhibit the secretion of glucagon, and it's glucagon that increases the liver's production of glucose (blood sugar). So, if amylin levels are lower than what they should be, glucagon will not be suppressed, and the liver will continue producing blood sugar, even when it is not needed. We manage patients on Symlin by continuing the drug until they can either be taken off insulin or until they are at doses of insulin that approximate what the body would normally produce in a day. Then, the Symlin can be stopped and the blood sugar level is watched closely.

High Blood Pressure Medications

Among the medications that may require an adjustment during the early stages of the 30-Day Diabetes Miracle program are blood pressure medications. There are too many blood pressure medications, used alone or in combination, for us to give specific guidelines concerning their management. We recommend, when you begin our program, that you monitor your blood pressure frequently. Furthermore, you should ask your physician for advice if you notice changes in your blood pressure readings or experience adverse symptoms. We frequently see *blood pressures go too low* in patients who are on medication and following our diet and physical activity recommendations, so your medication will probably have to be adjusted to a lower dose. This typically happens 7 to 10 days into the program and is caused by a variety of nutritional factors as well as the body responding to increasing activity. It's also important for you and your physician to keep in mind that, although many changes can and do occur in the early days of the program, changes will continue to occur weeks or even months down the road. So you need to stay vigilant as time goes on. It's entirely possible that many of you will be able to *get off blood pressure medication entirely.*

Lipid-Lowering (Cholesterol) Drugs

With proper lifestyle changes, medication for high cholesterol and/or high triglycerides often can be dramatically reduced or stopped. It's our experience at LCA that patients' triglycerides will drop by 20 percent and cholesterol by 12 to 15 percent over the first 2 weeks of the 30-Day Diabetes Miracle program. This is about what you can expect from taking any of the widely used statin medications, without the cost or adverse side effects. Many patients see quite dramatic results, as you'll see in later chapters. You should have your lipid profile monitored periodically after you begin following our recommendations, and many of you will be able to *discontinue your lipid-lowering medications entirely.*

ONE PILL MAKES YOU LARGER . . .

WE DOCTORS AND patients are guilty of wanting a magic bullet. Lifestyle medicine doctor Julian Whitaker, who runs a chronic disease prevention center in California, sums up this phenomenon perfectly: "Physicians are trained to prescribe. Doctors learn in medical school that drugs are the most powerful tools we have for treating disease." And because dietary changes and physical activity are "almost never presented as therapeutic tools . . . drugs are usually viewed as the only significant options available."[15]

We agree. The accepted way of doing things today is to prescribe first and recommend diet and physical activity as an *afterthought*. Listen carefully to all those television commercials advertising drugs: "When diet and exercise aren't enough" they say, "you need drug *x*." But we all know that's not the way it works in the real world. Most people opt for the pill first, and they'll never know the answer to the question of whether diet and exercise are enough. The answer is a resounding yes! Diet and physical activity usually are enough—almost always when it comes to type-2 diabetes.

Take diabetic neuropathy (nerve pain and numbness in the lower extremities)—just one diabetes complication that costs the United States $15 billion a year to treat.[16] All that pain and all that money—surely we should work on ways to alleviate, or better yet, prevent it. Now consider Lyrica (pregabalin), a new drug for diabetic nerve pain that is now being advertised in major diabetes magazines. The ads for Lyrica say it's specifically designed to treat diabetic nerve pain, but among its many common side effects is weight gain and swelling of the hands and feet ("You may have a higher chance of swelling or gaining weight if you are taking certain diabetes medicines with Lyrica."[17] Of course you *are* likely to be taking other diabetes drugs if your diabetes has progressed to the point at which you have diabetic nerve pain). Other side effects include "unexplained muscle pain, soreness, or weakness along with a fever or tired feeling"; "problems with your eyesight, including blurry vision"; dizziness ("Do not drive a car, work with machines, or do other dangerous things until you know if Lyrica makes you drowsy"); dry mouth; skin sores ("If you have diabetes, pay extra attention to your skin"); and trouble concentrating ("Lyrica may cause some people to feel 'high'"). Furthermore, "[i]t is not known if Lyrica may decrease male fertility, cause birth defects, or pass into breast milk."

Well, none of that sounds good, but the weight gain and swelling are particularly troublesome. The ads for Lyrica admit, quite transparently, that "[w]eight gain may affect control of diabetes. Weight gain and swelling can be serious for people with heart problems" (which, of course, are very common among people with advanced diabetes). So, to get this straight, you're supposed to take a drug to treat a symptom of uncontrolled diabetes that not only contributes to the cause of uncontrolled diabetes but also has some common side effects—blurred vision, trouble concentrating, swelling, pain, weakness, and skin problems—that pretty much mimic the symptoms of uncontrolled diabetes, too. Why would you do that?

Not to mention that we haven't even addressed the likelihood that when you report the side effects to your doctor, you will likely be given more medication to relieve the new symptoms (a water pill and potassium to treat the swelling, an anti-vertigo pill for the dizziness, and so forth). Of course, when these medications cause their own side effects, you will need even more pills. This causes a domino effect, creating a toxic chemical stew in your body. Surely it makes more sense to avoid the cost and possible misery of additional side effects, some of which could be dangerous, by working on the *cause* of the problem—or at least on not exacerbating the problems. Unfortunately the trend toward *polypharmacy*—the administration of excessive medication—continues unabated.

We want to point out that countless patients of ours have found great relief from their nerve pain by following the lifestyle recommendations in this book (and many other patients have benefited from other lifestyle treatments we offer in our residential programs).

This brings us to the enormous influence, relevant here, of pharmaceutical companies on the medical community and government policies. The practices of drug marketing and education to physicians and direct advertising to patients are very worrisome to us. The multibillion-dollar pharmaceutical industry is presented to physicians by competing armies of drug representatives (reps), whose job is to traverse the cities and small towns of America visiting doctors' offices. They usually come bearing free samples of medications for patients and other goodies for physicians and their staff (such as pens, magnets, note pads, and key chains). Despite American Medical Association guidelines prohibiting gifts of more than $100 to physicians, sometimes there are more lucrative offers (such as box seats to entertainment venues or trips to exotic locations) for doctors if they promote specific products. In fact, nearly

95 percent of physicians in the United States receive free meals, drug samples, sport tickets, and other gifts from the drug reps.[18] It's also fair to say that for some physicians the only continuing education they receive is presented to them directly (in the form of information they get from pharmaceutical reps) or indirectly (via seminars and meetings sponsored by drug companies) by the pharmaceutical industry.

Patients often ask their doctors for a specific medication as a result of television, newspaper, or magazine advertising. Although doctors might not believe the medication is necessary, they feel pressure to prescribe it because patients have been convinced by the advertiser they need the drug and will not feel satisfied until they obtain the prescription. This makes it a constant challenge for physicians to maintain the necessary objectivity and healthy perspective that puts the patients' best interests at the fore. Many of us, we fear, are unable to succeed in doing this.

In any case, it's safe to say that representatives for apricots, radishes, and flaxseed are not driving from practice to practice with briefcases full of free low-cal salad dressing for patients, cruise tickets for doctors, and the most recent research results demonstrating the benefits of a plant-based diet. How can wholesome lifestyle choices compete with Big Pharmaceuticals' marketing, advertising, and continuing education?

Now don't get us wrong. We count ourselves among those who believe that many drugs work very well. In fact, most approved drugs for cholesterol, blood sugar, and high blood pressure work just fine. But they shouldn't be used as the *primary* treatment modality. First of all, they're quite expensive, as you probably already know. They're usually focused on chasing some number; they're frequently not prescribed until the patient's condition has had plenty of time to mature to the point of causing symptoms; and, finally, they almost never address the *cause* of the disease. Indeed, many of the most popular drugs might actually be worsening the underlying condition—for example, some diabetes drugs, if taken without improved diet and physical activity, will cause weight gain, as we've already discussed. This ultimately worsens insulin resistance, which makes the diabetes condition worse, not better. This means you'll eventually need—you guessed it!—more drugs.

There are many other potentially bad side effects of common prescription drugs for diabetes, high blood pressure, and cholesterol, most of which are certainly more uncomfortable than the imagined side effects of the necessary lifestyle changes. Sure, you could sprain your ankle at the gym and you could initially get some gas from eating lots of fiber. But compare that to the potential side effects and complications of the drugs you're taking. Have you ever read the federally mandated insert that comes with each bottle of medication your pharmacist dispenses? Do that sometime. It's very scary.

The drugs used for treating blood pressure, obesity, diabetes, and heart disease are best used carefully, in conjunction with, or as adjuncts to, lifestyle and behavioral change. You'll see hundreds of studies in this book that back up that claim: Lifestyle is the keystone of good health. Even insulin—though life-sustaining for people with type-1 diabetes—is a double-edged sword. As we discussed earlier in this chapter, elevated insulin levels induce weight gain through promoting the storage of fat, and increased weight can make diabetes worse. Furthermore, extra weight drastically increases your chances of cardiovascular disease (remember, 65 percent of all people with diabetes die of heart disease).[19] So insulin, even among people with type-1 diabetes who need it to survive, should be taken in the *lowest dosage possible* along with intensive lifestyle changes, which we discuss in detail in the following chapters.

The SAD State of Our Diet

OBESITY IS NOW considered the second leading cause of death in North America. At the rate we're going, by 2025, 75 percent of the population on our continent will be overweight.[1] In 2000, the Worldwatch Institute indicated that, for the first time in history, as many people are overweight as are underfed—1.2 billion each.[2] Risk of diabetes is about doubled for those who are moderately overweight and tripled for those who are obese.[3]

So how did we get into this fine diabetic, overweight mess? One factor to blame is the standard American diet (SAD), the foundation of which is high in animal fat and protein, calories, sugar, and refined carbohydrates. Along with lack of activity, the SAD—not genetics, not heredity—is the chief cause of diabetes and many other chronic diseases. We know this is not what many other books on diabetes will tell you. They infer that it's not your poor lifestyle choices that caused your diabetes: They say it's genetics.

We disagree strongly. The fact is, even if you're loaded with genes that might predispose you to type-2 diabetes, your *lifestyle can alter the expression* of those bad genes. That means environment and lifestyle can trump genetics when it comes to diabetes. Yes, there are genetic factors that influence our weight and tendency toward diabetes. But if you take two people with identical sets of such genes and put one on a healthful diet along with physical activity and put the other on a fast-food diet along with no activity, doesn't it make sense that the latter person is creating a setting that enhances the effects of any diabetes genes? If diabetes is simply genetic, why is it spreading at such alarming rates? No genetic theory would allow for such a massive, swift genetic change across the entire globe. The problem is the SAD: too many calories, too much fat, too many refined carbohydrates (the staples of junk food and fast food), and—believe it or not—too much protein.

CALORIES, CALORIES, EVERYWHERE!

JUST ABOUT EVERYTHING you eat has calories—protein, fat, carbohydrate, and alcohol all contain them. Calories equal energy, which is a good thing because, of course, we need energy to live. But 5 pounds of spaghetti provides enough energy to brew a pot of coffee; one slice of cherry cheesecake could light a 60-watt light bulb for 90 minutes; and 217 Big Macs could power a car for 88 miles.[4] And in case you're wondering, there are plenty of people in America who eat 217 Big Macs in a year. The bigwigs at McDonald's call these folks "heavy users" in their internal documents.[5] The executives at Burger King call them "superfans."[6]

Calories will never pose a problem for you unless you consume more of them than you burn through physical activity. When that happens, those excess calories are stored as fat. In summary, to lose weight, you need to eat fewer calories and be more active.

The SAD News about Caloric Intake

Most of our patients report they're eating *at least* 3,000 to 3,500 calories a day. For many of them, it's more and often *much* more. Most health experts agree that an adult woman should be consuming no more than about 1,600 to 2,000 calories a day and adult men, 2,200 to 2,500 calories per day. And, by the way, those recommendations are for healthy people of normal weight, who are also regularly physically active. An overweight man who has diabetes and wants to lose weight should be consuming no more than 1,700 calories a day; an overweight woman with diabetes who wants to lose should stick to between 1,200 and 1,400 calories per day— and these patients still need regular physical activity if they expect to drop pounds. At the Lifestyle Center of America (LCA), our patients get between 1,250 and 2,100 calories a day. However, we don't teach them to count calories, and most of them have no idea they have reduced their calorie intake—it occurs because of the naturally high-fiber, lower-fat, and low-calorie content of the plant-based diet (PBD).

WEIGHT, WEIGHT, THERE'S MORE!

●

MOST people have to eliminate 3,500 calories from their diet (or burn them through increased physical activity) to lose about 1 pound. So if you want to lose 2 pounds a week, you'd have to raise your activity level enough to burn an extra 7,000 calories, or about 1,000 calories a day. That's possible, but not very easy. It would probably be easier to eliminate 1,000 calories a day from your diet. By the same token, if you eat just 500 extra calories a day (an order of Wendy's 10-piece Chicken Nuggets with Barbeque Nugget Sauce), you're going to gain about 1 pound each week. Better that you work against gaining weight from both sides of the equation: Burn more calories by increasing your activity and eliminate calories, especially the "empty" ones from junk food that come with no nutritional integrity.

LET'S GO TO FAT CAMP

WHEN IT COMES to calories, fat is a principal offender. There are more than twice as many calories in a gram of fat than in a gram of carbohydrate or protein. You can eat *twice as much carbohydrate and protein than fat*, for the same calories.

Eating low-fat foods is a good way to lose weight and improve your insulin resistance, which we explained in Chapter 3. It will help diminish diabetes and heart disease. But remember to look at the number of calories you're consuming, too, not just the fat intake. Eating low-fat processed foods often means you're taking in more sugar and more calories. Here you have to pay particular attention to the portion size listed on the package label. For example, you may think that a cup of whole milk would contain less fat than a scoop of ice cream. But the milk (8 grams [g] of fat per cup) actually contains about the same as the ice cream (8.3 g of fat per 1.9-ounce scoop).[7] Our preference would be to skip them both. Also remember that lots of fat-free foods, like soda, pasta, and beer, are still loaded with calories.

Nutrition authorities recommend adults consume no more than 20 to 35 percent of their total calories from fat. That's 44 to 77 g of fat or less per day if you eat 2,000 calories. We recommend staying as close as possible to the low end of that range and eating a maximum of 40–45 g of fat per day. Most of the fat you eat should be *unsaturated*, the type found most often in plant foods. *Saturated* fat is prevalent in animal products and junk food and should be avoided. About 80 percent of all saturated fat consumed in America comes from animal sources, and nearly a third of that comes from cheese, beef, and milk alone.[8]

Americans consume at least 40 percent of their calories from fat (lots of oils, butter/margarine, dairy, and meat are the main culprits). Many of our patients are on a 50 percent fat diet when they arrive at LCA, wondering why they're overweight and unhealthy. We put them on a wholesome plant-based diet. The formula is simple: Cut out the animal products, and you will cut out the fat.

The Atomic Skinny on Fats

All the popular news on fats can be confusing. What's important to get straight are the differences between saturated fats, unsaturated fats, and trans-fats. All fats are composed of a combination of saturated and unsaturated fatty acids. A saturated fatty acid is said to be saturated because it's jam-packed with hydrogen atoms, as many as will fit on the chain of carbon atoms. Saturated fats, like you'll find in steak, butter, and ice cream, are naturally occurring and come mainly from animal sources. They raise blood levels of triglycerides, total cholesterol, and low-density lipoprotein (LDL) cholesterol (aptly named the "bad" cholesterol because it blocks arteries). Because of this, including saturated fats in your diet will increase your risk of heart attack and other vascular diseases.

Unsaturated fats are also natural, and you can find them mainly in plant foods, like whole grains, avocados, nuts, olives, and canola oil. Their carbon atoms are not totally saturated with hydrogen. They're better for you and are even associated with lowering total and LDL cholesterol, thus reducing your risk of coronary and other artery blockages.

Trans-fats are those *unnatural*, manufactured fats that behave like saturated fats in our bodies. In fact, they are more dangerous, because not only do they raise triglycerides, total cholesterol, and LDL cholesterol but they also lower high-density lipoprotein (HDL) cholesterol (the "good" cholesterol). They also increase the risk of developing type-2 diabetes.[9] Trans-fats are a byproduct of a process called hydrogenation, or partial hydrogenation. Partially hydrogenated fats are more resistant to spoilage, are easier to ship and store, and last much longer on the grocery shelf. Partially hydrogenated oils also change the fundamental texture of foods to which they are added, so oils become spreadable, like margarine. Pie crusts are flakier, and puddings are creamier. So food manufacturers love it. Your body does not.

We suggest you keep your trans-fat intake as low as possible. Zero trans-fat intake would be fantastic but is likely not possible, owing to its nearly universal presence in processed foods. You will need to read labels and avoid any products that list trans-fat, or that mention the words *hydrogenated* or *partially hydrogenated* in the ingredient list. At most, your trans-fat intake should not exceed 2 g per day.

In some commercial food products, unhealthy trans-fats have now been replaced with another kind of synthetic modified fat called interesterified fat, which has been shown to be as dangerous to our health as trans-fat. So far in America, there's no legal requirement to list interesterified fat on the Nutrition Facts label along with the saturated fat and trans-fat, but you will be able to find it in the ingredient list: Look for the words *interesterified* or *fully hydrogenated* fat.

SUGAR SHOCK

NOW THAT WE'VE indicted the calorie and fat bandits robbing you of your health, let's look at sugar. How much sugar do you suppose you eat? Would it surprise you to learn that the average American consumes somewhere between 133 and 159 *pounds* of sugar per year?[10] This is equivalent to *40 to 50 teaspoons of sugar, or 500 to 600 calories, per day.*[11] Impossible, you say? That's not you, you say? Well, let's look at where sugar may be hiding.

The average American gets a third of their added sugar from soft drinks.[12] Can you guess how much sugar's in 32 fluid ounces of Coca-Cola? It's just shy of 1/4 *pound* (or 22 teaspoons). Many Americans consume up to 150 pounds of sugar per year from soft drinks alone.

If you think you're safe because you stay away from soft drinks, take a look at those upscale coffee and specialty drinks. A 24-fluid-ounce Starbucks Caramel Frappuccino Blended Coffee with whipped cream contains 14 teaspoons of sugar. A 16-fluid-ounce Dunkin' Donuts Tropicana Orange Coolatta—which might seem better for you because of all that "natural" orange—has 18 teaspoons of sugar! If you have one of these kinds of drinks every day but Sunday, you've just consumed 1 pound of sugar every week, which adds up to *52 pounds a year* just from your morning beverage alone.

So, how about juice, you ask? Don't go there if you have diabetes. The sugar in juice is concentrated and will raise your blood sugar faster and higher than the source food. A 15.2-fluid-ounce bottle of Welch's 100 percent grape juice, for example, has 80 g of sugar—even more than the Starbucks Frappuccino. The equivalent volume of whole grapes, on the other hand, has only about 30 g of sugar. It's *always* better to eat whole foods.

Don't forget that fructose is sugar, too. Fructose is relatively low glycemic, meaning it will not cause a huge, fast spike in your blood sugar the way regular table sugar might—but it's still sugar. In nature, fructose comes mostly from fruit, but scientists perfected a way to extract it from corn. This highly processed form of sugar in disguise, called high-fructose corn syrup (HFCS), is a ubiquitous and dangerous staple in most Americans' diet. HFCS is particularly bad for people with diabetes because it's high glycemic: It quickly and sharply raises blood sugar. There are studies that show a link between HFCS and development of central abdominal obesity, a major risk factor for insulin resistance, a precursor to diabetes and heart disease.

Just how much added sugar should you consume for optimal health? Our answer at LCA is unequivocal: None is best. If you already have type-2 diabetes, your sugar intake may be one major cause. If you don't yet have diabetes, there's a good chance you will soon if you subscribe to the SAD's sugar parameters. If you feel you *must* use some sugar (no one must, but you might feel that way), we make the following recommendations:

- Try to overcome your sweet tooth by using the cognitive behavior therapy (CBT) methods we discuss in Chapter 9.
- Use sugar in very small amounts: We mean no more than 1 teaspoon a day.
- Don't use any refined (white table) sugar or HFCS, at all. These products are so highly processed that not only do they provide no nutritional value but they also actually drain your body of other nutrients when they are metabolized; that's a net loss.

■ Use only low-glycemic sweeteners wherever possible (*low glycemic* means the food doesn't raise your blood sugar sharply or quickly). Good low-glycemic sweeteners include 100 percent pure floral honey (which raises blood sugar only half as much and half as quickly as processed commercial honey), pure fructose (not to be confused with HFCS), barley malt syrup, and agave nectar. Barley malt syrup is about 75 percent maltose, a more complex carbohydrate that the body breaks down more slowly than many other sweeteners. Agave nectar is a low-glycemic sweetener that has 16 g of carbohydrate per teaspoon and about the same number of calories per teaspoon as sugar, but it's much better for you if you have diabetes, because it is very high in natural fructose.

■ When you're reading labels, remember that all of the following ingredients fall under the category of sugar. They will all raise your blood sugar level to some degree:[13]

- beet sugar
- black-strap
- brown sugar
- carob
- chocolate
- confectioner's sugar
- corn sweetener
- corn syrup
- date sugar
- dextrin
- dextrose
- fructose
- fruit juice concentrates
- fruit sugar
- glucose
- golden syrup
- grape sugar
- high-fructose corn syrup
- honey
- honey maple syrup
- invert sugar
- lactose
- levulose
- malt syrup
- maltodextrin
- maltose
- mannose
- maple sugar
- milk sugar
- molasses
- powdered sugar
- raw sugar
- refiner's sugar
- saccharose
- sorbitol
- sorghum syrup
- sucanat (dehydrated cane juice)
- sucrose
- sugar
- sugar cane syrup
- syrup

- table sugar
- treacle
- turbinado

- xylitol
- xylose

Are You a Carbohydrate Addict?

Remember when you're reading labels for sugar content to check the listing for carbohydrates, as this is the most important thing for people with diabetes. Some carbohydrates (the natural, unprocessed ones like oatmeal, blueberries, and broccoli) are necessary and good for you in terms of your overall health and your blood sugar response. Others (the highly processed and refined kind, like candy, white bread, and chips) are unnecessary and risky if you're trying to keep your blood sugar low.

A 12-fluid-ounce can of Dr Pepper contains nearly half of the total carbohydrates that we recommend most male patients consume for an entire meal and almost 75 percent of what we recommend for most female patients. In LCA surveys, we find that the average new patient consumes 40 to 50 percent of their dietary intake in carbohydrates. You might assume that this is a medical disaster waiting to happen. However, it isn't necessarily bad to eat so much carbohydrate. In fact, the LCA diet contains 60 to 65 percent carbohydrates. And yet our patients are able to keep their blood sugars in better control than they were before entering the program. Sounds crazy? The key is in eating the *right kind* of natural, unprocessed, unrefined, high-fiber carbs.

Sugar Free Is a Trap!

We encounter so many people with diabetes who are convinced they're eating right because they eat only sugar-free desserts and breads. Please do not be fooled by this! It's just a nasty marketing ploy. While it might be true that there's no *added* sugar in most of these products, they are very often composed of nearly 100 percent carbohydrates, most often white, processed flour (that's why a muffin has more carbs than a doughnut—more flour). When it comes to the white flour that makes up most so-called sugar-free cookies and snacks, it really might as well be pure sugar, so quickly and dramatically will it raise your blood sugar.

The process of refining flour was just as devastating to our diet as the refining of sugar. To make soft, spongy white bread like classic Wonder

Bread, food manufacturers have to remove the whole grain's germ and bran layers. In doing so, they also strip the wheat of most of its vital fiber, B vitamins, and other crucial nutrients. This creates calories that are less beneficial. In the old days, only rich people could afford white bread, which was expensive to process and, therefore, a status symbol. Not anymore. The diseases of kings, like obesity and diabetes, have now become the diseases of everyone—the modern serf, all of us regular folks.

The second dangerous dietary trap is that most food manufacturers will up the fat content in sugar-free desserts and breads. They often use saturated fat and trans-fat oils because these fats extend products' shelf life and improve mouthfeel. The formula for processed and refined manufactured foods is simple: *The lower the sugar, the higher the fat*, and vice versa.

To quote Nancy Reagan, just say no.

Artificial Sweeteners

Artificial sweeteners may have no calories, but as far as the *long-term* safety of artificial sweeteners approved by the U.S. Food and Drug Administration (FDA), the jury's still out. But our own jury of experts has spoken: We believe artificial sweeteners are highly processed, non-nutritive chemicals that are unnecessary and don't fit into an optimal diet. We prefer our patients not consume artificial sweeteners at all and feel this is a reasonable recommendation.

This is our advice: Give your taste buds a chance to learn what the inherent sweetness of natural, honest-to-goodness food is like. This may take a few weeks. Then, if you still wish to sweeten some food, you should use small amounts of natural sweeteners like agave nectar, floral honey (the kind made by bees, not factories), and barley malt syrup.

If you find you have a problem with a sweet addiction, we recommend you wean yourself off sweeteners altogether. The craving for sweetness is not something you want to feed, even if you're not immediately raising your blood sugar or adding calories. Giving in to this craving can make you fat, even if you're consuming only no-calorie, low-glycemic sweeteners.

Did you know that drinking diet sodas can lead to weight gain? In one study, those who consumed one to two diet sodas per day over 8 years were 65 percent *more* likely to become overweight or obese than those who consumed the same amount of regular soda over the same period of time. How's that possible? The artificial sweeteners in diet soda seem to affect appetite, making us want to eat more. The sweetness somehow tricks the body into thinking it has consumed sugar (which has calories), but when no calories come, the body then craves calories from other food, resulting in overeating. Or those who consume diet soda may simply give themselves permission to indulge in other sweets and treats ("Two Whoppers with cheese and a Tab, please!").

It should be pointed out that you are not safe if you drink regular soda instead of diet, of course. There was a 33 percent chance of becoming overweight or obese in the group drinking one to two regular sodas per day over the 8 years. But note that your chances of getting fat drinking diet soda are actually considerably *higher* than if you drank only regular soda.[14]

PROTEIN

HUMANS REQUIRE PROTEIN. It's essential for our growth and continued existence. However, we don't need nearly as much as most people consume. And—this might come as a shock—we don't need to eat meat to get it.

The China Study, the most comprehensive nutritional study ever conducted, concluded that too much protein, not too little, is the source of our most dire diseases, from diabetes and obesity to cancer and heart disease. The study's lead researcher, T. Colin Campbell, blames a common assumption and a related cultural bias. Most people associate protein with meat and meat with wealth. Rich people are supposed to have that fatted calf on the table. It's only poor people who eat staple plant foods like potatoes and bread.[15]

Over the years, government authorities have substantially reduced the recommended daily allowance of protein (from 125 g in the early 20th century to 55 g today, according to the U.S. Department of Agriculture). But the American people and many doctors haven't gotten the message that "diets with more animal-based protein will create higher blood cholesterol levels and higher risks of atherosclerosis (hardening of the arteries), cancer, osteoporosis, Alzheimer's disease and kidney stones, to name just a few chronic diseases."[16] Of course, high cholesterol and atherosclerosis are strongly associated with diabetes and can certainly make matters worse if you have diabetes.

At LCA, our diet contains about 15 percent of the daily caloric intake from protein. And none of that protein comes from meat, dairy, or eggs. There are good plant sources of protein, such as beans, nuts, and tofu, that are better for you and are lower in calories than animal sources (the foods mentioned are only examples—all plant foods contain some protein, enough to provide more than adequate daily protein intake on a plant-based diet [PBD]). Don't be fooled by the term *incomplete protein* that you'll sometimes see associated with plant protein (as opposed to complete for animal sources). This has to do with the number and variety of amino acids that are in the protein, and nothing to do with the overall "quality" of the protein source. Food combining does not need to take place during the same meal. Simply eat a variety of plant-based foods, including a good selection of fruits, vegetables, whole grains, nuts, seeds, and beans, and you will be consuming all of the amino acids that your body requires to make the proteins it needs for optimal health. "There's a mountain of compelling research showing that . . . plant protein, which allows for slow but steady synthesis of new proteins, is the healthiest type of protein. Slow but steady wins the race."[17]

YOUR BRAIN AND EMOTIONS ARE YOUR DINNER COMPANIONS

IT OFTEN SURPRISES our doctors and nutritionists to find out how much people are consuming at home by way of desserts and junk food, even though they have diabetes. This really comes down to *emotional* eating issues for many people—"confusing food with feelings."[18]

The SAD has built-in ingredients guaranteeing it continues to be self-sustaining. Because of its very low fiber, high-sugar, high-fat, high-calorie foundation, it may give immediate pleasure, but doesn't provide long-lasting satisfaction. It can leave you constantly scrounging for a snack to quiet your need for more of the same. Studies have shown these cravings are not unlike what drug addicts experience when jonesing for a fix of their favorite poison. Then most of us, when we see the scale moving up, get frustrated and disappointed with ourselves. Those two emotions lead to more of you know what: emotional eating. On top of this, many authorities believe that sugar itself can contribute to depression.[19]

Highly processed, high-calorie, high-fat foods were simply not meant to be accessed so easily—and in such bulk. At LCA, we believe psychologist Douglas Lisle when he asserts that humans allowed our advances in food-innovation science to short-circuit nature. We've found a magic button to access the pleasure centers of our brain, those that alert us to a sense of security amid our natural fear of famine. Like cats chasing balls of yarn, we're only following our instincts when we stalk, hunt, and wolf down Cinnabons at the local mall (two Caramel Pecanbons have a shocking 2,200 calories, 162 g of fat, and 282 g of carbs; the average total *daily* calorie intake in Vietnam, India, Peru, and Haiti[20]). This is very similar to the process of alcohol or drug addiction: The pursuit and acquisition of the sought-after caloric prize becomes paramount as the brain seeks ever-more quick fixes for its insatiable desire. A doughnut can trigger a dopamine reaction in the brain just like any other stimulus the brain treats as "pleasure," whether it's good for you or not. When you combine this instinct with our mixed-up way of emotional eating (food = love; food = reward; food = comfort), it's clear that we must work on ways to shut off this gluttony circuit.

People on the LCA diet are able to break this cycle. They report that their thinking gets clearer; they feel more satisfied and less hungry. Most don't experience extreme highs and lows in blood sugar, so they don't snack as much between meals. The change occurs as a result of the lack of refined sugars, starches, and junk in their diet as well as the high fiber content (40 to 50 g of fiber makes one feel full, but passes through the body instead of staking a claim on the thighs). The 30-Day Diabetes Miracle diet and the rest of our program will help you lose weight and conquer diabetes: You won't feel the need to eat as much, you'll feel better (not deprived) about your food choices, and you won't suffer the yo-yo effect of high and low blood sugars that compel you to eat poorly.

MEAT AND MILK:
Worth the Risk?

THE EVIDENCE IS overwhelming that a diet high in animal protein, saturated fats, and cholesterol will increase your risk of diabetes, heart disease, high blood pressure, osteoporosis, and some cancers. But there is another hazard that many people do not often think about. It is the danger of catching a communicable illness from the animal foods you eat—in other words, getting food poisoning. Consider these sobering facts concerning the U.S. food supply:[21]

- There are about 76 million individual cases of illness due to contaminated food *each and every year*!
- Approximately 325,000 people are hospitalized annually because of food poisoning.
- Every year, 5,000 individuals die as a result of food-related illness.

The overwhelming majority of these illnesses are related to foods derived from animal products. This is because the bacteria involved are normally found in the intestinal tracts of animals, and during slaughter these organisms can contaminate the meat. In the case of dairy products, bacteria can be shed directly into the milk, but more commonly they are present because of direct manure contamination. Eggs can be tainted either from bacteria entering through a crack in the shell or incorporated into the egg itself from a healthy-appearing infected hen, before the shell is formed.[22]

Raw foods of animal origin are the most likely to be contaminated. Food processing that mixes products of many animals can also dramatically increase chances of infection. For example, milk is usually "pooled" from scores of dairy cows; a pound of ground beef can contain meat from hundreds of cows; a broiler chicken carcass can be exposed to the drippings and juices of many thousands of other birds that went through the same cold water tank after slaughter[23]—you get the idea.

Yes, plant foods can also be a potential source for foodborne illnesses. Outbreaks can, and do, occur, but the bacteria responsible for such infections are not organisms normally found on plants. Instead, they are *bacteria found in the intestinal tracts of animals*. The contamination can usually be traced to contaminated water or manure sources. However, the odds of purchasing a carrot or head of lettuce that is contaminated with bacteria is infinitely less than your chances of buying a contaminated piece of meat. One recent study revealed that 83 percent of fresh broiler chickens purchased nationwide contained one or both of the two most common bacteria associated with food poisoning.[24]

One of the last animal foods given up by most people is dairy. Part of this is because of acquired tastes for these products, but undoubtedly much is also related to the immense marketing done by the dairy industry, stressing to the public that milk and cheese are essential to our health. If you ask anyone older than a first- or second-grader where people get calcium for strong bones, the answer will be milk. There is calcium in milk, of course, but cows get their calcium from eating green plants. People can get all the calcium they need from eating green plants, too.

Along with calcium, you can get infections from milk. In a 1997 study, between 20 and 40 percent of U.S. dairy herds were infected with a bacterium called *Mycobacterium paratuberculosis*. This organism is resistant to pasteurization and can be secreted directly into milk or be present because of manure contamination. There is much evidence to support the theory that this bacteria may cause Crohn's disease, a painful inflammation of the small intestine affecting a half million Americans, many of whom are younger than 30 years old.[25] Other bacteria that can be present in milk include salmonella, *Campylobacter*, *Escherichia coli*, listeria, and shigella.[26] Pasteurization will kill most of these bacteria, but the pasteurization process is not 100 percent effective (if it were, pasteurized milk would not have to be refrigerated and would have an infinite shelf life!). As if all of this were not enough, about 90 percent of U.S. dairy herds are infected with bovine leukemia virus,[27] an organism that is also found in the milk of the infected animal. This virus has been shown to cause cancers in sheep and monkeys. It has also been found in human breast cancer specimens.[28]

Let's also not forget mad cow disease. Milk may not be free of the infectious particle for this mysterious ailment, and in fact recent research indicates it likely is present.[29] If it's present in milk, pasteurization will certainly not inactivate it, owing to its extremely high heat tolerance. Remember the old advertising slogan, "Milk. It does a body good"? We disagree.

WRAP THAT UP TO GO

THE STANDARD AMERICAN diet is truly SAD. It's literally killing us. But because it usually looks, smells, and tastes good to most of us (food manufacturers spend a lot of money to pull off that magic), we go willingly to our deaths. All our major chronic diseases can be linked to the SAD state of affairs on our plates. Diabetes is definitely a direct result, and it's crippling individuals and families at an alarming rate. As baby boomers age, the diabetes brought on by the SAD will soon weaken our already straining health-care system and, eventually, our entire economy. The increase in adult-onset diabetes contributed to a whopping 64 percent rise in diabetes treatment from 1987 to 2002.[30] Since then, the numbers have sharply risen. We wouldn't be surprised if the real annual cost of diabetes is already close to $200 billion.

But you can't put a price on a lost limb, can you?

Or a lost grandma.

Is that cupcake *really* worth it?

5

The Edible Antidote to Diabetes

CHOOSING WHAT YOU eat when you have diabetes can be one of the most frustrating aspects of living with the disease. Eating is, after all, one of the most enjoyable activities in life. We're designed, hardwired, to enjoy it. But we absolutely shouldn't eat mindlessly.[1] At Lifestyle Center of America (LCA), we promote what we call *The Big Three Goals* in planning your diet if you have diabetes:

1. *Eat to keep your blood sugar levels in a low, healthy range and as tightly controlled as you can.* The American Diabetes Association (ADA) is as emphatic as we are that the number one priority for people with diabetes is to try to maintain normal or near-normal glucose levels. Why should this be a priority? We base this imperative not only on all our clinical experience but also on two landmark diabetes studies,[2] both of which have provided unequivocal evidence that chronically high blood sugar levels—that means blood sugar levels that are high pretty much all the time—are responsible for the gruesome long-term complications of diabetes: the destruction of your eyes, your kidneys, and your nerves. But the good news is that the opposite is also true. *If you maintain tight blood sugar control, you can delay, avoid, and in some cases even reverse the devastating complications of diabetes.* According to the largest, most comprehensive study ever done on diabetes,[3]

if you have diabetes, tight control of your blood sugar will greatly reduce your risk of major diabetes complications.

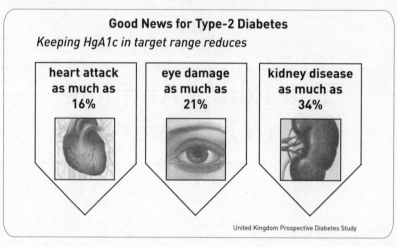

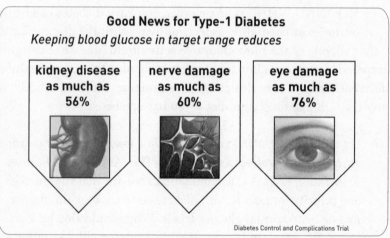

2. *Keep your overall fat and calories down.* Weight gain and diabetes very often go hand in hand, usually through the process of insulin resistance. Remember there are slightly more than twice as many calories in a gram of fat as there are in the same amount of carbohydrates.

3. *Try to eat about the same amounts and types of food at each meal, and try to eat each meal at about the same time every day.* Your life is not like a "metabolic laboratory" where you can control every jot and tittle of everything you eat and when you

eat it. But if you simply eat mindfully, aware of what you're consuming and when, you'll be ahead of those masses engaged in what Cornell University food scientist Brain Wansink has called "desk and dashboard dining."[4]

There is a diet that covers all these bases. It's not even close to the diet recommended by the American Diabetes Association or the American Dietetic Association, and that's probably one reason that most people with diabetes in the United States are not getting better, but getting worse. In short, this diet is plant based. Most people with type-2 diabetes who stick to a plant-based diet (and the right kind of physical activity, which we'll talk about in Chapter 8) are able to stay off their oral diabetes medicines and insulin for the long term.[5] And even people with type-1 diabetes can significantly reduce their insulin intake with our diet.

Our diet takes care of the first goal of keeping blood sugar levels tight—and not merely by "covering" what you eat with enough insulin or oral medicine. After all, you could eat two boxes of Girl Scout cookies and then take enough insulin to cover all those carbohydrates, which would keep your blood sugar levels tight. Obviously, that's a terrible idea. Instead our diet handles the *causes* of diabetes and the metabolic syndrome. When you work on the source, the blood sugar will eventually take care of itself.

THE SIX PROTECTIVE HEALTH FACTORS OF A PLANT-BASED DIET

DESPITE THE INCORRECT old assumption that vegetarians are weak, feeble, and pale from lack of protein,[6] many studies have drawn exactly the opposite conclusion. Vegetarians are among the healthiest and longest-lived Americans. Just look at members of the Seventh-Day Adventist (SDA) church, co-founded by Ellen G. White in the mid-19th century. The SDA church has been a principle proponent of a plant-based diet (PBD), mainly for health reasons. White writes, "Grains, fruits, nuts, and vegetables constitute the diet chosen for us by our Creator. These foods prepared in as simple and natural a manner as possible, are the most healthful and nourishing."[7] About 40 percent of today's SDA members are still vegetarian. The School of Public Health at Loma Linda University in California has conducted three huge studies of members of the SDA church. Two previous studies involved 24,000 and 34,000 Californian Adventists over 40 years. Adventist Health Study-2 is a new and even bigger study that began in 2001 and will include more than 100,000 Adventists from the United States and Canada. Over the past 50 years, hundreds and perhaps thousands of researches have looked at all the data Loma Linda collected. Their studies found that certain aspects of the Adventist lifestyle, in particular vegetarianism, protected people in the study group from early death and poor health. Both men and women practicing the plant-based lifestyle live longer than their carnivorous counterparts. Those on the strictest plant-based diet have a 63 percent lower risk of early death than those eating the least amount of plant-based foods,[8] and suffer far less from diabetes and other chronic diseases.[9]

For the sake of transparency, we should note that while LCA is not officially affiliated with the SDA church, our founders and many of our staff are members. Much of what we practice in terms of diet and lifestyle is consistent with the SDA church's philosophy on healthcare.

PLANT-BASED DIET BEST FOR DIABETES HEALTH

●

A vegetarian diet reduces the occurrence of diabetes. In a study begun in 1960, 25,698 white adult Adventists were followed for 21 years. Results showed that the Adventists' risk for developing diabetes was about *half* that for all U.S. whites. And the vegetarians in the study had substantially lower risk than did the meat eaters of dying from diabetes.[10]

In the following sections, we introduce the six best health-protecting factors of a PBD, in no particular order.

A Plant-Based Diet Has More Dietary Fiber Than Does an Animal-Based Diet

When the deer munch on brush on the LCA grounds each morning, their systems can break down the cellulose fiber into energy and make use of it. But we humans can't. Yet dietary fiber—the part of fruits, vegetables, nuts, and whole grains that is not broken down in the human digestive system—is the bedrock of the LCA diet. Over the years, fiber's been like the Rodney Dangerfield of nutrition: It doesn't get any respect.

This is unfair, because fiber lowers our risk for diabetes, heart disease, strokes, appendicitis, and even some cancers.[11] Our colleague and former staff physician Dr. Tim Arnott used to say, "Fiber is everyone's friend." A high-fiber diet can actually help patients with diabetes reduce their insulin intake, even when lots of fruits are eaten,[12] which surprises many people with diabetes who assume all fruits are "bad." One study found that 21 of 23 patients on oral medications and 13 of 17 patients on insulin were able to get off their medications after 26 days on a near-vegetarian diet with lots of fruits and a physical activity program.[13]

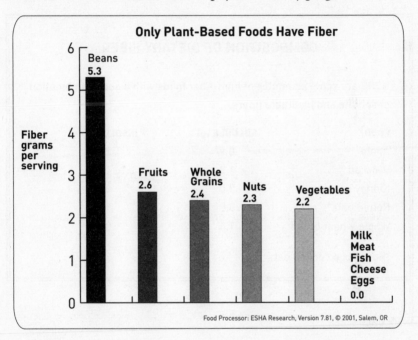

Only Plant-Based Foods Have Fiber

Fiber grams per serving

Beans 5.3
Fruits 2.6
Whole Grains 2.4
Nuts 2.3
Vegetables 2.2
Milk Meat Fish Cheese Eggs 0.0

Food Processor: ESHA Research, Version 7.81, © 2001, Salem, OR

Soluble Versus Insoluble Fiber: What's the Difference?

Why would we want to eat a substance that we can't digest or absorb? The answer has to do with the two kinds of fiber: soluble and insoluble.

SOLUBLE FIBER

Soluble fiber (such as gums and pectins) dissolves in water. It's found mainly in fruits, vegetables, oats, barley, and legumes. Think of Metamucil: It takes only 1 teaspoon dissolved in 8 fluid ounces of water. It'll stay watery for a while, then start thickening, becoming a jellylike mass. In foods, think of the gummy, sticky consistency of oatmeal or blueberry pie. It's that gummy consistency that requires you to stay well hydrated when you're on a high-fiber diet. You need enough water to make sure all the soluble fiber doesn't sit like a plug in your digestive tract. Soluble fiber can also bind things like cholesterol, so that it doesn't wind up getting absorbed into the bloodstream where too much of it can do damage. Our lifestyle medicine colleague Dr. Neal Nedley tells patients, "Fiber from plant foods helps dilute, bind, inactivate, and remove toxic substances and carcinogens found in our food supply."[14]

COMPOSITION OF DIETARY FIBER

•

HERE are some examples of high-fiber foods with a good combination of soluble and insoluble fibers:

FOOD	SOLUBLE (g)	INSOLUBLE (g)
Apple	0.9	2.0
Broccoli	1.3	1.4
Kidney beans	3.0	3.5
Rolled oats*	0.9	1.1
Whole wheat bread	1.4	0.3

*For ½ cup cooked oats

INSOLUBLE FIBER

Insoluble fiber (such as cellulose and lignin) does not dissolve in water. It makes the cell walls of plants rigid, structuring wheat as a stalk instead of a puddle. Insoluble fiber *absorbs* water and expands in volume (think of a dry sponge placed in a shallow dish of water). Wheat bran is the classic example of insoluble fiber, so think crunchy-chewy like All-Bran cereal. Insoluble fiber adds bulk to our intestinal contents, acting like a scrub brush when it gets to the large intestines and colon. It's the insoluble fiber that absorbs the fluid of the intestinal contents, expands, and provides the bulk that keeps the waste products moving out of the body. It's the insoluble fiber that helps keep us regular.

Most foods with fiber have a combination of both insoluble and soluble fiber. An apple has 0.9 grams (g) of soluble fiber and 2.0 g of insoluble fiber. A half cup of cooked kidney beans, a fiber superfood, has 3.0 g of soluble fiber and 3.5 g of insoluble fiber. Raspberries also go to the head of our fiber class: 1 cup has 11 g of fiber (as a result, they don't raise blood sugar as quickly as many other fruits).[15]

Friendly Fiber

Fiber is everyone's friend—especially those with diabetes, for four reasons:

- Fiber does *not* contribute to raising blood glucose levels. That means people with diabetes could eat something high in fiber and not have to worry about it raising their blood sugar as much as when they eat the same food without fiber. For example, a whole orange won't raise your blood sugar as much as that same orange made into orange juice. Though fiber is one of the three main types of carbohydrates in our diets (the other two are starches and sugars), we don't have the enzyme to free the glucose molecules from fiber, *so we can't absorb the glucose.* That's not true for starch and sugars; those glucose molecules can be freed and then absorbed and thus will affect blood sugar levels.
- The soluble types of fiber, especially pectins and gums, increase the viscosity (thickness) of the food in our stomach and small intestines by their gel-like action. This actually slows down digestion and the time it takes to empty the stomach.[16] In turn, this slows down the rate of absorption of glucose into the bloodstream. So a high-fiber meal means that the glucose in the food moves slowly into the blood, thus keeping the rise in blood sugar after eating more gradual. This has the added benefit of requiring less insulin to bring that blood sugar back down.[17] This is the opposite of what happens after a high-fat meal containing carbohydrates (think cheese and pepperoni pizza). While there will probably not be a big blood sugar spike 2 hours after eating that pizza, the blood sugar will spike 3 to 4 hours later and can remain high for hours.[18] A high-fiber, high-whole grain diet can lower your insulin levels and raise your insulin sensitivity, which is good news if you're trying to reduce your insulin resistance, a leading factor in diabetes.[19]

- Fiber decreases the amount of available carbohydrates in a given food. In other words, the more fiber in food, the less of the other kinds of carbs (starch and sugars) there are for you to worry about.
- Because the glucose in fiber is not digested and absorbed into the bloodstream, fiber does not in general provide calories. Yet we get a wonderful sense of fullness when we eat fiber-rich foods. We wind up eating less of everything else and therefore take in fewer calories.

Most important, dietary fiber is found *only* in plant-based foods. There is no fiber in animal products (meat, fish, milk, cheese, eggs). As a result, people on a PBD consume 50 to 100 percent more fiber than nonvegetarians. We recommend at least 35 g of fiber per day. Some of our patients eat 45 g per day. The average American probably gets only 10 to 15 g a day, and half the country eats less than 10 g of fiber daily.[20] For reference, a high-fiber diet means more than 16 g, and we're talking about doubling that—at least.

The bottom line: A high-fiber diet protects us against diabetes.

Make Sure You're Getting the Whole (Grain) Truth

Here's a counterintuitive proposal for those who continue to associate grains with diabetes: studies show the opposite is true. *Whole* grains decrease your risk for diabetes, and the more you eat them, the more they can start to reverse the diabetes you already have. The secret to the benefit of grains is in the word *whole*. That's the grain with all its parts. That means the fiber and other nutrients are still there. Dr. Teresa Fung from Simmons College in Boston and Dr. Jukka Montonen at the National Public Health Institute in Helsinki, Finland, have found that those eating the most whole grains are at 30 to 61 percent lower risk of developing type-2 diabetes than those eating the least amount of whole grain foods. And the more you eat whole grains in place of refined (processed) grains, these researchers found, the lower your risk.[21] The important part of these studies is that they show if you want to lower your diabetes risk, it's not necessarily enough to avoid only refined (white) flour—you also have to *increase your intake of whole grains*. So, if, like most people, you like carbohydrates, you're in luck. Just make sure you eat them whole, not processed.

When searching for bread, cereal, and other whole grain products, you should strive to avoid the *Great Imitators:*

- *100 percent wheat* doesn't mean whole wheat.
- *Stone-ground* might mean something about the processing of the wheat, but it doesn't mean whole.
- *Multigrain* sounds healthful, but it doesn't mean whole; most times it means white wheat flour–based bread with refined flours from several other grains added.
- *Hearty grain* sounds nice, but the term means nothing.
- *Bromated flour* has just enough of a twinge of the exotic to sound like it might be good for you, but all it means is that the flour's been bleached with bromine and not chlorine or other agents.
- *Degermed, milled,* and *refined* are definitely not whole grains.
- *Enriched* might be the worst lie foisted on unsuspecting consumers in search of whole grains. Enriched flour means they take out 20 to 25 important nutrients and most of the fiber and then put back 6 or 7 nutrients in a different, usually less natural form. Dr. Seale puts it this way: "It's like a guy mugs you and takes your last twenty bucks. But right before he runs away, he tosses you a five and says, 'I want to leave you *enriched.*'" Here's what gets mugged out of enriched flour:[22]

  - 100 percent of phytochemicals
  - 98 percent of vitamin E
  - 78 percent of fiber
  - 78 percent of vitamin B_6
  - 72 percent of chromium
  - 72 percent of magnesium
  - 62 percent of zinc
  - 50 percent of folic acid

What exactly do all these missing nutrients do? They boost the immune system, remove dangerous free radicals from the body (discussed later in this chapter), control appetite, assist in fetal brain development, and help cellular metabolism and vital chemical reactions. But . . . who needs 'em? Food manufacturers will just "enrich" the flour after they rob it.

Remember: 100 percent *whole* grain is the only one you need![23]

A Plant-Based Diet Is Lower in Fat Than an Animal-Based Diet

Plant-based diets have less total fat, less saturated fat, and much less or no trans-fat. About 70 percent of the calories in cheese come from fat. In meat, milk, and eggs, about 50 percent of calories are from fat. Most fruits and vegetables have practically no fat, and the fat they do have is beneficial to us.

As you already know, high-fat food—especially food high in saturated fat and trans-fat—is linked to an increase in the risk for diabetes, heart disease, and obesity. It's no surprise most adults with diagnosed diabetes are overweight or obese—and so many have heart disease. The 1976 Adventist Health Study found that adult vegetarian Adventists were 13 pounds lighter than their nonvegetarian counterparts of the same height.[24] And this much should be obvious by now: If you lose weight, you will lower your risk of diabetes and you'll likely live longer.[25]

The foods with the highest proportion of saturated fat include beef, pork, poultry, full-fat dairy (not low-fat or fat-free), chocolate (sorry!), and most tropical vegetable oils (palm, palm kernel, and coconut oil).

A PBD, on the other hand, has little saturated fat and practically no trans-fat.[26] If you eat only a whole food (unprocessed) plant-based diet, it's possible to eliminate *all* trans-fat. Trans-fat (like those created by partial hydrogenation of vegetable oils) promotes insulin resistance and is, therefore, a contributing factor to diabetes.[27] Trans-fat also increases your total cholesterol at twice the rate of saturated fat; increases your low-density lipoprotein (LDL), or "bad," cholesterol; decreases your high-density lipoprotein (HDL), or "good," cholesterol; and increases your triglyceride (fat in the blood) levels.

Look at the differences in fat levels among the following foods:

- 1 Marie Callender's chicken pot pie has 20 g of saturated fat and 16 g of trans-fat.
- 1 serving of Entenmann's crumb coffee cake contains 2.5 g of saturated fat and 2.5 g of trans-fat.
- 1 cup cooked butternut squash has less than 0.2 g of unsaturated fat, 0.3 g of saturated fat, and 0 g of trans-fat.
- 1 medium cucumber has 0.4 g of unsaturated fat, 0.1 g of saturated fat, and 0 g of trans-fat.
- 1 cup blueberries has 0.6 g of unsaturated fat, less than 0.1 g of saturated fat, and 0 g of trans-fat.[28]

You get the idea.

Even a short time off saturated and trans-fat can have a remarkable effect: While we were working on this chapter in January 2007, one of our residential patients, Chuck, a 56-year-old overweight Oklahoman with type-2 diabetes, dropped his triglycerides by an astounding *800 points*, from 1,100 to 300—in just 15 days on the 30-Day Diabetes Miracle program, which includes a PBD with moderate activity. We were also able to take him off his blood pressure medicine and oral diabetes medicine, and halved his daily insulin intake starting in the first week (cutting his insulin was probably a major factor in the reduction of his triglycerides). Steep drops like Chuck's are not infrequent here, but it's not about the numbers; it's about hope. How much do you suppose Chuck's hope for the future improved when he saw the benefits brought on by changing his diet? Chuck told us the answer: 100 percent. Now *that's* a number we can be proud of.

It's very important that we point out that Chuck was able to do this because of the pristine diet he ate. We want our readers to get the same benefits as the patients who have been treated at LCA. And the only way is to strongly encourage you to follow the same diet and to tell you that if you don't do this, you can't expect the same sort of miracle. Your level of improvement will be commensurate with how faithfully you follow our recommendations.

The connection between a high-fat diet and diabetes goes deeper than the obvious benefits of losing weight. Fat affects blood sugar, too.[29] That's right. For a long time, we've found that a higher carbohydrate diet that is also lower in fat tends to get more people off insulin and more blood sugar levels under control. Among people with diabetes who still need to inject insulin, we've found that those on the highest fat diet don't reduce their insulin intake nearly as much as those on the lowest fat diet. Keep in mind this is true even for those eating a high-carbohydrate diet.[30] Keeping insulin levels as low as possible is important because too much insulin in the system is itself a problem, as you recall. Remember, insulin is a growth hormone, so it actually forces weight gain. It also causes the body to make more cholesterol, and it tends to turn off the receptors on the cells so that they no longer respond appropriately to glucose. Excess insulin is one of the causes of insulin resistance and loss of blood sugar control. All of these things make diabetes worse. It's great to know—especially for those of us who love fruits and grains in our diet—that we can keep blood sugar, insulin, and cholesterol down while still enjoying good carbohydrates, even in amounts as high as 75 percent or more[31] of our calories. So, the take-away message here is, eliminate the harmful fats from your diet and reduce the beneficial ones every chance you get. The best way to do this is with a whole grain, high-fiber, plant-based diet with no processed foods.

One U.S. Army study[32] conducted in the 1970s looked at a group of men who did not have diabetes. The men were put on a high-fat diet and then their fat intake was gradually lowered in several steps. After each step, the men took a glucose tolerance test to see how well their bodies were dealing with the sugar in their diets. At 30 minutes after eating the food with the lowest amount of fat, the dieters had an average blood sugar level of 134. At 2 hours, their blood sugar had come down to about 116. In other words, the low-fat dieters' blood sugars did not go up very high and came back down quite quickly. But when the men ate the highest amount of fat, the researchers found very different results in the processing of blood sugar. At 30 minutes after eating, the mens' blood sugar level was 155; at 2 hours, it was 184. That's close to a 70-point difference in the same men. The researchers concluded that the worsening glucose tolerance seemed to be related to the high fat intake. Meal after meal over the long haul, that 70-point difference will have catastrophic effects on people eating a high-fat diet but will protect people eating a low-fat diet.

How Does Fat Affect Blood Sugar?

It's clear there's something about eating a lot of fat—especially saturated animal fat—that affects blood sugar. But what is it?

In Chapter 3 we talked about how glucose gets into busy cells. Glucose needs a key, called insulin, in order to enter the cells and be used for energy. However, the metabolism of fat is different. Fat does not need a key to get into cells. In fact, it doesn't even need to go through the door. Instead, it just pushes right through the cell wall. As fat keeps filling cells, they get stuffed. All the biochemical mechanisms in the cell get plugged up with all the fat, so that metabolism actually decreases. Later, when glucose tries to enter the cells for energy, it can't get in. There's just no room because of all the fat. This means the blood sugar is going to get elevated, of course. And it will report back to the pancreas that it couldn't get into the cells. The pancreas will assume that the problem was just not enough keys (insulin). You know what that means: more insulin to unlock those doors.

So you can see how too much fat can create the nightmare scenario for diabetes: high blood sugar *plus* high insulin levels. The high blood sugar will keep causing higher insulin in a vicious circle. The insulin will force us to gain weight; and as long as insulin remains high, it will be nearly impossible to lose any of that weight. Notice that none of this has anything to do with carbohydrates! Yet, astoundingly, so many diabetes prescriptions call for increasing fat and decreasing carbohydrates, based on unbridled enthusiasm for an erroneous assumption.[33]

How do you break this cycle? Imagine a cell that's not stuffed so full of fat that no glucose can fit. Picture a busy, active muscle cell instead. It's busy and active because its owner has started to walk every day. These cells are happy about this development. Why? You already know that glucose is a primary fuel for energy in the cell. But there's another energy source inside a cell: fat. Muscle cells in particular like to burn fat. That's how you lose weight when you exercise. There's a lot of fat readily available for burning in your cells. So your metabolism increases as you get more active. You start burning that excess fat mucking up the biomechanisms of your cells. If you're also eating less fat, then less is going into your cells. The glucose that might otherwise have had no place to go but the bloodstream can now fit into the cells. Your blood sugar goes down and your diabetes process begins to reverse. Now that's exciting news—many would call it a miracle!

A lower-fat diet even improves insulin sensitivity in patients with type-1 diabetes. Remember insulin sensitivity is a measure of how well the cells listen to the pancreas' call, "The energy's coming!" Dr. A. M. Rosenfalck and colleagues at Hvidovre University Hospital in Denmark did a 3-month study, concluding that subjects eating a low-fat diet saw "a significant improvement in insulin sensitivity . . . compared with the standard diabetes diet," which is higher in fat.[34]

Just how fast can you see improvements by lowering your fat intake and starting to get active? You don't have to wait 3 months, like those Danish test subjects. It can happen within 3 *days*. Simply by starting to get physically active and by eating a diet that's lower in fat and higher in those good whole grains, vegetables, fruits, and beans, your diabetes will start to reverse. The effect can be so dramatic, so fast, that you should not do it without first consulting your doctor.

LIFESTYLE RECOMMENDATIONS FOR CONTROLLING CHOLESTEROL, TRIGLYCERIDES, BLOOD SUGAR, AND WEIGHT

●

- Achieve your ideal body weight.
- Get physically active five to six times a week (see Chapter 8).
- Eat a plant-based diet of whole grains, vegetables, fruits, beans, and limited amounts of nuts and seeds (a healthy serving is about 1 ounce, or a small, cupped handful; approximately 20 almonds = 1 ounce).
- Limit your intake of saturated fat.
- Avoid ingesting trans-fat by eliminating animal products (meat and dairy), fast food, and all products containing hydrogenated oil, partially hydrogenated oil, interesterified fat, shortening, or margarine.
- Limit your intake of total fat and primarily use monounsaturated fats (olives and olive oil, canola oil, avocado, nuts, and seeds).
- Increase your intake of legumes (pinto beans, lentils, black beans, garbanzo beans [chickpeas], black-eyed peas, soybeans, split peas).[35]
- Increase your intake of dark green, leafy vegetables (spinach, kale, collards, turnip greens, Swiss chard, mustard greens, beet greens, sweet potato greens) and vegetables that grow above the ground (broccoli, cabbage, green beans, squash, cauliflower, onions).
- Increase your intake of fiber (fruits, vegetables, whole grains, beans, and limited nuts and seeds). There is no fiber in any animal products.
- Avoid drinking caffeinated sodas, coffee, and tea. Caffeine not only can raise stress and blood pressure[36] but can also raise cholesterol and arterial inflammation related to atherosclerosis, which can exacerbate diabetes in several ways.[37] Caffeine also increases the circulating amount of fat in the blood, making more fat available to plug up cells.
- Avoid ingesting refined, processed (white) flour products.
- Avoid eating sweets (soda pop, fruit juices, candy). This includes products that are sweetened artificially. Limit desserts to one small serving (think 1/16 of a pie) once or twice per week. Better yet, eat three or four servings of northern-hemisphere grown fruits daily (apples, pears, berries, cherries, apricots, peaches, plums, nectarines) and let them satisfy your sweet tooth.
- Avoid drinking alcohol. Alcohol, even in small amounts, can raise triglycerides significantly, according to the U.S. Surgeon General.[38] Alcohol can also raise serum cholesterol.
- If you smoke, quit. Smoking, too, is linked to higher cholesterol and blood pressure.

A Plant-Based Diet Contains No Cholesterol

Cholesterol is a critically important substance for human life. It's a waxy, fatlike compound that is a necessary structural component of cell walls as well as certain hormones. But *all the cholesterol we need is manufactured by our liver,* which cranks out millions of molecules a day. Dietary cholesterol is found only in foods that came from organisms with a liver. (A cow has a liver. A turnip does not.) So the good news is that there is no dietary cholesterol in plant foods. Dietary cholesterol has been implicated in raising blood cholesterol and increasing the risk of heart disease. Although health experts advise limiting cholesterol intake, we recommend avoiding it altogether. You simply don't need it. Eating a PBD high in whole grains, vegetables, fruits, and beans with limited nuts and seeds will eliminate dietary cholesterol because *plant foods do not contain cholesterol.*

Now it's important to differentiate between two main components of our total cholesterol (TC): the "heavenly darling," or "good," HDL, and the "little devil," or "bad," LDL. Simply put, LDL cholesterol is the component that is deposited *into* our artery walls and causes blockages. HDL cholesterol is the component that carries cholesterol *out* of our blood stream to the liver to be excreted, thus helping prevent artery blockages. So we want our HDL to be as high as possible. Remember, *H* = high. We want our LDL to be as low as possible. Remember, *L* = low.

Many doctors and healthcare agencies still fail to consider the difference between HDL and LDL and make recommendations solely on the basis of total cholesterol, which can be a grievous mistake. A much more sensible approach is to consider the ratio between the total cholesterol and HDL cholesterol. Find out from your doctor what your TC:HDL ratio is. You want it to be as low as possible. The average marathon runner has a ratio of 3.4. That's pretty good, considering the typical man with coronary artery disease has a ratio between 5.5 and 6.1. But this is worth looking at twice: Total vegetarians (people who eat nothing but plants) have an average ratio of only 2.8![39]

Patients treated at LCA see cholesterol reductions of approximately 15 percent in just 2 weeks. Our patients obtain these results by eating more good-quality carbohydrates and less fat than they did previously and by ingesting no cholesterol.

A Plant-Based Diet Has All the Protein You Need, Without Animal Protein

Adequate dietary protein is essential for normal growth. That's why rat's milk has more than 10 times the amount of protein than human milk. Human babies double their birth weight in about 120 days, but rats double theirs in about 4.5 days. Because adults are no longer growing, their need for protein is less. Whenever the body is repairing or replacing tissue (think physical trauma like a burn), protein needs are increased, sometimes to regulate the process, sometimes to become part of a body structure. Proteins form the basis of most body structures, including muscle, blood, skin, nails, hair, bones, and teeth. Protein is also vital for muscle function, hormone synthesis (including the manufacture of insulin), and enzyme production.

In 1960, the head of the Nutrition Division of the Food and Agriculture Organization of the United Nations (U.N.) declared that protein deficiency was the most "serious and widespread problem in the world." In 1968, the U. N. bemoaned an "impending protein crisis." But by 1974, it was concluded that much scientific thinking about protein had been dead wrong. The U.N. had realized that science was not on their side.[40] Most nutritional problems were not the fault of too little protein. Instead, it was *too much protein* that was the problem—especially animal protein. T. Colin Campbell's massive China Study proved this, with dramatic and disturbing findings about protein's bad influence on serious diseases.[41] We should repeat here that it's *animal* protein that causes problems, not *plant* protein (especially when it comes to cancer).[42]

It's a myth, pure and simple, that vegetarians don't get enough protein. The fact is quite the opposite: Nonvegetarians get *too much* protein—and from less healthful animal sources. Such concentrated protein comes with high fat, especially saturated fat, dietary cholesterol, trans-fat, no fiber, and high calories. The U.S. government advises us to eat 0.8 g of protein per kilogram of body weight (1 kilogram is about 2.2 pounds). So, according the U.S. Department of Agriculture (USDA), the average American woman should be eating about 46 g of protein a day, and the average American man, 56 g of protein per day. But that's based on the weight they assume we *should* be. Let's take a "real" American, though. One of our patients, Betty, weighs 170 pounds. Divide her weight in pounds by 2.2 to get her weight in kilograms (77.27 kilograms). Now multiply that weight by 0.8 g to determine the USDA's recommendation: Betty should eat 61.8 g of protein per day. The World Health Organization (WHO) takes a less strident view for the rest of the planet's population. The WHO says 37 to 40 g of protein a day is enough.

Just how much protein does the average American actually consume? Women are eating an average of 70 g and men 100 g per day.[43] Why so much? Ever since German scientists discovered protein in the 19th century, there's been a long, unfortunate legacy of belief that we need this much protein ("Eat your meat!") for strength and endurance. Those scientists recommended eating up to 250 g of protein a day![44] Nineteenth century German cows must have been shaking in their hooves.

The notion that meat equals strength and endurance is a great fallacy. In fact, carbohydrates are much better than protein and fat for endurance. Even already-fit, peak-performance athletes—even well-trained soldiers—can substantially improve their fitness, strength, and endurance levels after switching from a meat diet to a PBD.[45] Just think about it: In the animal kingdom, it's plant eating that leads to endurance. Vegetarian elephants and horses can run fast for hours, carrying their massive bulk for 25 miles or more, whereas carnivorous cheetahs and panthers are most effective in short bursts, but tire out in mere minutes.[46] And among humans, there's lots of proof, too: There have been many peak-performing vegan and vegetarian athletes. In fact, the original Olympics of ancient Greek included vegetarian athletes.

Speaking of Greece, *protein* means "of the first quality" in Greek. This still makes sense, despite the great value of carbohydrates as a primary energy source. We reiterate that we do *need* protein, we just *don't need it in such abundance or from animal sources*. Yet the first thing your friends and family are going to confront you with when you tell them you're leaning toward a plant-based diet is, "Where are you going to get your protein?" The answer? It's almost impossible to become protein deficient. Especially when we eat enough calories to maintain a healthy weight and include servings of whole grains, beans, and vegetables on a daily basis.[47]

Do you know how much protein we actually need to survive and thrive? We need only about 26 g a day of good-quality protein (5 to 6 percent based on a 2,100-calorie diet)—three to five times less than the average American consumes. In fact, if you consume any animal products, it's almost impossible not to eat too much protein. It's even hard to stay at or below the USDA guidelines. Just 3 ounces of pot roast (about the size of a deck of cards) has about 25 g of protein.[48] And most meat eaters would eat a larger portion than that.

Another way to realize that we're eating way too much protein for the growth and development we require is to analyze a very widely consumed food from our early days. When is it that you are growing the most, developing the most, and thus needing the most protein? It's when you're a baby. From ages 6 to 9 months, you double your birth weight. And breast milk is your primary source of food. Yet a mere 5 percent of the calories in breast milk come from protein.

So how can you get the needed 5 to 6 percent of calories from protein? First, remember that protein provides the building blocks of life. That means that anything once alive has protein in it. So you can forget the meat altogether and start with some brown rice: 8 percent of its calories are from protein. Same with oranges: 8 percent. Potatoes (Russet) have even more protein: 11 percent. Beans are the big daddy of plant-based protein, though: 26 percent of their calories come from protein—that's the same percentage as beef rib roast (fat trimmed to 1/8 inch)! We'll do one better—did you know there's 30 percent more protein per calorie in soybeans than there is in beef roast?[49]

People with diabetes should be especially cautious about too much protein in their diet. One major complication of long-term, uncontrolled diabetes is kidney malfunction (nephropathy). Many people with diabetes suffer from nephropathy, and many go on dialysis:[50]

- In 2002, diabetes was the leading cause of kidney failure, accounting for 44 percent of new cases; 44,400 people with diabetes began treatment for end-stage renal disease (ESRD); and 153,730 people with ESRD caused by diabetes were living on chronic dialysis or with a kidney transplant.
- Therapy that keeps blood glucose levels as close to normal as possible in people with type-1 diabetes reduces damage to the kidneys by 35 to 56 percent.[51] Experts believe that these results can also be applied to those with type-2 diabetes.

Diabetes and Your Kidneys

What exactly does diabetes have to do with the kidneys? The kidneys' job is to filter impurities from the blood and send them out of the body through the urine. The diabetic process, because of high blood glucose, taxes the kidneys by damaging the small blood vessels that do the filtering work. Studies show that when people with diabetes switch to a low-protein diet, their kidneys' ability to filter waste greatly improves; this function is maintained as long as the person remains on the low-protein diet.[52] That's very good news.

A sign of kidney dysfunction is protein in the urine. Protein molecules are too large to be routinely passed through the kidney filters into the urine. When the small blood vessels in the kidney are damaged, the filters get leaky and let the protein molecules through. Studies show that when such damage has occurred, a high-protein diet will accelerate further damage. A diet *adequate but not excessive* in protein is kidney protective.[53] In fact, a low-protein diet can reduce urine protein in diabetes patients by a factor of 20 after 1 year of eating a healthful, plant-based diet.[54]

All this despite Dr. Robert Atkins's, of Atkins diet fame, very unscientific assertion: "I have yet to see someone produce a study for me to review, or even cite a specific case, in which a protein-containing diet causes any form of kidney disorder"[55] (more on this later in this chapter).

And the reasons keep piling up for eliminating our animal protein intake: Switching from animal protein to vegetable protein also lowers cholesterol—up to 100 points after 6 weeks.[56]

Protein Quality

We need to say a word about *protein quality*, which you might have heard about. Some protein sources have more or less of the essential amino acids that are necessary for human survival. The relative quality of a protein is determined by how many grams of each of the eight essential amino acids can be found in a 100-g serving of a given food. On this scale, milk, beef, eggs, and chicken are all considered high-quality proteins because they offer high levels of a good mix of all the essential amino acids. This makes sense, because the sources of those products are made from similar biochemical stuff as we are. It seems logical for people to assume animal proteins are superior to plant proteins because, after all, a cow or chicken is biologically closer to a human than is a zucchini or bell pepper.

But this is where many nutritionists and doctors fall into a trap, believing that a PBD cannot provide adequate quality protein. How do they think the cows managed to grow and survive with enough essential amino acids, even though *they* don't eat meat?[57] There are two answers, both of which should be fairly obvious. First, all a vegetarian (human or cow) needs to eat is a *variety* of plant-based protein sources. When proteins are consumed, they're digested and disassembled into their individual amino acid components. Your body then takes these available amino acids and reassembles them into the proteins needed for daily function. Not all dietary proteins need to be individually complete (contain all of the essential amino acids)—all you need to do is consume a variety of proteins, which, when combined, will contain all of the amino acids you need. Just be sure you eat a good variety of beans, whole grains, vegetables, fruits, nuts, and seeds and you'll have no protein concerns. A classic example of a good protein meal without meat is beans and rice, a staple of the traditional Mexican diet. You don't have to do any math calculations to get enough protein: Just mix it up. You don't even need to mix every meal, just be sure you're getting a good *daily* balance. Remember: *Variety* is the key.

The second way to ensure you're getting enough quality protein is even simpler. Consider how the determination is made for oatmeal, for example, which is not considered a quality protein source. Although 14.2 percent of the calories in oatmeal come from protein, this cereal is high in some essential amino acids, like leucine, but somewhat lower in others, like lysine. Because every essential amino acid doesn't quite make the ideal level, oatmeal is not considered high-quality protein on this scale. But that determination is based on only a 100-g serving (about 7 tablespoons). So if you want to solve this "problem" of low quality, just eat a little more oatmeal.

The bottom line is that high-quality and low-quality protein lists are arbitrary, artificial, confusing, and not at all helpful. But, sadly, many doctors and nutritionists from the old school still don't get that. When it comes to getting enough necessary protein on a plant-based diet, *size matters*—portion size, that is, as well as *variety*. The automatic assumption by health professionals and government agencies that you need meat, milk, and eggs to get enough protein is incorrect and is contributing to chronic diseases that are responsible for nearly 1.5 million deaths each year in the United States alone.[58] A PBD is rich in the right amount of protein, which, in combination with high fiber, actually protects you from diabetes and its major complications, like cardiovascular disease and high cholesterol.[59]

Atkins and His Ilk: Deadly Diet Myths

What about the hugely popular high-protein, high-fat, low-carbohydrate diet sold to the American public by Dr. Robert Atkins?[60]

Among us three authors, we managed to agree unanimously on just about every point we make in this book. Not so when it came to how to regard Atkins. As a person with diabetes who experimented with an Atkins-like diet (and suffered disastrous effects), Ian, along with Drs. House and Seale, agrees with Campbell's assertion that Atkins "became one of the richest snake oil salesmen ever to live"[61] by foisting his deceptive, unscientific, and dangerous diet recommendations on America and the world. However, Seale, while not at all a proponent of the Atkins diet, was concerned about judging the deceased doctor's personal health history and was adamant about us not dredging up the controversy over how Atkins died or drawing conclusions based on his physical condition.[62]

Here's also where we agree: There's no credible evidence from any *long-term* study showing that low-carbohydrate diets work for good health. In fact, just about every study shows that long-term carbohydrate restriction is associated with serious complications, from cancer, increased serum cholesterol, osteoporosis, kidney stone formation, and even sudden death.[63]

Will such diets help you to lose weight? In the short term, probably yes. But as Campbell writes, so will undergoing chemotherapy or a stint of heroin addiction.[64]

Sadly, even some diabetes doctors have fallen for the low-carb, high-fat, high-protein myth. Dr. Richard Bernstein, who has type-1 diabetes, writes, "Protein will become the most important part of your diet if you are going to control blood sugars."[65] We searched for the clinical data to support Bernstein's claim (along with his assertion that "eating fat will make you fat is about as scientifically logical as saying that eating tomatoes will turn you red"[66]). We were out of luck—Bernstein's book has no references to scientific studies. Are you going to believe Atkins and Bernstein, who provide no proof, or Campbell, who spent the better part of 30 years studying thousands of people and interpreting thousands of other studies in what the *New York Times* called the "Grand Prix of epidemiology"?[67]

We've had lots of patients come to us either mid- or post-Atkins. The less said here about their condition when they arrived, the better. And

Ian came to us in 2004 after having suffered on Bernstein's extremely restrictive and nutritionally bereft diet for a year. Ian had never enjoyed eating meat before his diabetes diagnosis. But, desperate to get better, he tried Bernstein's diabetes "solution," which consisted of lots of salami and cheese; whole-fat cream mixed with water; very, very little whole grains; and no fruits. He was particularly crestfallen when he read Bernstein's instruction to "limit yourself to . . . a single cherry tomato per cup of salad."[68] After a year, Ian, who had been really motivated to get better, had instead gained 20 pounds, become insulin resistant, and was still not in control of his blood sugar. When he first came to LCA, he couldn't believe the gorgeous salad bar. Still holding on to the fallacy of the low-carbohydrate diet, he shook his head at us and said, "You guys must be crazy. Look at all those berries! And how can I eat oranges? Dr. Bernstein says he hasn't eaten fruit in 30 years!"[69] Just 18 days later, Ian's blood sugar was totally under control, and his LDL cholesterol had dropped substantially, along with his triglycerides. He even managed to lose some of the weight he'd put on before coming to LCA—no small feat for a person with type-1 diabetes and a level of insulin resistance. After a few more months, he'd lost all the weight and then some.

A Plant-Based Diet Has Many More Antioxidants Than an Animal-Based Diet

The theory regarding the power of antioxidants states that chronic disease is caused by internal imbalances that weaken the body and makes it susceptible to germs and other environmental factors. To fight disease, to get your health restored, you need to think about balancing the *whole body*.[70] And that's where the antioxidant properties of certain vitamins, minerals, and enzymes come in. Here's a quickie review of some ninth-grade science that just might save your life:

All matter is made up of atoms. The nucleus of each atom is made up of protons and neutrons, and electrons orbit the nucleus in the way that planets orbit the sun. Usually, those orbiting electrons are in pairs: Electrons are strongly attracted to each other and usually find another to make a pair. When the electrons are paired, the atom is chemically stable (balanced). But sometimes, those electrons are single or unpaired, and their atoms, called *free radicals*, are therefore highly unstable.

Here's where it gets interesting. Unpaired electrons are desperate to find mates. But they're not too particular. Unpaired electrons tend to just grab any old electron they can get their hands on, without much discrimination, even when this means they snatch that electron off a nearby stable molecule. The important thing to know is that this filching of electrons, called *oxidation*, happens in the blink of an eye and, in the process, renders the hijacked molecule into another, unstable free radical. Now *that* free radical's unpaired electron will go on to pilfer its neighbor's in a chain reaction of oxidation that can damage the body unless something—an *antioxidant*—interrupts the process.[71] Some well-known antioxidants are beta-carotene, vitamins C and E, and melatonin. There are many more.

The lion's share of antioxidants comes from plant-based foods. Dr. James F. Balch, one of the world's only urologists with a master's degree in theology, puts it this way: "Counterfeit foods, those created by man, are unable to supply what the body needs to maintain this stability and wholeness . . . (only) God's food (plant-based food) contains the life force—the essential nutrients, enzymes, et cetera—that are necessary to maintain the body's healing force within. Without them, the body perishes before its time."[72] Antioxidants are an ideal example of this balance: When you take them in supplement form, they don't perform nearly as well as when you consume them in their natural state. They're more than the sum of their parts. It seems they work *with each other* for optimum health when consumed in our food. People on a PBD have higher intakes of antioxidant-rich foods than those on the SAD and, therefore, have higher levels of antioxidants in their blood.

Keep in mind that some oxidation is natural and necessary in the body's normal processes—in destroying germs and poisons, for example, in pursuit of that elusive balance—but too much of it can wreak havoc. Free radicals that exist outside the body's normal destructive processes have been associated with more than 50 diseases.[73] It is possible, but unlikely on a typical PBD, to get too many antioxidants. Let's review just a few that are most relevant to people with diabetes:

- *Alpha lipoic acid* is an antioxidant that seems to improve insulin sensitivity and glucose disposal in people with type-2 diabetes.[74] It has been shown to be very useful for painful diabetic neuropathy (nerve pain).[75] It also appears to help protect diabetes patients from diabetes-related kidney damage.[76] Alpha lipoic acid is produced in our bodies and is also found in spinach and broccoli.

- *Vitamin E* is an antioxidant that can help prevent vascular disease, eye damage, and kidney damage in diabetes patients.[77] It also helps slow the aging of tissues, which can be accelerated by diabetes. The best dietary source is wheat germ. Other good sources are nuts, seeds, and dark green leafy vegetables.

- *Coenzyme Q10* is an antioxidant with properties similar to vitamin E. It helps improve heart health and blood sugar control and also lowers blood pressure and cholesterol levels.[78] Whole grains are a good dietary source.

- *Beta-carotene* is an antioxidant that you can find in the humble carrot (although it's not an above-the-ground vegetable, it's still very healthful if eaten in moderation). Beta-carotene is converted to vitamin A, which helps maintain good vision.[79] It also helps prevent heart disease and cancer.[80] Other good dietary sources are yellow, orange, and green leafy vegetables.

- *Vitamin C* is an antioxidant that can help lower cholesterol and prevent vascular damage that can lead to blockages.[81] It also helps boost the immune system.[82] It is found in citrus fruits, red and green peppers, strawberries, kiwifruit, melons, and many other fruits and vegetables.

- *Zinc* is a trace mineral that aids in absorption of other vitamins. It is helpful in the production and storage of insulin.[83] Its deficiency has been associated with diabetes.[84] You can find it in beans, whole grains, pumpkin seeds, and sunflower seeds.

A Plant-Based Diet Has Many More Phytochemicals Than an Animal-Based Diet

In addition to the well-known list of antioxidants that includes beta-carotene and vitamins C and E, scientists have discovered a whole other class of life-enriching, health-giving compounds abundant only in plant foods. These compounds are called *phytochemicals*. While some vitamins are themselves phytochemicals, only those nutrients that have been proven to prevent diseases of deficiency (like scurvy and rickets) are considered *necessary* nutrients. But there might be literally thousands of biologically active components in plant foods that provide the kind of important health benefits we know vitamins do.[85]

Many of these compounds, after more study, might become necessary nutrients of the future.

Phytochemicals are those substances in plants that give them color, flavor, and aroma. They also protect plants against environmental insults and diseases. For example, a plant might manufacture a chemical to protect itself against the damaging ionizing radiation from the sun or to fight against mold, bacteria, or insects. So when we eat these plant foods, we can expect that, in many cases, those same phytochemicals will protect us, too, against environmental insults and disease.

Beta-carotene is a good example of a useful phytochemical. It is in the carotenoid family of plant pigments (there are about 500 more),[86] and it's what makes carrots and sweet potatoes orange. When we ingest it, it can provide vitamin A for the body. And like many phytochemicals, it's also known to be a strong antioxidant.

Isn't it interesting that the powerful ammunition for stimulating the immune system, repairing damage, and otherwise fighting diseases comes from the very same substances that make the source foods so attractive to us? Eating a ripe beefsteak tomato wouldn't be nearly as rewarding or fun if it weren't for its color and unique, robust flavor. And those same properties are what help protect us from disease. Did you know that in addition to beneficial lycopene, tomatoes alone are believed to contain about 10,000 different phytochemicals![87] You'll never get that from a cupcake—no matter how hard the food manufacturers try.

Phytochemicals are found only in plants (*phyto-* comes from the Greek prefix for "plant"). You can find phytochemicals in every whole grain, fruit, vegetable, legume (sprouts, beans, peas, soybeans), seed, and nut in a PBD. Although you can take phytochemical supplements, you won't get the same positive effect. These substances are meant to be ingested in their natural state, in combination with each other, and in some abundance. Besides, wouldn't it be easier and more satisfying to eat a tomato instead of 10,000 supplements or one giant pill? This is why we recommend *eating by color*: In other words, when you shop for produce (or graze at the salad bar), you should eat a variety of colors to ensure you're getting a good mix of phytochemicals. By the way, studies show that phytochemicals usually remain intact through cooking and other processing.

Another class of antioxidant phytochemicals, the *flavonoids*, has been getting a lot of press lately because of their presence in red wine, which has been associated in some studies with health benefits if used

COFFEE, DIABETES, AND STRESS

●

CAFFEINE is the most widely used drug in the world and 90 percent of Americans consume caffeine daily.[90] Yet medical research has linked caffeine with higher rates of certain cancers, miscarriages, low birth weight babies, worsening depression, anxiety, fatigue, elevated blood pressure, heart palpitations, heart disease, bone loss, and osteoporosis—even frontal lobe disorders.[91] Studies show higher blood sugar, decreased insulin sensitivity, and impaired glucose tolerance after caffeine consumption, all of which adversely affect diabetes control.[92] Caffeine raises stress hormone levels, a primary risk factor for diabetes, and increases vascular resistance, in which blood vessels constrict and circulation is reduced, which is bad for diabetes. Caffeine also raises the level of homocysteine (a toxic waste product) as well as fatty acid levels in the blood, which greatly increases the risk for cardiovascular disease and degeneration of blood vessels in the eyes.[93]

In very large doses (10 g), caffeine is lethal.[94] But way before that, serious problems occur, notwithstanding the possibility of benefits. Caffeine increases dopamine (a neurotransmitter) levels just like amphetamines, cocaine, and heroin do. Then you get a jolt of adrenaline. Finally, caffeine blocks the reception of the brain chemical adenosine, which makes you more alert and less sleepy. All this makes you feel good[95]—but it's only temporary. When the caffeine wears off (its half-life is about 6 hours), you start to feel bad—fatigued, depressed, even anxious. The solution? More caffeine. However, the process of breaking the cycle can be very unpleasant. Exhaustion, depression, lethargy, irritability, and an extreme headache from blood vessel dilation in the brain can result.[96]

We suggest that you gradually taper your caffeine intake to prevent these side effects. If you drink coffee or caffeinated tea or soda, use a blend of 25 percent decaffeinated and 75 percent regular for a few days, followed by a few days of 50/50, and finally a few days of 75 percent decaffeinated and 25 percent regular. By the end of 2 weeks, you should be able to discontinue caffeine altogether. There's much more information about coffee and diabetes as well as suggestions for healthful coffee substitutes, on our website (www.diabetesmiracle.org).

in moderation. Despite this possibility, we don't recommend you drink wine if you have diabetes, because in addition to raising triglycerides, it can dangerously lower your blood sugar if consumed on an empty stomach. But we do recommend flavonoids, which are abundant in berries, apples, onions, green beans, and grapes.[88] Flavonoids are associated with decreased risk of stroke and heart attack and are, therefore, of benefit to people with diabetes.

When it comes to the enormously beneficial potential of phytochemicals, we think, as does Dr. Walter Willet of Harvard Medical School, that perhaps "we should just consider whole fruits and vegetables as vitamins, given their already proven ability to prevent . . . diseases."[89]

D IS FOR "DESIRABLE"

THIS IS PROBABLY a good time to talk briefly about one of two nutrients *not* adequately available in a total PBD. It's vitamin D (the other is vitamin B_{12}, which we discuss in Chapter 10). While vitamin D is not found in significant amounts in plant foods, it's a unique substance in that humans can manufacture it, provided they have adequate sunlight exposure. Therefore, those who get plenty of sunshine do not need any dietary source of this valuable nutrient. Because Americans live a largely sedentary and indoor lifestyle, with many people working in offices, and because we widely use sunscreen, it's very common for us to have suboptimal levels of vitamin D. This can create problems.

An adequate amount of vitamin D is necessary for optimal insulin production and effectiveness.[97] One study of people with type-2 diabetes and vitamin D deficiency found a 60 percent improvement in both pancreatic production of insulin and insulin sensitivity when vitamin D was replaced.[98] Because people with type-2 diabetes often have significant risk factors for vitamin D deficiency—such as obesity and not enough outdoor activities—it's reasonable to request that your doctor measure your serum level of 25-hydroxy vitamin D (it is important to get this specific test done and *not* a 1,25-dihydroxy vitamin D level; be sure your doctor orders the correct test). A minimum level of 30 nanograms per milliliter or higher is necessary for maximal health benefits. These benefits likely include protection from infections, cancers, and osteoporosis as well as some autoimmune diseases like rheumatoid arthritis, lupus, Hashimoto's thyroiditis, and even type-1 diabetes.[99]

ALCOHOL:
DOES IT FIT ON THE LCA PLAN?

●

TO use alcohol or not will be your choice, but we recommend you eliminate or reduce alcohol consumption:

- Alcohol is perceived by the body to be toxic (ethanol, the basis of alcoholic beverages, is a toxic chemical in the human body). The liver's responsibility is to detoxify alcohol by changing it into other substances that are less dangerous. Part of it gets converted by the liver to fat. The fat gets deposited locally, which is why the term *beer belly* is appropriate.
- Alcohol is high calorie (7 calories per gram), so if you're trying to lose weight, you will have to ask yourself whether it's really worth it.
- Alcohol's intoxicating effects can loosen inhibitions (including the inhibition against overeating) and impair judgment (including the judgment to test your blood sugar and to determine whether you're hypoglycemic).
- Most important, alcohol can affect blood sugar—drastically in some individuals.

If you choose to use alcohol, we suggest you use in moderation. Consider the words of the Harvard Medical School: "Alcohol's effects depend on the dose. A little bit can be beneficial. A lot can destroy the liver, lead to various cancers, boost blood pressure, trigger bleeding (hemorrhagic) strokes, progressively weaken the heart muscle, scramble the brain, harm unborn children, and damage lives."[101]

Vitamin D is safe unless levels exceed 150 nanograms per milliliter (ng/mL). When low levels are identified, your doctor can "aggressively" supply you a boost of 50,000 Internation Units (IU) orally once or twice a week—we do this regularly at LCA. Levels should be rechecked in a month or two to ascertain whether toxicity (more than 150 ng/mL) is being approached. In the absence of adequate sunlight exposure, taking a daily supplement of 1,000 IU is a reasonable thing to do. You will likely not get adequate sun exposure during the months of October through April if you live at a latitude north of Oklahoma City.

Recommendations have now been made that the upper safe daily intake level of vitamin D should be 10,000 IU per day. This might seem excessive to some, but the mounting evidence of health benefits to the immune and skeletal system have made it clear that we need more vitamin D than simply enough to avoid rickets or osteoporosis.[100]

PARTING SHOT

YOU MIGHT BE wondering, with all this overwhelming evidence about the great benefits of a plant-based diet for people with diabetes, why hasn't the word spread? Well—it has. The lifestyle approach to the treatment of diabetes has taken off in the past few decades and become much more widely accepted by the old-guard establishment. Recently, a study at Georgetown University, in Washington, DC, was conducted with the Physician's Committee for Responsible Medicine—these are two serious heavyweights of research science. The study looked at a low-fat, vegan diet versus a standard diet recommended by the American Diabetes Association (ADA) for people with type-2 diabetes. The study found that the plant-based participants dropped their glucose levels by 28 percent (nearly 60 percent more than the control group), decreased their medicine (the control subjects did not), substantially dropped their cholesterol levels (more than the control group), and lost an average of about 16 pounds in 3 months (doubling that of the control group's weight loss).[102] An even more recent study had similar results.[103] Work at Harvard University's School of Public Health, Loma Linda University, and many other prestigious institutions has backed the benefits of a vegetarian diet for diabetes control.

PLANT-BASED DIET LOWERS BLOOD SUGAR

●

FOR 6 months starting in March 2002 we followed 58 patients who had attended our residential program for either 12 or 18 days. Those patients who stayed on a PBD for 6 or more days a week saw blood sugar improvements that were five times better than those who managed to stay on a PBD for only 2 days or fewer per week.[104]

Many of the chronic diseases associated with lifestyle factors like the SAD can be considered challenges to our immune systems. In a broad sense, our bodies are constantly fighting off threats (like unhealthy food) that come from our environment. Or at the least, our bodies are trying to balance damaging external stimuli with a need for internal equilibrium, or *homeostasis*. We're trying to achieve health and ease despite living in an environment and making certain choices that often make such a state elusive. Seen in this way, *dis-ease* and its symptoms are merely signs of the body doing maintenance work on itself. The pancreas struggles to pump out enough insulin to cover all the blood sugar in a fast-food meal. The kidneys and liver grapple to filter out toxins entering our bodies through junk food. You have to give your body the break it needs. You alone—not doctors, not nutritionists, not best-selling diet books or even huge epidemiologic studies, but *you*—have the power to ease your dis-ease.

A PBD high in carbohydrates of the whole grain variety and low in fat is the perfect place to start. To summarize, diets rich in fiber and complex carbohydrates and restricted in fat:

- Improve control of blood glucose concentration up to 27 percent
- Delay glucose absorption
- Lower insulin requirements by an average of 40 percent
- Increase peripheral tissue insulin sensitivity
- Decrease serum cholesterol and triglyceride values up to 32 percent
- Aid in weight control
- Lower blood pressure in patients with diabetes[105]

As one of our doctors, Teresa Sherard, says, "A plant-based diet agrees with the palate, the pancreas and the pocketbook."[106]

The Right Kind of Carbs

WHEN DR. CHRISTIAN Roberts and coworkers at the University of California, Los Angeles (UCLA) published a study in 2006 that showed type-2 diabetes and its precursor, the metabolic syndrome, could be reversed within 3 weeks,[1] some in the medical establishment were shocked and dismissive. But at Lifestyle Center of America's inpatient programs, we see such "impossible" outcomes at the end of every 18-day session, 14 times a year. That's when our patients stand up at their graduation ceremonies and usually have to wipe away tears. They stand with the results of their latest laboratory tests in hand, and they tell their stories. Many have found relief from the pain of diabetic neuropathy (nerve pain and numbness in the legs and feet). Many have reduced or even eliminated their diabetes medications, including their insulin. Many have gotten out of their wheelchairs or dismissed their walkers and canes. Most marvel in and relish their newfound vigor and hope. Many of our guests who come back for their "Return Care" visits 6 months or 1 year later tell us their doctors at home were baffled by their improvements. Some even reversed their clinical diagnosis of type-2 diabetes.

The secret to the 30-Day Diabetes Miracle program is a total plant-based diet (PBD) and an increase in activity level[2]—of course, it doesn't hurt that our residential program makes adherence to the diet and activity plan easier and less stressful than it might be at home. Despite what many doctors and nutritionists (usually well meaning, but misinformed) proclaim, you do not have to eliminate or severely restrict your carbohydrate intake to conquer diabetes. In fact, studies show it's probably the low–saturated fat, high-fiber, high–whole grain diet that offers the most protection against diabetes.[3]

In this chapter, we review one of the cornerstones of the 30-Day Diabetes Miracle program: the counterintuitive proposal that *most of a diabetes patient's calories should come from carbohydrates*, specifically plant-based carbohydrates, including whole grains. We review the function and process of carbohydrate breakdown and hammer home the point that not all carbs are created equal. Then we outline a simple method for calculating carbohydrate intake and predicting how different kinds of foods might affect your blood sugar according to the *glycemic index* (GI). For example, we show you that an apple is a better choice of carb than a watermelon if you're trying to keep your blood sugar low.

We know you don't intentionally search for foods that will cause your blood sugar to go up. But you do look for goodies that satisfy your appetite or cravings. We show you that some goodies really are good, and some might better be called *baddies*. You may seek foods you think are going to gratify your palate, and most of the time you probably don't consider what they might do inside your body once you consume them. The reality is that you need to think about the consequences of your diet if you want to prevent diabetes or help improve your diabetes if you already have it. You need to have food work *for* you, not *against* you.

FROM FRUSTRATION TO FREEDOM

ONE THING WE'VE learned guiding diabetes patients at Lifestyle Center of America (LCA): Ignorance is *not* bliss when it comes to your blood sugar. It's important to know how to keep it as low as possible while still enjoying the foods you eat. If you're like many of our patients, every time you go to your doctor and hear the lecture about keeping your blood sugar down, you *try* to be conscientious for a while. But you don't always know what to eat or why to eat it and what to avoid and why to avoid it, do you? "Whattya mean that sugar-free chocolate cake is going to raise my blood sugar?" In the end, you might have just thrown up your hands and said, "Oh, forget it. I'm just gonna eat what I want."

So in response to this very common and exhausting frustration, we've developed a relatively easy meal plan that people with diabetes can practice at home. We believe it's the most important dietary key for achieving optimum control over your diabetes. This plan has three parts:

- *Carbohydrate counting.* The goal is to control your carbohydrate intake by eating the same amount of carbs at the same mealtime from day to day.
- *Glycemic control.* The basis is the GI, developed by nutrition researchers to determine a given carbohydrate's relative effect on blood sugar after eating. What will spike your blood sugar faster: a cup of white rice or a cup of pearled barley?[4]
- *Blood sugar monitoring.* This is not about something you put in your body, but something you take out: teeny drops of blood.

CARBS:
The Basics

NOT ALL CARBOHYDRATES are bad simply because they raise blood sugar. You *need* carbs to survive and thrive! You just don't need to get them from doughnuts and candy. So we'll say it again, emphatically: *Carbs are not the enemy.* First of all, carbs are the most efficient source of glucose, a nutrient that is absolutely critical to life. The reason for this is that every cell in the body can run on glucose for energy. The brain uses glucose as its *only* fuel. All things being equal, a brain cell uses twice the amount of carbs for energy than other body cells do. This is why very low-carbohydrate diets like the Atkins diet have been associated with impaired mental ability (for more on this diet, see Chapter 5). Your need for glucose is like your car's need for gas. If you're planning a trip and you notice your gas tank's empty, you have to fill the tank with energy (gas) to keep the motor running. Your body is the same way; you must give it glucose to keep your engine from dying and you along with it. Carbs happen to be the easiest way to get glucose, because they're made of glucose molecules linked together in long chains. The other two macronutrients—fats and proteins—are not.

We should also point out that carbs have been the foundation of the human diet since the beginning of time. And if you look at societies all over the world, this is still the case. Carbs are the most widely consumed substance in the world after water. Beans, grains, vegetables, seeds, and nuts are the dietary foundation for billions of the Earth's inhabitants.[5] There are two important caveats to that assertion. One is that there are a few places, America being one of them, where there is a strong (very strong!) economic basis of support for animal consumption. The second point is that there are cultures, such as America's, where the bulk of the diet still comes from carbs but in grossly altered forms—not in a whole, natural, unadulterated, unrefined state. Heavily processed white flour and multiple corn byproducts are still the basis of the Western diet. This is not the way carbs were meant to be eaten.

One of the most valuable things we can impart through this book is that the bulk of human calories should come from *plant-based carbohydrates in a form that is as natural and unrefined as possible.* Life-sustaining carbohydrate energy, fiber, vitamins, minerals, phytochemicals, the right kind of protein, and the healthiest kind of fat: a PBD has it all. So the key is not to eliminate carbs from your diet or even greatly reduce them, as many fad diets suggest. Instead, you just need to eat the right quantity and differentiate between the best- and worst-*quality* carbs. This is easier than it might sound.

CARB ACTION

Why do we put so much focus on carbohydrates? What about fat? What about protein? Fats and proteins do influence blood sugar and diabetes (see Chapters 3 and 5), but we're focusing on carbohydrates because they are the primary nutrient responsible for raising blood sugar levels most quickly and dramatically right after eating.

DIETARY CARBOHYDRATES

There are three main types of dietary carbohydrate: sugar, starch, and fiber.

Sugar

Sugars are referred to as "simple" carbohydrates, because their chemical structures are simple in comparison to starch and fiber. The simplest of the sugars are single molecules, and several are found in nature. You're already familiar with one of them: glucose, which we also know as blood sugar. It's the fuel our body's cells require for energy production. There are others, such as fructose and galactose, which are also common in food. Even though dietary fructose and galactose are absorbed into the bloodstream through the intestine, they cannot be used for energy until they are chemically converted into glucose.

Two individual sugar molecules can be linked together to form a more complex sugar. Sucrose (table sugar), for example, is made when a glucose and fructose molecule are linked together. When sucrose is eaten, it must first be *digested*, or broken down into the individual glucose and fructose molecules. The molecules (glucose and fructose) can then be absorbed into the blood, where fructose is converted into glucose before it can be entirely used for energy.

Starch

Starches, on the other hand, are referred to as "complex" carbohydrates because they are composed of long chains of glucose molecules. These chains can be several thousand glucose molecules long. Starch is the storage form of energy used by plants. When ingested, our digestive system must break down the chemical bonds between each glucose molecule before the molecules can be absorbed into our bloodstreams. This will begin rather quickly—within minutes after you start eating. Once absorbed, they are already in the form needed (glucose, or blood sugar) to be used for energy. Think of a potato, a very starchy carb, as a very large version of a glucose tablet in terms of what it might do to your blood sugar levels.

A simple concept to remember is that the closer a food is to a simple glucose molecule, the faster it will be absorbed by the intestine and the faster it will raise your blood sugar. It's easy to see that consuming pure glucose (also called dextrose on food labels) will act the fastest on blood sugar. Fructose will not act so rapidly, because it has to first undergo chemical changes to be made into glucose. The glucose-fructose mixture called sucrose will also act more slowly, because it must be digested and absorbed, and the fructose portion must then be chemically changed. Because starches must first have the glucose molecules "cut" away from them, it takes even longer for them to raise blood sugar than if you ate an equivalent amount of pure glucose (dextrose). This is a bit of a generalization, but we hope you get the picture. This concept comes into play when, later in this chapter, we discuss the GI of a food—its ability to raise blood sugar levels compared to eating an equivalent amount of glucose.

Fiber

Fiber is the last type of dietary carbohydrate. Like starch, fiber is a complex carbohydrate, made up of long chains of simple sugars. But, unlike sugar and starch, fiber cannot be digested by humans, so it adds no calories to the diet. *All plant foods contain both soluble and insoluble fiber.* Foods that come from animals have absolutely no fiber at all. Not so long ago, the instructors in medical schools taught that because fiber had no nutritional value, it could be ignored. That's certainly not the case in today's nutritional world. But not understanding how fiber works (or at least underestimating its power to transform our diet) is where many otherwise brilliant diabetes experts got their early diet prescriptions wrong.

But attitudes are changing. In March 2007, the American Diabetes Association's flagship magazine, *Diabetes Forecast*, reported a recent study that pitted its own 2003 dietary guidelines against the kind of low-fat, low (but adequate) protein, vegan (plant-based) diet we promote at LCA. The study participants in each group, all with type-2 diabetes and most overweight, stayed on their respective diets for 22 weeks. As expected, the researchers concluded that both diets were associated with significant improvements in diabetic health markers. The vegan group did better across the board. Those on a PBD saw improvements in blood sugar nearly *twice* that of the traditional dieters: They lost about 50 percent more weight, and improvements in their blood pressure, low-density lipoprotein (LDL), or "bad," cholesterol, high-density lipoprotein (HDL), or "good," cholesterol, and triglycerides were all better than those on the ADA standard diabetes diet. And here's the kicker: People in the vegan group were more likely to stick to their diet than those assigned to the standard diabetes diet. The researchers credited the drops in hemoglobin A_{1c} (HgA_{1c}; a long-term blood sugar marker) to weight loss, which occurred in the vegan group even though they were allowed to eat as much as they wanted.[6]

The thing is, when you're on a diet full of whole grains and healthful, filling fiber, you don't *want* to eat as much as you do when you consume junk food and animal products. Patients at LCA, even those with type-1 diabetes, eat *no snacks* during the day and no midnight snacks full of extra calories. And they don't experience hypoglycemia nearly as much as some doctors and nutritionists worry about. Again, a big part of the secret is the amount of diabetes-friendly fiber in our meals.[7]

CARB COUNTING 101

YOU NEED TO concentrate on both the *amount* of carbohydrate you're consuming, as well as the *type* of carb (quantity and quality). Let's start with the quantity. Step one to mastering the LCA diet is to count how much carbohydrate you're eating at each meal. With the guidelines in this chapter and help from your doctor or nutritionist, you should strive to keep your daily carb intake reasonable and consistent from meal to meal.

Carb counting has been around since the 1920s,[8] but it really took off after a major study called the Diabetes Control and Complications Trial proved it was effective.[9] This dietary strategy has been tested in many clinical trials and has been shown to work for all ages and all types of diabetes. For instance, children,[10] the elderly,[11] pregnant women,[12] and those with special dietary challenges can all learn to use it and implement it.

- *Carb counting is practical and simple.* Once you learn the basic principle of what constitutes a carb choice, there's very little math, and there are few of the complications of more cumbersome diabetic exchange lists.
- *Carb counting is effective* in helping people with diabetes achieve optimal blood sugar goals.[13] The goals are to *control blood sugar naturally*, not through reliance on medication, and to reduce or eliminate the process of insulin resistance that underlies diabetes. Remember that simply covering your carb intake with enough insulin or oral diabetes medicine will make your diabetes worse.

- *Carb counting is flexible.* You can use it to calculate your intake from all kinds of carbs, from the produce section of an organic market to a cruise ship buffet. Carb counting has been used in hospitals, prisons,[14] nursing homes, and even among competitive athletes with diabetes, and it's been proven the best method to provide adequate energy with minimal risk of either high or low blood sugar.[15]

To master the basics of carb counting, you're going to have to learn a little carb-counting lingo. Everything has its jargon—computers, sports, politics—and medicine is at the top of that heap. That's why most of us don't understand what our doctors are telling us half the time. But you're going to understand carb counting, because it's much simpler. All you need to know are these four things:

- What foods contain carbs?
- What is a carb choice?
- How many carb choices per meal are appropriate for me?
- What portion size equals a carb choice?

What Foods Contain Carbs?

Very simply put, all of the foods recommended in the 30-Day Diabetes Miracle program are carbohydrate based, because they're plant foods. Fruits, vegetables, grains, beans, seeds, and nuts all contain carbs. Some contain more than others. Green, leafy vegetables and vegetables that grow above the ground tend to have fewer carbs. This often allows you to eat more with less of a spike in your postprandial blood sugar. On the other hand, grains and starchy root (below the ground) vegetables contain more carbs and, therefore, require more portion control. This is why we often repeat the mantra to eat mostly above-the-ground vegetables. Not to say that their underground fellows like radishes, carrots, potatoes, turnips, and the like are bad for you—you simply need to pay attention to how much of them you're eating if you have diabetes.

The total carbs in a food equal the sum of the sugar, starch, and fiber. But it's not so much the total you have to worry about. You might have heard the term *net carbohydrates*, or seen it on a food label. Think of the total amount of carbs in your diet as your *gross* carbs—like your paycheck before taxes are deducted. Net carbs include only the glucose that is available from sugar and starch during the process of digestion. Remember, the glucose from sugar and starch can be absorbed from the digestive tract into the bloodstream and thus can raise the levels of sugar in your blood after you eat. While fiber is also a carb, it's not digestible, so its glucose is not available to you (like that percent of your gross pay the government makes unavailable to you). Fiber is everyone's friend, and this is why fiber is an especially good friend to people with diabetes.

Because of this, when you determine the grams of carb you eat at a meal, it's only the *net* carbs that you need to consider. You can determine the amount of net carbohydrates in food by subtracting the grams of fiber from the total grams (g) of carbohydrate:

Total carbohydrates (g) — Fiber (g) = Net carbohydrates (g)

What Is a Carb Choice?

Here comes pretty much the only math necessary to figure carb choices. All you have to commit to memory is that *15 g of net carbohydrates equals 1 carb choice*. You just have to remember that, as if it were your anniversary or your pay day:

15 g Net carbohydrate = 1 Carb choice

How Many Carb Choices per Meal Are Appropriate for Me?

On *average*, if you have type-1 or type-2 diabetes, we recommend 3 to 5 carb choices for breakfast (45 to 75 g), 3 to 5 for lunch (45 to 75 g), and 0 to 3 for supper (0 to 45 g). Keeping supper's carb choices as low as possible will help with your overnight and morning blood sugar levels (more on that in Chapter 7). We find that patients who stay within the range of 9 to 13 carb choices (135 to 195 g) per day tend to experience the best blood sugar control, weight loss, and overall resolution of their diabetes problems.

It's best to count your carb choices *per meal*, not *per day*. In other words, we don't suggest saving up all your carb choices for dinner and consuming your daily quota of carbs all at once. Having said that, if you are *planning* a high-carb meal—say it's a very special occasion, such as your wedding, and you really want to have a piece of cake—it's not a bad idea to eat less in the previous or subsequent meal. (We should note that many of our patients, even those with type-1 diabetes, don't experience hypoglycemia when they skip meals, probably thanks to all the fiber in our diet.)

BRAIN FOOD

●

REMEMBER when we said that glucose is the only fuel the brain can use? Research tells us that the brain needs *at least* 130 g of carbohydrates per day to work properly. Contrast this with the super-proscriptive diet regimens recommended by some diabetes doctors that limit carbohydrates to no more than 6 g for breakfast, no more than 12 g for lunch, and 12 g for dinner.[16] That's a *total* of 30 g of carbs per day (the equivalent of ¼ cup boiled buckwheat). Does that sound like a healthful, balanced diet to you?

If the food you're eating has *5 g of net carbs or less* (like ½ cup asparagus) you can consider it a *free food*. That means you don't count that serving when totaling your carb choices for that meal. Just remember that if the amount you are eating is more than one serving, the amount of carb you are eating will increase. That means what started out as a free carb choice can end up actually counting as 1 carb choice if your portion size increases.

Finally, remember that the *kinds* of carbs matter, too. Carb counting should not be the only tool you use to plan your meals: To work properly, it needs to be combined with the GI, which we'll discuss later in this chapter.

CARB COUNTING 101

●

	BREAKFAST	LUNCH	SUPPER
Number of carb choices*	3–5	3–5	0–3
Number of grams of carbs	45–75	45–75	0–45

*These are averages; consult your doctor or nutritionist.

What Portion Size Equals a Carb Choice?

Just how much of your favorite foods can you eat to get 1 carb choice? Well, 1 medium apple or orange is about 15 g of carbs, or 1 carb choice. The same for one slice of whole wheat bread and ½ cup of corn flakes or cooked beans.

Unfortunately, there is no shortcut to using the "Carb-Counting Guide" in Appendix 2 (pp. 281–286). But the more you use it, the easier it will be to carb count. In this process, we recommend you take time to learn what the various portions look like on your plate. For example, measure out ½ cup beans, put it in the bowl or on the plate you usually use, and see what that amount looks like. Think of it as a form of behavior modification. Just practice the behavior, and soon you'll become comfortable with it.[17] Remember: The carbohydrate content of foods varies with brand and portion size, so *always read labels.*

THE CARB-COUNTING GUIDE

●

SEE the "Carb-Counting Guide" in Appendix 2 for examples that will help you plan your meals. You can also go to our website (www.diabetesmiracle.org) for a much more comprehensive carb-counting guide. Also, keep track of your daily carbohydrate intake. Sample logs are provided in Appendix 1.

THE GLYCEMIC FACTOR:
A Tale of Two Cities

YOU MIGHT STILL be wondering how we could propose a high-carb diet for people with diabetes. It sounds like an oxymoron (like *jumbo shrimp*)! Most doctors and nutritionists still get caught in that same trap of thinking: high carbohydrates = lots of glucose = high blood sugar = high insulin levels = diabetes. Seems like a no-brainer. Well, it turns out that not all carbs are created equal.

Dr. Zeno Charles-Marcel, the first medical director at LCA, explains carb quality in a way our patients say makes a lot of sense: When we eat carbohydrates, they're broken down into single glucose molecules, which are absolutely critical for life because nearly all the cells in the body require glucose as their energy source. But then, why is it that some carb foods cause us to have too much of this sugar in our blood? There's a tale about two cities that might help you understand. We'll call one city Petersville and the other one Paulsville.

Petersville and Paulsville are two beautiful cities. Last year Petersville had a rainfall of 21.3 inches, and Paulsville had a rainfall of 21.2 inches. Now, you might think that those two cities sound like they had very similar weather last year. But actually, Petersville had a practically rain-free year except during Labor Day weekend. The rain started to fall Friday evening, and it went all the way through until Tuesday morning. It poured cats and dogs all weekend, and Petersville ended up with its total rainfall for that year, 21.3 inches, all occurring in one wet weekend.

In Paulsville, however, the weather was quite different. There it seemed to rain all year. Rain, rain, rain, all the time. It drizzled one day. It piddled the next day. It was more like a mist sometimes, and once in a while it came down pretty hard, but not all day. The people of Paulsville considered it a lousy, wet year. But it turns out the people of Petersville had a lot more to complain about—and not just that their Labor Day weekend was ruined. They suffered severe flooding, followed by a serious drought.

These two cities, even though they had similar rainfalls, experienced very different *consequences*. In Petersville, because the rainfall occurred all at once, the riverbanks overflowed, the levees were breached, and there was a lot of flooding; after Tuesday, much of the city was in ruins. But in Paulsville, even though it rained nearly every day, it rained only a little bit, allowing the water to flow naturally down the river, where it was carried out to sea.

We can use this allegory as a model for what happens in our bodies when we eat carbohydrates. There are some carb foods whose characteristics will cause us to have a flood of blood sugar after we eat them. The blood sugar will go up too high and fast with some foods, because the carbohydrates are rapidly digested, releasing a lot of glucose into the bloodstream in a short period of time. That's what's known as a *high-glycemic* food—it causes a blood sugar flood. It gives you a lot of sugar in a short period of time, like the rainfall in Petersville. On the other hand, some carb foods will be digested more slowly, releasing glucose into the bloodstream gradually over several hours. This causes the blood sugar to go up gradually and not too high. That's what a *low-glycemic* carb is like. Think of it as *slo-o-o-o-o-ow* carb or a time-release carb, like the rainfall in Paulsville was time released.

What's the actual process that causes the change in blood sugar so dramatically in some foods and more gently in other foods? In the past, we used to focus only on characterizing carbs as chemically simple or complex. The thinking was that simple sugars, like those found in table sugar, candy, white bread, and soda, tend to raise blood sugars more rapidly and higher than complex carbohydrates, like whole wheat bread, brown rice, vegetables, and beans. That analysis is valid, but it doesn't tell the whole story. Even though some carbs may be complex, they still cause the blood sugar to rise rapidly. White potatoes are a good example. On the other hand, some simple carbs don't cause a high, fast spike in blood sugars. Floral honeys (those made by bees, not food processors) are a good example of these. So just deciding whether a carb is complex or simple isn't enough to determine the quality of the carb for a diabetic diet.

Instead, we ought to look at the physiological process of food breakdown—otherwise known as digestion—how different carbs break down in the body, and what impact they have on the blood sugar. The glycemic index (GI) is a good tool to help with this. The GI is a measure of how rapidly and how high the blood sugar will go up when a certain food is consumed. It's just a basic, useful way to characterize foods' effects on blood sugar.

Now we can think about it in terms of those two cities: Petersville and Paulsville. We don't want a flood of high blood sugar, because high blood sugar causes damage to our bodies. We want to limit high-GI foods that will bust through the levees. Instead we want to eat low-GI foods, so that we can experience the great benefits of healthful carbs without the serious drawback of high blood sugar responses. In fact, it seems that eating a high-GI diet can actually lead to the development of diabetes[18] and the metabolic syndrome, whereas eating a low-GI diet can take your body in the opposite direction, away from insulin resistance.[19]

The Glycemic Index

It's important for people with diabetes to keep their after-meal (postprandial) blood sugars as low as possible because this correlates with long-term avoidance of diabetes complications.[20] Since about 1980, we've known that different foods with carbs affect the body differently in terms of postprandial blood sugar.[21] The GI measures the *quality* of a carb, which means the effect of a food's carbs in comparison to a standard amount (50 g) of a reference food, which is pure glucose. With pure glucose, there's no digestion required before the glucose gets into the bloodstream. When someone consumes 50 g of glucose, his or her blood sugar will go up in a pretty predictable fashion: fast and high.

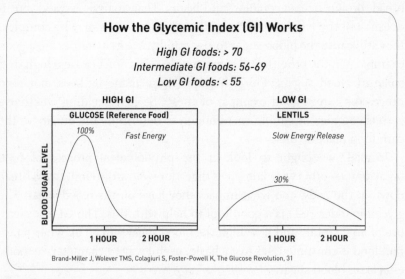

The glycemic index (GI) measures carbohydrate quality. The numerical ranking (0 to 100) of foods is based on how they affect blood sugar levels.

To calculate the quality of carbohydrates, scientists use standardized testing procedures to determine their effect on blood sugars. They, might, for example, give people who are fasting 50 g of banana or 50 g of sesame bagel, and then test blood sugars at regular intervals. Foods are then given numbers, either the same or lower than the number for pure glucose, which is 100. Foods containing carbs that break down quickly during digestion have the highest GI rating and, therefore, the highest numbers. Low-GI foods, on the other hand, break down more slowly and thus affect the blood sugar more slowly. High-GI carbs can spike your blood sugar, but low-GI foods cause slower, more subtle increases.

Eating low-GI foods in the short term will help your immediate blood sugar levels. And if you follow through in the long term, frequently substituting low-GI food for high-GI food, you will see an improvement—sometimes a dramatic improvement—in your blood sugar, which can lead to a lessening of complications.[22]

A slice of 100 percent whole wheat bread has a low GI (43) but a white flour dinner roll has a much higher GI (73). What's interesting about that is that they both have about the same number of grams of carbs—they're both 1 carb choice (14 g and 16 g, respectively).[23] Remember that the GI is not about the *amount* of carbohydrates, but the *quality*, in terms of effects on your blood sugar.

There are a few stipulations concerning the GI:

- The GI should not be the *only* tool you use to determine healthfulness of food. A Betty Crocker chocolate cake mix with frosting has a low GI (38). Nutella chocolate hazelnut spread is even lower (30). Salted corn chips are also low (42).[24] But we wouldn't consider any of these foods healthful by any standard. So remember to also keep your eyes on saturated fat, trans-fat, calories, processing, and so on when you choose foods. Large amounts of fat (and protein) in food tend to slow the rate at which the stomach empties. That means that high-fat foods usually have lower GI values than their low-fat equivalents. Here's another example: Potato chips have a lower GI value (54) than potatoes baked without fat (85). Many cookies have a lower GI value (55 to 65) than bread (70). The fat in these foods, especially saturated fat, trans-fat, and/or interesterified fat (see Chapter 5), will have negative effects on heart health and the overall diabetes process that far outweigh the short-term benefit on immediate blood sugar levels.

- Some foods that would otherwise seem very healthful have high GIs. For example, ¾ cup of watermelon has a GI of 76, about the same as 2 ounces of licorice or 1 ounce of jelly beans. That doesn't mean watermelon is inherently bad, it just means it will raise blood sugar much faster and higher than, say, grapefruit, which ranks very low at 25.

- Some low-GI foods (bananas, grapes, mangoes, unsweetened fruit juice, pastas) and intermediate-GI foods (pineapple, cantaloupe, raisins) may *not* be low glycemic *for you*. The GI for these foods was scientifically determined with real people,[25] but everyone's different. Experiment to see what your personal blood sugar response is to these foods after you eat them.

GET A LOAD OF THIS

●

ALONG with the quality of carbs as measured by the glycemic index, we can't forget about quantity. Researchers at Harvard University discovered that the real effect on blood sugar (how high it gets and how long it stays high) is determined by the GI of the foods we eat in a given meal combined with *how many* carbs we consumed in that meal. They dubbed this measure the glycemic load (GL). You don't need to know the math behind this—all you need to know is two things:

- Diets with a high GL are associated with an increased risk of type-2 diabetes and cardiovascular disease.[26]
- The best strategy for keeping the GL as low as possible is to keep your per-meal carb count in the range we suggest, plus keep it relatively consistent from day to day and substitute as many low-GI foods for high-GI foods as you can.

- There are lots of foods that have not been tested yet for their GI. Testing foods is expensive and time consuming, and only authorized laboratories can do it. You have the option of doing an informal test to develop your personal GI list of the foods you most enjoy. Here's one example of what you might do. Say one of your standard breakfasts is 1 cup of cooked oatmeal, ½ cup beans, ½ ounce of nuts, ¼ cup of unsweetened soy milk, and 1 cup of fresh berries. Almost every time you eat this meal you get a similar 2-hour postprandial sugar around 140. Now you want to find out if half a cantaloupe in place of those berries is still going to give you that good postprandial blood sugar. So the next time you eat this meal you decide to substitute the half of cantaloupe for the cup of berries. You check your blood sugar 2 hours later and find it's 200. You might conclude that the cantaloupe tends to be high glycemic for you in the context of that meal. Maybe you could have some cantaloupe, but a much smaller portion; or maybe you can have cantaloupe at a different time of day, with different foods. Experiment and see how it works for you.

- Watch portion sizes! Sweetened fruit-flavored soy yogurt might be low GI, but if you have three containers of it, you've just consumed an entire meal's worth of carbs. The good news is that portion control should be easier if you eat low-GI foods. One interesting study at Children's Hospital in Boston showed rapid absorption of glucose after consumption of high-GI foods causes a series of hormonal and metabolic changes that might promote excessive eating, at least in the short term.[27] This makes sense physiologically. Insulin is a growth hormone. Low blood sugar causes hunger. High-GI foods stimulate the production of an insulin spike more quickly and more intensely than low-GI foods. That spike is usually followed by a rapid drop in blood glucose, which is accompanied by hunger, the body's cry for needed energy.
- Don't forget: High-GI foods contribute to more frequent eating and thus weight gain.

GLYCEMIC INDEX GUIDES

●

SEE Appendix 3, "Glycemic Index Guidelines for a Plant-Based Diet," for the GI ratings of many foods, or go to our website (www.diabetes miracle.org) for a much more comprehensive guide.

Strategies for a Low-GI PBD

Using Appendix 3:

- Choose most of your food from the low-GI choices (under 55).
- Choose food occasionally from the intermediate-GI choices (56 to 69).
- Eliminate (or greatly minimize) foods from the high-GI choices (above 70).
- Replace high-GI foods with low-GI foods.
- If you decide to include a high-GI food in the meal (white potatoes, for example):

  - Eat a smaller portion of the high-GI food.
  - Add lower-GI choices to balance the meal (beans,

steamed broccoli with lemon juice, raw salad, nuts,
and/or seeds). This will lower the glycemic load (GL) for
the entire meal.

- Include an acid food with the meal, such as fruit, lemon
  juice, or tomatoes. Acids in food slow down stomach
  emptying, slowing the rate of carbohydrate digestion,
  and thus slowing the rate glucose (blood sugar) enters
  your bloodstream.

- Use cornstarch or Thicken Up brand instant food thickener
  rather than flour to thicken foods.[28]
- Remember that a GI value was never meant as the *only* crite-
  rion for healthy food.

A LOW-GI DIET IS BEST AT REDUCING WEIGHT

●

A diet rich in carbohydrates with a low GI appears to be more effective
in reducing fat mass than diets with a high GI or high in protein, Dr.
Jennie Brand-Miller and her Australian research team reported in
2006. In two high-carb diets, those eating the lower-GI diet lost twice
as much fat as those on a higher-glycemic diet. The investigators also
found that total and LDL "bad" cholesterol levels increased in the
high-GI diet and decreased in the low-GI diet.[29]

TESTING, TESTING, 1, 2, 3

FINALLY, WE STRONGLY urge you to test your blood sugar regularly. In a
weird way, blood testing can be fun and interesting, if you treat it like
your own personal science experiment. Remember, ignorance of your
blood sugar levels can (eventually) mean the difference between losing
your feet to amputation or running your first 10K race—or at least playing a few rounds of golf again. You should test yourself six to eight times
a day, at least for the next several months until you've got a good handle on it. See Chapter 3 for our recommendations on glucose meters.
Ideally, use your meter to test:

- When you wake up (*fasting* blood sugar)
- Before meals (*preprandial* blood sugar)
- Two hours after the *start* of meals (*postprandial* blood sugar)
- Before you go to bed
- Once in the middle of the night when you first change your diet and activity levels substantially. We especially recommend this for people on insulin who experience ups and downs in their blood sugar levels.

Have fun with it! It's actually quite interesting to see how certain foods affect your blood sugar. Do oranges and grapefruits have different effects? Will two pieces of toast have exactly twice the effect as one piece of toast? If you're hypoglycemic (have low blood sugar), what will bring your sugar up faster, a half of a banana or five pineapple chunks? As you discover results and glean new insights, adjust your eating accordingly. Remember, not every person's body will react the same way to the same input. For example, some people report little or no blood sugar changes from moderate amounts of alcohol, whereas some people report dramatic changes. Also remember that not every input is the same every time. That 1 cup of Bing cherries today will not *ever* have *exactly* the same effect as another cup eaten tomorrow (but it should be close enough to predict within reason).

If you follow our diet, you'll have another good reason to test your blood sugar regularly: to congratulate yourself on the lowest numbers you've seen in years.

And there's also a serious reason to test frequently. When you're following the LCA diet, you're likely to require less oral diabetes medicine and/or less insulin than you're used to taking on your current diet (see Chapter 3). After a while, many of you will need *no medicine at all*. This is particularly true if you've been diagnosed recently. So, if you're still taking diabetes medicine of any kind, you must test religiously to ensure that you're not hypoglycemic. We reiterate that you should be in regular communication with a trusted physician and/or nutritionist as you follow the 30-Day Diabetes Miracle program. There's a checklist in Chapter 10 that you can take to your physician.

*   *   *

FIBER, CARB COUNTING, the glycemic index, and regular testing are what make the difference. If you focus your diet choices on high-fiber, low-glycemic carbs and if you control the quantity of carbs you consume, you will feel satisfied, while avoiding a big blood sugar spike 2 hours after eating. No need for the prescription one of our patients got from an endocrinologist after getting a diabetes diagnosis: "You should be eating every few hours at the least. And if you're doing any activities like walking, you should eat a half a sandwich every half hour." This is a recipe for making diabetes much worse. It's whole grain, high-fiber carbs that make diabetes better, by increasing insulin sensitivity and helping promote weight loss, which works especially well among the heaviest people.[30]

7

Menus and Recipes

BREAKFAST LIKE A KING!

AS YOU PREPARE the menus presented in this chapter, keep in mind that a simple lifestyle habit can have a profound effect on your health. Do you remember your mom, a teacher, or a public service announcement advising you that breakfast is the most important meal of the day? Well, we agree with that advice. At Lifestyle Center of America (LCA), we like the saying:

Eat breakfast like a king, lunch like a prince, and supper like a pauper.

In other words, you should eat more food earlier in the day and less at the end of the day. That's the opposite of what most of us are used to. But if you really ponder it, this counterintuitive idea starts to seem much more intuitive. Food is energy—calories are used as fuel to get you through the day. If you want the most energy to get you through the day, you should logically consume the most early in the day.

But most Americans have it backward when it comes to fueling their daily journeys with food. They typically skip breakfast and have their largest meal at the end of the day, when they're least likely to use that energy through their daily physical demands. Sometimes they get a huge input of energy in the form of a heavy meal right in front of the TV, just before going to bed. That's a recipe for packing on the pounds through the dynamic of too much energy in, not enough energy out.

This prescription of eating most of your food early in the day holds true especially for people with weight to lose. In a healthy person, glucose tolerance, the body's ability to handle sugar, decreases as the day progresses.[1] This suggests that the body is better able to handle larger meals at the beginning of the day rather than at the end of the day. All you need to know is that eating breakfast is associated with successful weight loss maintenance in national studies[2] as well as in our own follow-up data.[3]

On the other side of the equation, we recommend you don't eat a dinnertime (evening) meal—or you eat a very small one, such as some steamed vegetables, a small cup of plant-based soup, or a small salad. We also think it's best not to snack at all at night. The idea behind eating nothing or very little after lunch is to put your body into a fasting state while you sleep until you break the fast at breakfast. Remember, overnight fasting increases insulin sensitivity, which is good.

This is a sensible way to sleep better, lose weight, rest your pancreas, and lower your diabetes medicine needs. Leaving off that midnight snack will prevent another midnight ride of the Paul Revere Hormone shouting, *"The Energy's Coming!"* to an inactive body. Bedtime snacking in people with diabetes is associated with obesity, elevated hemoglobin A_{1c} (HgA_{1c}) levels, and an increased number of complications related to diabetes.[4] Just try it for a few days. Eat a nice high-fiber, plant-based lunch, then stop eating for the day and see how much lower your morning (fasting) blood sugar levels are the next day.

Best of all, not eating late in the day means you wake up hungry! You won't *want* to skip breakfast, and you'll be more inclined to load up on those high-fiber good carbs from a big bowl of oatmeal, whole wheat toast, and fruit. This, in turn—thanks to the filling effect of fiber—will make it much easier for you to forgo snacking. That's good news for several reasons. We have another saying at LCA:

The bigger the snacks, the bigger the slacks.[5]

Not only do many of us tend to eat *too much* while snacking, but we so often eat the worst kinds of snacks. High-sugar, high-fat foods (cakes, cookies, candies, chocolate, and desserts) are the things we crave, and these—not celery sticks—are the kinds of snacks that contribute considerably to caloric intake[6] and, of course, higher insulin needs as well as higher blood sugar. Very few healthy people are snackers.[7] Did you know that increased frequency of meals and snacks is even associated with increased risk of colon cancer?[8] At LCA, we find that eating small, frequent meals throughout the day—such as the American Diabetes Association (ADA) recommends—increases the number of times your pancreas is stimulated and thus aggravates the diabetes process rather than improves it.

It takes at least 3 to 4 hours for your food to properly digest. We recommend you give yourself about 5 hours between meals (eat breakfast at, say, 7:30 a.m. and lunch at 1 p.m.). Eating regular meals using low-glycemic, high-fiber foods will keep your blood sugar controlled and keep you satisfied so that you're not hungry until your next meal. With two good meals at breakfast and lunch, you can have a light supper, or even skip it, and not feel hungry.

That leads us to the question of how you should think about lunch. We say "eat lunch like a prince" because the meal should be a full one, but not as big as breakfast's king-size meal. If you eat a plant-based, high-fiber lunch (heavy on the salad, veggies, beans, and whole grains), you'll be surprised to discover what many of our patients have: *You won't be hungry between meals.*

Because we recommend you eat light at night, if at all, our lunches tend to be more elaborate than you might be used to—more like traditional dinners. But we recognize that not everyone has a lot of time to whip up lunch. To make this important meal more convenient and portable, we recommend you make batches of the entrees and sides, then store them in individual containers that are microwave safe.

Skipping or significantly reducing supper, which is traditionally the highest-calorie meal (and doing so without feeling hungry or restricted) is a great secret to weight loss and morning blood sugar control. Avoiding caloric excess is associated with prolonged life. In fact, restricting caloric intake to 60 to 70 percent of the normal requirement for weight maintenance prolongs the lifespan across a broad range of species, from rats to humans.[9] Caloric restriction in adult men and women results in decreased metabolic, hormonal, and inflammatory risk factors for diabetes, cardiovascular disease, and possibly cancer.[10] Some researchers have found that caloric restriction showed benefits on insulin resistance; blood lipid levels; blood pressure; asthma; seasonal allergies; infectious diseases of viral, bacterial, and fungal origin; rheumatoid arthritis; osteoarthritis; and other conditions.[11]

MENUS AND RECIPES

THE REST OF this chapter presents a week's worth of menus. If a meal is printed in bold type or italics, the recipes are included in this chapter. Carb counts can be found in the nutritional analysis accompanying the recipes. Please note that some recipes are higher in fat than others, so watch portions to ensure an overall low-fat diet. For more recipes, go to our website (www.diabetesmiracle.org).

Sunday

MEAL	PORTION SIZE	CARB CHOICES (number)
Breakfast		
Old-Fashioned Rolled Oats	1 c	1½
Fresh blueberries	1 c	1
Walnut halves	½ oz (7 halves)	free
Breakfast Beans	1 c	2
Milk, unsweetened soy or almond	½ c	free
Whole Ground Flaxseed	1–2 Tbsp	free
Lunch		
Haystacks	1 haystack	3
Dinner		
Garden Minestrone Soup	1 c	⅔
Caesar Salad	2 c	½
Pear	1 medium	1⅓
Total Carb Choices		10

Old-Fashioned Rolled Oats

YIELD: 4 CUPS

4 c water   2 c old-fashioned rolled oats
¼ tsp salt

IN a medium saucepan, bring the water and salt to a boil. Add the oats and stir briefly. Reduce the heat, cover, and simmer for 20 minutes, or until the water is absorbed.

Note: Overstirring during cooking may cause oatmeal to become gummy.

———

ANALYSIS FOR 1 SERVING: 1 CUP COOKED OATMEAL
Calories: 156, Fat: 2.6 g, Total carbohydrates: 27.1 g, Protein: 6.5 g, Dietary fiber: 4.3 g, Sodium: 150 mg, Net carbs: 22.8 g, Carb choice: 1½

———

Breakfast Beans

YIELD: 5½ CUPS (11 ½-CUP SERVINGS)

6 c canned beans, drained (use pinto or Great Northern beans)

1½ c water

1 tsp onion powder

½ tsp garlic powder

1 tsp cumin

1 tsp nutritional yeast flakes

COMBINE all ingredients in a saucepan and heat through. Smash about ⅓ of beans against side of pot to make recipe thick and saucy.

———

ANALYSIS FOR 1 SERVING, WITH PINTO BEANS: ½ CUP

Calories: 131, Fat: 0.5 g, Total carbohydrates: 24.4 g, Protein: 7.9 g, Dietary fiber: 8.1 g, Sodium: 151 mg, Net carbs: 16.3 g, Carb choice: 1

ANALYSIS FOR 1 SERVING, WITH GREAT NORTHERN BEANS: ½ CUP

Calories: 137, Fat: 0.4 g, Total carbohydrates: 24.7 g, Protein: 9.7 g, Dietary fiber: 6.2 g, Sodium: 235 mg, Net carbs: 18.5 g, Carb choice: 1

———

Whole Ground Flaxseed

YIELD: 3 TABLESPOONS + 1½ TEASPOONS

2 Tbsp whole flaxseed, light or dark

MEASURE whole seeds and put in seed grinder, small coffee grinder, or mini food processor, and grind fine, about 10 to 30 seconds. Eat after grinding by adding to hot or cold cereal, breads, soups, or salads. Once ground, don't leave flaxseed at room temperature or it will spoil—always refrigerate or freeze in a sealed container, where it will keep for up to 6 months.

Caution: As outstanding as flaxseed is, don't have more than 3 tablespoons whole seeds per day, because the husks of the seeds contain compounds that can be toxic in high doses.

———

ANALYSIS FOR 1 SERVING: 1 TABLESPOON GROUND FLAXSEED
Calories: 35, Fat: 2.4 g, Total carbohydrates: 2.4 g, Protein: 1.4 g, Dietary fiber: 2 g; Sodium: 2 mg, Net carbs: 0.4 g, Carb choice: free

———

Haystacks
A MEAL IN ITSELF

YIELD: 1 SERVING

1 c *Kickin' Western Chili* (p. 131)

1 oz (18 chips) Guiltless Gourmet Baked Yellow Corn Tortilla Chips or other low-fat, whole grain baked corn chips

1½ c lettuce, shredded

½ c tomato, diced

2 Tbsp onion, diced

⅛ avocado, sliced

1 Tbsp black olives, chopped or sliced

Salsa—optional

Soy sour cream—optional

HEAT the chili. Layer ingredients on a plate in the following order: chips, chili, lettuce, tomato, onion, avocado, salsa (if using), and soy sour cream (if using).

Variation: Add or substitute any other vegetables. For a lower-fat version, use fat-free baked tortilla chips.

ANALYSIS FOR 1 SERVING: 1 HAYSTACK
(WITHOUT SALSA OR SOY SOUR CREAM)

(The analysis amounts in this recipe are higher than for most recipes because this is designed to be a complete meal.)

Calories: 396, Fat: 9.7 g, Total carbohydrates: 63.8 g, Protein: 18 g, Dietary fiber: 15.5g, Sodium: 740 mg, Net carbs: 48.3 g, Carb choice: 3

Garden Minestrone Soup

YIELD: 7 CUPS

⅓ c onion, diced

1 tsp olive oil

4 c water

1 c carrots, cut in ½-inch slices

⅓ c celery, cut in ½-inch slices

1 c zucchini, cut in ¼-inch slices

1 c fresh or canned tomatoes, diced

⅔ c cooked whole grain macaroni, elbows, or shells

1 c canned low-sodium red beans, drained

1½ tsp McKay's Beef Style Seasoning, vegan

1 tsp salt

1 tsp dried sweet basil

½ tsp dried oregano

⅛ tsp garlic powder

1 bay leaf

IN a soup pot, sauté the onion in the olive oil over medium-high heat until tender, about 3 to 4 minutes. Add the water, carrots, and celery. Cook until tender, about 15 minutes. Add the remaining ingredients and simmer until done, 15 to 20 minutes. Remove the bay leaf before serving.

———

ANALYSIS FOR 1 SERVING: 1 CUP

Calories: 89, Fat: 2.3 g, Total carbohydrates: 14.6 g, Protein: 3.9 g, Dietary fiber: 3.4 g, Sodium: 442 mg, Net carbs: 11.2 g, Carb choice: ⅔

———

Caesar Salad

YIELD: 7½ CUPS

1 c *Seasoned Croutons* (recipe
follows)

½ c *Caesar Salad Dressing*
(recipe follows)

6 c Romaine lettuce, coarsely
chopped

½ c onions, sliced

¼ c pitted black olives

PREPARE the *Seasoned Croutons*. Prepare the *Caesar Salad Dressing*.
Put the lettuce in a bowl. Add the onions, olives, croutons, and salad
dressing. Mix all together well.

———

ANALYSIS FOR 1 SERVING OF SALAD: 1 CUP

Calories: 61, Fat: 3.3 g, Total carbohydrates: 6.0 g, Protein: 3.2 g, Dietary fiber:
1.8 g, Sodium: 180 mg, Net carbs: 4.2 g, Carb choice: free

———

▶ Seasoned Croutons

YIELD: 7½ CUPS

12 slices whole grain bread, cut
  into ½-inch cubes

1 Tbsp olive oil

1½ Tbsp onion powder

1½ Tbsp garlic powder

1½ tsp dried oregano

2 tsp dried sweet basil

1 Tbsp dried parsley

½ tsp salt

Preheat the oven to 225°F. Place the bread in a large bowl. Add the remaining ingredients and gently mix together well. Spread the cubes on a cookie sheet and bake for 40 minutes, or until completely dry, checking every 10 minutes.

_____

ANALYSIS FOR 1 SERVING: ½ CUP

Calories: 81, Fat: 2.1 g, Total carbohydrates: 11.5 g, Protein: 4.8 g, Dietary fiber: 1.8 g, Sodium: 157 mg, Net carbs: 9.7 g, Carb choice: ⅔

_____

▶ Caesar Salad Dressing

YIELD: 1 CUP

½ c *Low-Fat Tofu Mayonnaise* (recipe follows)

2 Tbsp canola oil

2 Tbsp lemon juice, freshly squeezed

2 whole garlic cloves

2 Tbsp nutritional yeast flakes

½ tsp salt

¼ tsp citric acid (can be purchased as a powder at most drugstores); or 1 crushed vitamin C tablet

Prepare the *Low-Fat Tofu Mayonnaise* and put ½ cup in a blender. Add the remaining ingredients and blend until creamy, about 1 minute. Chill in a covered container before serving.

———

ANALYSIS FOR 1 SERVING: 2 TABLESPOONS

Calories: 52, Fat: 4.4 g, Total carbohydrates: 1.9 g, Protein: 2.2 g, Dietary fiber: 0.6 g, Sodium: 195 mg, Net carbs: 1.3 g, Carb choice: free

———

▶ *Low-Fat Tofu Mayonnaise*

*You can use a prepared tofu mayonnaise, such as Vegenaise
or Nayonaise, or make your own with this simple recipe.*

YIELD: 2 CUPS

1 (12.3-oz) pkg extra-firm silken
  Mori-Nu Lite tofu

⅓ c water

½ tsp salt

1½ tsp onion powder

⅛ tsp garlic powder

2 Tbsp canola oil

1 Tbsp lemon juice, freshly
  squeezed

In a blender, blend all the ingredients together until creamy, 1 to 2
minutes. Store chilled in a covered container.

———

ANALYSIS FOR 1 SERVING: 2 TABLESPOONS

Calories: 24, Fat: 1.9 g, Total carbohydrates: 0.5 g, Protein: 1.4 g, Dietary fiber:
0.02, Sodium: 93 mg, Net carbs: 0.48 g, Carb choice: free

———

Monday

MEAL	PORTION SIZE	CARB CHOICES (number)
Breakfast		
Traditional Scrambled Tofu	1 c	½
Kickin' Western Chili	¾ c	1
Orange	1 medium	1
Ezekiel 4:9 Sprouted Grain Bread toast (bread can be found in frozen food section)	1 slice	1
Peanut butter, natural unsalted	1 Tbsp	free
Whole Ground Flaxseed	1–2 Tbsp	free
Lunch		
Grilled Portabello Mushroom	1 mushroom (3 oz)	free
Baked Sweet Potato	½ medium	⅔
Green beans	1 c	⅓
Saucy Red Kidney Beans	1 c	½
Strawberry Spinach Salad with **No-Oil Raspberry Dressing**	2 c 2 Tbsp	⅔ free
Dinner		
White Bean and Kale Soup	1 c	1
Salad of leafy greens and raw vegetables	2 c	free
Salad dressing	2 Tbsp	free
(We recommend *No-Oil Raspberry Dressing* or Newman's Own Lighten Up Raspberry & Walnut Dressing.)		
Apple	1 medium	1
Total Carb Choices		9

Traditional Scrambled Tofu

YIELD: 3 CUPS

1 (12-oz) pkg water-packed firm or extra-firm tofu

1½ tsp olive oil

½ c onions, chopped

2 Tbsp chives or scallions, sliced

2 tsp McKay's Chicken Style Seasoning, vegan

⅛ tsp turmeric powder (or less for lighter yellow color)

½ tsp salt

½ tsp onion powder

¼ tsp garlic powder

2 Tbsp nutritional yeast flakes

RINSE the tofu in a colander and drain. In a large skillet, sauté the onions and chives in the olive oil over medium-high heat until soft, about 3 to 4 minutes. Crumble the tofu into skillet with onions. Add the remaining ingredients to the tofu and stir together well. Cook over medium heat for 5 to 10 minutes, until heated through. The tofu will turn a golden yellow color.

Variation: You may add ¼ cup chopped bell peppers and ½ cup chopped fresh tomatoes to the dish; they will not significantly change the nutritional analysis.

———

ANALYSIS FOR 1 SERVING: ½ CUP

Calories: 82, Fat: 4.4 g, Total carbohydrates: 5.0 g, Protein: 7.7 g, Dietary fiber: 1.2 g, Sodium: 215 mg, Net carbs: 3.8 g, Carb choice: free

———

Kickin' Western Chili

YIELD: 18 CUPS

1 Tbsp olive oil

3 c yellow onions, chopped

½ c green bell pepper, chopped

6 garlic cloves, minced

¼ c chili powder

1 Tbsp ground cumin

¼ tsp oregano

1½ tsp sweet paprika

6 c Morningstar Farms Grillers Recipe Crumbles (one and a half 12-oz bags) or other meatless burger crumbles

3 c canned pinto beans, drained

3 c canned red kidney beans, drained

3 c canned black beans, drained

26 oz canned diced tomatoes

½ c tomato paste

¼ c canned mild green chilis, chopped

3 c water

Soy sour cream—optional

Fresh cilantro, chopped—optional

IN a large saucepan over low heat, warm the oil. Add the onions, bell peppers, and garlic. Sauté, stirring until the onions are soft. Add the seasonings, burger crumbles, canned products, and water. Bring to a boil, reduce heat, and simmer until the flavors are blended, 30 to 40 minutes. Serve in a bowl. Garnish with soy sour cream (if using) and cilantro (if using).

———

ANALYSIS FOR 1 SERVING: ½ CUP (WITHOUT THE SOY SOUR CREAM AND CILANTRO)

Calories: 97, Fat: 1.5 g, Total carbohydrates: 15.7 g, Protein: 6.4 g, Dietary fiber: 4.5 g, Sodium: 237 mg, Net carbs: 11.2 g, Carb choice: ⅔

———

Grilled Portobello Mushroom

YIELD: 4 SERVINGS

4 (3-oz) large Portobello
mushrooms

5½ Tbsp Italian vinaigrette
dressing, reduced calorie

4 Tbsp *Mustard Sauce* (recipe
follows—prepare before
grilling Portobellos)

CUT the stems off of the mushrooms and wash thoroughly. Place the mushrooms in the vinaigrette and let marinate, turning to ensure both sides are covered. Meanwhile, place oven rack 4 to 5 inches from broiler unit and preheat to medium-high.

When the broiler is heated, place the mushrooms on a baking sheet, gill side up. Broil until brown and softened, about 4 to 5 minutes. Turn the mushrooms over and brush marinade onto each one. Broil until brown and tender, 4 to 5 minutes more. Serve hot, topping each mushroom with 1 tablespoon of *Mustard Sauce*.

———

ANALYSIS FOR 1 SERVING: 1 GRILLED MUSHROOM (WITHOUT SAUCE)

Calories: 50, Fat: 3.0g, Total carbohydrates: 4.7 g, Protein: 2.6 g, Dietary fiber:
1 g, Sodium: 142 mg, Net carbs: 3.7 g, Carb choice: free

———

▶ Mustard Sauce

YIELD: ¾ CUP

2 Tbsp minced shallot or green onions

½ tsp olive oil

2 Tbsp prepared mustard

½ c Nayonaise

¼ c water

1 tsp cornstarch

In a small pan, sauté the onions in the oil over medium-high heat until tender. In a small bowl, whisk the remaining ingredients together, and add to the onions. Cook on medium heat 12 to 15 minutes, until thick.

———

ANALYSIS FOR 1 SERVING: 1 TABLESPOON

Calories: 29, Fat: 2.6 g, Total carbohydrates: 1.3 g, Protein: 0.4 g, Dietary fiber: 0.2 g, Sodium: 105 mg, Net carbs: 1.1 g, Carb choice: free

———

Baked Sweet Potato

YIELD: 2 SERVINGS

Vegetable cooking spray
1 medium (2-by-5-inch) sweet potato

PREHEAT the oven to 350°F. Spray a baking sheet with cooking spray. Peel the potato and cut it into 4 pieces. Place the pieces on the baking sheet. Spray the potato pieces with cooking spray for about 3 seconds. Bake for 30 to 35 minutes, or until tender.

———

ANALYSIS FOR 1 SERVING: ½ OF POTATO

Calories: 65, Fat: 0.8 g, Total carbohydrates: 13.8 g, Protein: 1.0 g, Dietary fiber: 1.7 g, Sodium: 6 mg, Net carbs: 12.1 g, Carb choice: ⅔

———

Saucy Red Kidney Beans

YIELD: 4½ CUPS

⅓ c onions, chopped

⅓ c green bell pepper, chopped

¼ tsp garlic powder

2 tsp olive oil

3½ c canned kidney beans,
drained

1 c water

⅔ c tomatoes, diced

⅛ tsp ground oregano

½ tsp dried sweet basil

⅛ tsp salt

IN a medium saucepan, sauté the onion, bell pepper, and garlic powder in the oil until tender, 4 to 5 minutes. Add the remaining ingredients and simmer until heated through, about 10 minutes.

———

ANALYSIS FOR 1 SERVING: ½ CUP

Calories: 99, Fat: 1.4 g, Total carbohydrates: 16.5 g, Protein: 5.9 g, Dietary fiber: 4.6 g, Sodium: 191 mg, Net carbs: 12.1 g, Carb choice: 1

———

Strawberry Spinach Salad
with No-Oil Raspberry Dressing

YIELD: 9½ CUPS

15 *Roasted Garlic Cloves* (recipe follows)

¼ c *Toasted Pecans* (recipe follows)

⅓ c *No-Oil Raspberry Dressing* (recipe follows)

12½ c raw packed baby leaf spinach

½ c red onion, slivered

1½ c strawberries, sliced (or sliced pears, with skins on)

PREPARE the *Roasted Garlic Cloves*. Prepare the *Toasted Pecans*. Prepare the *No-Oil Raspberry Dressing*. Mix all ingredients together and serve immediately.

___

ANALYSIS FOR 1 SERVING: 1 CUP

Calories: 91, Fat: 6.8 g, Total carbohydrates: 7.4 g, Protein: 2.4 g, Dietary fiber: 2.7 g, Sodium: 120 mg, Net carbs: 4.7 g, Carb choice: ⅓

___

▶ Roasted Garlic Cloves

Garlic cloves
Cooking spray
Salt, to taste

Preheat oven to 300° F. Prepare roasted garlic cloves by spraying garlic for 3 seconds with vegetable cooking spray and place in an aluminum foil pouch. Bake in preheated oven for 10 to 12 minutes.

▶ Toasted Pecans

1 c chopped pecans

Preheat oven to 275° F. Spread pecans on unsprayed baking sheet and toast in preheated oven for 10 minutes. No need to turn. Immediately remove from baking sheet and store in covered container.

▶ *No-Oil Raspberry Dressing*

YIELD: 3 CUPS

3 (0.7-oz) pkg dry Good Seasons Italian dressing mix

½ c plus 1 Tbsp lemon juice, freshly squeezed

2 c water

6 Tbsp white grape raspberry juice frozen concentrate

⅓ c Resource (Novartis) Thicken Up, or other instant food thickener

Blend all ingredients in a blender on high setting until smooth, about 20 seconds. Chill in a covered container until ready to serve.

Note: For a low-fat, lower-sodium dressing, use Newman's Own Lighten Up Raspberry & Walnut Dressing.

———

ANALYSIS FOR 1 SERVING: 2 TABLESPOONS
Calories: 21, Fat: 0.0 g, Total carbohydrates: 5.2 g, Protein: 0.1 g, Dietary fiber: 0.1 g, Sodium: 314 mg, Net carbs: 5.1 g, Carb choice: ⅓

———

White Bean and Kale Soup

YIELD: 10 CUPS

1 c onion, diced

1 garlic clove, minced

1 Tbsp extra-virgin olive oil

6 c water

2 c carrots, cut into ¼-inch slices

¾ c celery, cut into ¼-inch slices

2 c fresh kale, chopped

⅛ tsp garlic powder

1 Tbsp seasoned salt

⅛ tsp dried thyme

2 bay leaves

½ tsp dried rosemary

2 c canned tomatoes, diced

2 Tbsp chopped fresh parsley

2 c canned low-sodium small white beans, drained and rinsed

SAUTÉ onion and garlic in the oil until golden brown and tender, 3 to 4 minutes. Add the water, carrots, celery, kale, and seasonings. Cook until the vegetables are tender, about 15 minutes. Add the tomatoes, parsley, and beans. Simmer for 10 minutes. Remove the bay leaves before serving.

———

ANALYSIS FOR 1 SERVING: 1 CUP

Calories: 96, Fat: 1.7 g, Total carbohydrates: 16.6 g, Protein: 5.0 g, Dietary fiber: 4.3 g, Sodium: 504 mg, Net carbs: 12.3 g, Carb choice: 1

———

Tuesday

MEAL	PORTION SIZE	CARB CHOICES (number)
Breakfast		
Oat Bran Cereal	1 c	1
(with optional Smart Balance Light Buttery Spread and sprinkle of cinnamon added to the top)	1 tsp	free
Breakfast Beans	1 c	2
Almonds	½ oz (11 nuts)	free
Whole Ground Flaxseed	1–2 Tbsp	free
Blackberries	1 c	⅔
Lunch		
Tofu Egg Salad	½ c	⅓
served in Ezekiel 4:9 pita pocket with green leaf lettuce, slice of tomato, slice of red onion in each half pocket	2 half pockets	1
Raw vegetables (broccoli, cauliflower, cucumber, grape tomatoes)	1 c	free
Classic Hummus, for dipping	¼ c	⅔
Oatmeal Cranberry Cookie	1 cookie	1
Dinner		
Roasted Red Pepper Bisque	1 c	1
Salad of leafy greens and raw vegetables	2 c	free
Salad dressing	2 Tbsp	free
Ryvita Dark Rye Crackers	3	1½
Total Carb Choices		9

Oat Bran Cereal

YIELD: 3 CUPS

3 c water   1 c dry oat bran
¼ tsp salt

IN a medium saucepan, bring the water and salt to a boil. Add the oat
bran and stir briefly. Cover, reduce heat, and simmer about 30 minutes,
until thickened.

———

ANALYSIS FOR 1 SERVING: 1 CUP
Calories: 77, Fat: 2.2 g, Total carbohydrates: 20.8 g, Protein: 5.4 g, Dietary fiber:
4.8 g, Sodium: 199 mg, Net carbs: 16 g, Carb choice: 1

———

Tofu Egg Salad

YIELD: 2 CUPS

1½ c *Traditional Scrambled Tofu* (p. 130), may use leftover

¼ c plus 1 Tbsp Nayonaise

1 tsp prepared mustard

1 Tbsp plus 1 tsp Mt. Olive No Sugar Added Sweet Relish or ½ cup chopped celery

COMBINE all the ingredients in a small bowl and mix well. Serve ¼ cup in a ½ pocket of pita bread or use as a sandwich spread.

———

ANALYSIS FOR 1 SERVING: ¼ CUP, MADE WITH RELISH (WITHOUT THE BREAD)
Calories: 61, Fat: 4.4 g, Total carbohydrates: 3.0 g, Protein: 3.6 g, Dietary fiber: 0.6 g, Sodium: 196 mg, Net carbs: 2.4 g, Carb choice: free

ANALYSIS FOR ONE SERVING ¼ CUP, MADE WITH CELERY (WITHOUT THE BREAD):
Calories: 55, Fat: 3.9 g, Total carbohydrates: 2.8 g, Protein: 3.2 g, Dietary fiber: 0.7 g, Sodium: 166 mg, Net carbs: 2.1 g, Carb choice: free

———

Classic Hummus

YIELD: 2½ CUPS

2½ c fresh cooked or canned low-sodium garbanzo beans, drained

½ c tahini (sesame seed butter)

6 Tbsp lemon juice, freshly squeezed

4 garlic cloves

1 tsp salt (see note)

1½ tsp onion powder

4 oz canned green chilis, chopped—optional

COMBINE all the ingredients, except the chilis, in a blender and blend on high speed for 1 to 2 minutes until smooth and creamy. Pour into a bowl and stir in the chilis. Chill before serving. Spread on bread, crackers, pita pockets, or serve as a dip for chips and raw vegetables.

Note: Use half the salt if using canned beans.

———

ANALYSIS FOR 1 SERVING: ¼ CUP

Calories: 146, Fat: 7.6 g, Total carbohydrates: 15.6 g, Protein: 5.9 g, Dietary fiber: 5.4 g, Sodium: 182 mg, Net carbs: 11.1 g, Carb choice: ⅔

———

Oatmeal Cranberry Cookies

YIELD: 14 COOKIES

Vegetable cooking spray

½ c garbanzo bean flour

¼ c whole wheat pastry flour

1½ c old-fashioned rolled oats

¼ tsp salt

¼ tsp ground cinnamon

¼ c dried cranberries

⅔ c Smart Balance Light Buttery Spread, room temperature

⅔ c fructose

1½ tsp Ener-G Egg Replacer

3 Tbsp soy milk

1 tsp vanilla extract

PREHEAT the oven to 375°F and spray a cookie sheet with cooking spray. In a small bowl, stir together the flours, oats, salt, cinnamon, and cranberries; set aside. In a medium bowl, cream together the spread and fructose. In a small bowl use a fork to stir together the egg substitute and soy milk until fluffy. Add to the fructose mixture along with the vanilla. Add the dry ingredients to the creamed mixture and stir well. To make a cookie, pack the mixture into a 2-tablespoon measuring scoop. Place on the cookie sheet and flatten.

Bake 15 to 20 minutes, or until slightly brown.

ANALYSIS FOR 1 SERVING: 1 COOKIE

Calories: 135, Fat: 4.8 g, Total carbohydrates: 20.8 g, Protein: 2.6 g, Dietary fiber: 1.7 g, Sodium: 111 mg, Net carbs: 19.1 g, Carb choice: 1

Roasted Red Pepper Bisque

YIELD: 7½ CUPS

2½ c water

1 tsp McKay's Beef Style
Seasoning, vegan

1 tsp McKay's Chicken Style
Seasoning, vegan

1 c red potatoes, peeled and
diced

1 c onion, diced

½ c celery, chopped

2½ c fire-roasted red peppers
(or pimientos), canned or
jarred

2 Tbsp cornstarch

2 c soy milk

¼ tsp dried marjoram

1½ Tbsp low-sodium soy sauce

¾ tsp salt

Pinch (¹⁄₁₆ tsp) cayenne pepper

IN a large saucepan, bring the water, beef-style seasoning, and chicken-style seasoning to a boil. Add the potatoes, onion, and celery and simmer for 15 minutes. Add the red peppers and cook for an additional 15 minutes. Place the mixture in the bowl of a food processor and add the cornstarch. Pulse until smooth. Return the mixture to the saucepan. Add the remaining ingredients, and simmer until the soup thickens. Serve immediately.

―――――

ANALYSIS FOR 1 SERVING: 1 CUP

Calories: 89, Fat: 1.4 g, Total carbohydrates: 16.6 g, Protein: 3.9 g, Dietary fiber:
2.9 g, Sodium: 506 mg, Net carbs: 13.7 g, Carb choice: 1

―――――

Wednesday

MEAL	PORTION SIZE	CARB CHOICES (number)
Breakfast		
Baked Apple Oats	1 serving	1
Kickin' Western Chili	1 c	1⅓
Ezekiel 4:9 toast	1 slice	1
Almond butter	1 Tbsp	free
Milk, unsweetened soy or almond	½ c	free
Whole Ground Flaxseed	1–2 Tbsp	free
Lunch		
Lemon Basil Kabobs	2	1
Wild Rice (see package instructions)	⅓ c	1
Steamed fresh broccoli	1 c	free
Tossed garden salad	2 c	free
Salad dressing	2 T	free
Tortilla chips	1 oz (16 chips)	1
served with **Classic Hummus**	1/4 c	⅔
Dinner		
Mediterranean Barley and Lentil Soup	1 c	1
Salad of leafy greens and raw vegetables	2 c	free
Salad dressing	2 Tbsp	free
Total Carb Choices		9

Baked Apple Oats

YIELD: 16 SERVINGS

1½ c apple, chopped

3 c old-fashioned rolled oats

5 c unsweetened soy milk

1 tsp vanilla extract

¾ tsp salt

2 Tbsp unsweetened shredded coconut

½ c walnuts, chopped

½ tsp cinnamon

PREHEAT the oven to 350°F. Spread the apples in the bottom of 9-by-13-inch baking dish. Distribute oats evenly over the apples. In a bowl, quickly blend the soy milk, vanilla, and salt, and pour slowly over the apples and oats. Sprinkle the coconut, walnuts, and cinnamon on top. Bake for 45 minutes, or until golden brown.

ANALYSIS FOR 1 SERVING: $\frac{1}{16}$ OF THE RECIPE

Calories: 136, Fat: 5.1 g, Total carbohydrates: 18.0 g, Protein: 5.7 g, Dietary fiber: 3.1 g, Sodium: 192 mg, Net carbs: 14.9 g, Carb choice: 1

Lemon Basil Kabobs

YIELD: 16 SERVINGS

Kabob Marinade (recipe follows)

2 large carrots, cut into 1-inch wedges

1 large onion, cut into 2-inch dice

1 large green bell pepper, cut into 1-inch dice

12 medium button mushrooms

1 large red pepper, cut into 1-inch dice

3 Roma tomatoes, quartered and seeded

1 large zucchini, cut into 1¼-inch slices

1 large yam, peeled and cut into 1-inch dice

1 (12-oz) pkg water-packed extra-firm tofu, cut into 1-inch cubes

16 skewers

PREPARE the *Kabob Marinade.* Assemble the kabobs by placing one piece of each item listed on a metal or wooden barbecue skewer, and place in a baking dish. Pour the marinade over, cover, and let marinate overnight in the refrigerator. When ready to cook, preheat the oven to 400°F. Place the kabobs on a baking sheet and bake for 12 to 15 minutes, until vegetables are just cooked through. No need to turn while baking. Kabobs can also be grilled instead of baked. Serve immediately.

ANALYSIS FOR 1 SERVING: 2 KABOBS

Calories: 202, Fat: 9.0 g, Total carbohydrates: 24.6 g, Protein: 10.4 g, Dietary fiber: 5.8 g, Sodium: 239 mg, Net carbs: 18.8 g, Carb choice: 1

▶ *Kabob Marinade*

YIELD: 4½ CUPS

3 c onion, coarsely chopped

½ c Bragg Liquid Aminos (can be purchased at health-food stores or well-stocked grocery stores)

1 c lemon juice, freshly squeezed

1 Tbsp dried basil

¾ c canola oil

1 tsp salt

Place the onion in a blender container and blend until liquefied. Add the remaining ingredients and blend until creamy.

───────

ANALYSIS FOR 1 SERVING: 1 TABLESPOON

Calories: 25, Fat: 2.4 g, Total carbohydrates: 0.8 g, Protein: 0.3 g, Dietary fiber: 0.2 g, Sodium: 107 mg, Net carbs: 0.6 g, Carb choice: free

───────

Mediterranean Barley and Lentil Soup

YIELD: 6 CUPS

1 c water

½ c dry French lentils, cleaned and rinsed

2 Tbsp pearl barley

2 tsp olive oil

¾ c onion, chopped

3 large garlic cloves, minced

2 tsp ground cumin

½ tsp ground coriander

¹⁄₁₆ tsp ground cayenne pepper

¼ tsp salt

½ tsp onion salt

1 cinnamon stick

1 c plus 2 Tbsp can low-sodium diced tomatoes

5 c water

1 Tbsp plus 2 tsp McKay's Chicken Style Seasoning, vegan

IN a large soup pot, combine 1 cup water, lentils, and barley. Bring to a boil uncovered and cook for 20 minutes. The water should be nearly gone. While the lentils and barley are cooking, in a medium skillet heat the olive oil, add the onion and garlic and sauté 10 minutes. When lentils and barley are done cooking, add sautéed onion and garlic to the soup pot along with the remaining ingredients. Bring to a boil again, reduce the heat, partially cover, and simmer for 40 minutes. Remove the cinnamon stick and serve hot.

———

ANALYSIS FOR 1 SERVING: 1 CUP

Calories: 116, Fat: 2.1 g, Total carbohydrates: 20.1 g, Protein: 5.5 g, Dietary fiber: 5.4 g, Sodium: 265 mg, Net carbs: 14.7 g, Carb choice: 1

———

Thursday

MEAL	PORTION SIZE	CARB CHOICES (number)
Breakfast		
Groats and Oats	1 c	2
Breakfast Beans	½ c	1
Fresh strawberries	1 c	½
Pecans	½ oz (10 halves)	free
Milk, unsweetened soy or almond	½ c	free
Whole Ground Flaxseed	1–2 Tbsp	free
Lunch		
Quick and Easy Eggplant with **Chunky Marinara Sauce**	1 serving	1
Asparagus spears	1 c	⅓
Saucy Red Kidney Beans	1 c	2
Caesar Salad	2 c	½
Raspberry Swirl Cheesecake	¹⁄₁₆ pie	1
Dinner		
Indian Lentil Soup	2 c	2
Salad of leafy greens and raw vegetables	2 c	free
Salad dressing	2 Tbsp	free
Total Carb Choices		10⅓

Groats and Oats

YIELD: 2⅔ CUPS

2½ c water   ½ c dry steel-cut oats

½ c dry buckwheat groats   ¼ tsp salt

IN a medium saucepan, combine all the ingredients. Bring to a boil, then immediately reduce the heat to low. Partially cover, until the boiling subsides to a simmer. Simmer, covered, about 20 minutes, until the water is absorbed.

———

ANALYSIS FOR 1 SERVING: ½ CUP

Calories: 113, Fat: 1.4 g, Total carbohydrates: 22.0 g, Protein: 4.3 g, Dietary fiber: 3.2 g, Sodium: 114 mg, Net carbs: 19.9 g, Carb choice: 1

———

Quick and Easy Eggplant

YIELD: 9 SERVINGS

2 c *Eggplant Breading Mix*
(recipe follows)

Vegetable cooking spray

1 large eggplant

½ c Nayonaise

2¼ c *Chunky Marinara Sauce*
(recipe follows), or Classico
Roasted Garlic spaghetti
sauce

PREPARE the *Eggplant Breading Mix*. Preheat the oven to 350°F and spray a baking sheet with cooking spray. Peel the eggplant and slice it into ½-inch-thick crosswise slices. Lightly coat both sides of each eggplant slice with Nayonaise and dip the slice into the breading. Place the breaded slices on the baking sheet and bake for 10 minutes, turn the slices over and bake another 10 minutes to brown evenly. Meanwhile, heat the *Chunky Marinara Sauce* or Classico spaghetti sauce in a saucepan. To serve, make eggplant stacks by stacking 2 slices on a plate and topping with ¼ cup of the sauce.

———

ANALYSIS FOR 1 SERVING: 2 SLICES WITH ¼ CUP CHUNKY MARINARA SAUCE
Calories: 122, Fat: 4.4 g, Total carbohydrates: 19.5 g, Protein: 3.4 g, Dietary fiber:
3.8 g, Sodium: 324 mg, Net carbs: 15.7 g, Carb choice: 1

ANALYSIS FOR 1 SERVING: 2 SLICES
WITH ¼ CUP CLASSICO SPAGHETTI SAUCE
Calories: 161, Fat: 5.8 g, Total carbohydrates: 26.7 g, Protein: 3.5 g, Dietary fiber:
3.9 g, Sodium: 453 mg, Net carbs: 22.8 g, Carb choice: 1½

———

▶ Eggplant Breading Mix

YIELD: 2 CUPS

5 slices Ezekiel 4:9 bread

½ tsp sweet paprika

½ tsp onion powder

¼ tsp garlic powder

1 tsp Italian seasoning

Break 2 slices of bread into 4 pieces each and put into a blender. Blend until bread crumbs are formed and transfer to a medium bowl. Repeat with the remaining bread. Add the remaining ingredients and stir well.

Note: We use Ezekiel 4:9 bread because it is flourless and contains beans, making it more diabetic friendly. Flour-based products tend to have a higher GI. You may use any whole grain bread.

——

ANALYSIS FOR 1 SERVING: 2 CUPS
Calories: 45, Fat: 0.3 g, Total carbohydrates: 9.3, Protein: 1.8 g, Dietary fiber: 1.1 g, Sodium: 41 mg, Net carbs: 8.2 g, Carb choice: ½

——

▶ *Chunky Marinara Sauce*

YIELD: 4 CUPS

1 c onion, chopped

1 or 2 cloves garlic, minced

1½ tsp extra-virgin olive oil

3 c diced canned tomatoes, with liquid

½ c Hunt's Tomato Sauce, No Salt Added

1 tsp dried basil

½ tsp dried oregano leaves

½ tsp dried thyme

½ tsp salt

1 Tbsp lemon juice, freshly squeezed

In a saucepan, sauté onion and garlic in oil until tender, 3 to 4 minutes. Add the rest of the ingredients and bring to a boil. Reduce heat and simmer 10 minutes.

——

ANALYSIS FOR 1 SERVING: ½ CUP MADE WITH 2 CLOVES GARLIC
Calories: 39, Fat: 1.0 g, Total carbohydrates: 7.3, Protein: 1.3 g, Dietary fiber: 1.6 g, Sodium: 286 g, Net carbs: 5.7 g, Carb choice: ⅓

——

Raspberry Swirl Cheesecake

YIELD: 16 SERVINGS

¼ c fresh or frozen raspberries

1 plus ⅓ (12.3-oz) pkgs extra-firm silken Mori-Nu Lite tofu

½ c Tofutti cream cheese, nonhydrogenated (yellow container)

½ c fructose

2 Tbsp cornstarch

3 Tbsp lemon juice, freshly squeezed—optional

½ tsp vanilla extract

1 (9-inch) Arrowhead Mills graham cracker crust

PREHEAT the oven to 350°F. Place the raspberries into a blender container and blend to form a puree. Strain puree to remove seeds and set aside. In a blender on high speed, blend the tofu, cream cheese, fructose, cornstarch, lemon juice (if using), and vanilla until creamy. Put half of the mixture into the crust and smooth with a rubber spatula. Place half the raspberry puree in dollops on top of filling. Swirl the puree into the filling with a toothpick or fork. Top with the remaining cheese mixture, smooth, and top with the remaining raspberry puree, swirling it into the filling as before. Bake 40 minutes or until golden brown.

──────

ANALYSIS FOR 1 SERVING: ¹⁄₁₆ OF THE PIE

Calories: 118, Fat: 4.6 g, Total carbohydrates: 17.2 g, Protein: 2.6 g, Dietary fiber: 0.9 g, Sodium: 90 mg, Net carbs: 16.3 g, Carb choice: 1

──────

Indian Lentil Soup

YIELD: 8 CUPS

1 c dry red lentils

5 c water

1 garlic clove, crushed

1 Tbsp olive oil

1 c onion, chopped

½ c celery, thinly sliced

1 c carrots, finely diced

1½ c canned chunky tomatoes

1½ Tbsp tomato paste

1 bay leaf

⅛ tsp chili powder

1½ tsp salt

½ c fresh parsley, chopped

COMBINE the lentils, water, garlic, oil, onion, celery, and carrots in a soup pot and bring to a boil; reduce the heat, cover, and let simmer for about 2 hours. Add the tomatoes, tomato paste, bay leaf, chili powder, and salt and let it simmer a few more minutes. Just before serving, add the parsley and remove the bay leaf.

———

ANALYSIS FOR 1 SERVING: 1 CUP

Calories: 120, Fat: 2.1 g, Total carbohydrates: 19.9 g, Protein: 7.1 g, Dietary fiber: 6.9 g, Sodium: 550 mg, Net carbs: 13 g, Carb choice: 1

———

Friday

MEAL	PORTION SIZE	CARB CHOICES (number)
Breakfast		
Golden Soy Oat Waffle	1 waffle	1⅓
topped with **Very Berry Topping**	⅓ c	½
and toasted almond slivers	1 Tbsp	free
Breakfast Beans	½ c	1
Whole Ground Flaxseed	1–2 Tbsp	free
Lunch		
Veggie burger (Boca, Gardenburger, or other)	1 patty	2½
on Ezekiel 4:9 whole grain burger bun with green leaf lettuce, slice of tomato, slice of Vidalia onion, mustard, low-carb ketchup	1 bun with fixins	2
Sweet Potato Fries		
Black beans (Use **Breakfast Beans** recipe)	½ c	1
Celery sticks	½ c	free
with peanut butter	1 Tbsp	free
Dinner		
Our Favorite Split-Pea Soup	2 c	2
Salad of leafy greens and raw vegetables	2 c	free
Salad dressing	2 Tbsp	free
Total Carb Choices		10⅓

Golden Soy Oat Waffles

YIELD: 4 (6-INCH) WAFFLES

1 c soaked soybeans (see note)

1⅔ c water

1 Tbsp floral honey

2 tsp canola oil

1 tsp vanilla or maple flavoring

½ tsp salt

1⅓ c old-fashioned rolled oats

PLACE all the ingredients in a blender and blend on high until smooth, 1 to 2 minutes. Pour the batter into a bowl. Preheat the waffle iron to medium-high. (The batter will thicken as it sits and will be the right consistency by the time the waffle iron is hot. You will not need to thin the batter.) Use ¾ cup of batter per waffle, and bake 4 to 5 minutes.

———

ANALYSIS FOR 1 SERVING: ½ OF A 6-INCH WAFFLE
Calories: 109, Fat: 3.9 g, Total carbohydrates: 13.4 g, Protein: 5.7 g, Dietary fiber: 2.7 g, Sodium: 149 mg, Net carbs: 10.7 g, Carb choice: ⅔

———

Note: To soak soybeans: Rinse the dry soybeans in a colander. Place the beans in a covered container in a generous amount of water and refrigerate. Soak the beans overnight, about 9 hours. (Assume ½ cup dry beans of any kind results in at least 1 cup soaked beans.) When ready to use, drain the beans in a colander and measure the amount needed. Put any remaining beans in water in a covered container and keep refrigerated. Soaked soybeans keep in the refrigerator for about 10 days. Change the water once during the week.

▶ Very Berry Topping

The brilliant colors of berries make this sauce as beautiful as it is delicious.
It's the perfect low-glycemic topping for waffles, pancakes, and desserts.

YIELD: 2 CUPS

1 c fresh sliced or frozen
    unsweetened strawberries,
    separated

½ c fresh or frozen
    unsweetened blueberries

½ c fresh or frozen
    unsweetened blackberries

½ c fresh or frozen
    unsweetened sweet cherries

2 tsp floral honey

Thaw berries if frozen. In a blender on high setting, blend ½ cup of strawberries until creamy, about 1 minute. Pour into a bowl, add remaining ingredients, and stir together. Serve over waffles as is or slightly warm in a saucepan or microwave before serving.

ANALYSIS FOR 1 SERVING: ⅓ CUP

Calories: 44, Fat: 0.4 g, Total carbohydrates: 10.8 g, Protein: 0.6 g, Dietary fiber: 2.3 g, Sodium: 2 mg, Net carbs: 8.5 g, Carb choice: ½

Sweet Potato Fries

YIELD: 3 CUPS

Vegetable cooking spray

3 c peeled sweet potatoes,
    sliced into ½-inch-thick
    French fries

¼ tsp salt

PREHEAT the oven to 350°F. Spray a baking sheet with cooking spray. Lightly spray the potatoes with cooking spray. Bake for 30 to 35 minutes, or until tender, turning the potatoes over halfway through baking.

ANALYSIS FOR 1 SERVING: ½ CUP

Calories: 92, Fat: 0.2 g, Total carbohydrates: 21.4 g, Protein: 1.5 g, Dietary fiber: 2.6 g, Sodium: 107 mg, Net carbs: 18.8 g, Carb choice: 1

Our Favorite Split-Pea Soup

YIELD: 10 CUPS

2 c dry green split peas

8 c water

1 c celery, cut into ¼-inch dice

1 c carrots, cut into ¼-inch dice

½ c onions, cut into ¼-inch dice

2 Tbsp McKay's Chicken Style Seasoning, vegan

¼ c dried onion flakes

2 tsp extra-virgin olive oil

1 tsp salt

¼ c nutritional yeast flakes

COOK the split peas in 8 cups of water until almost tender, about 30 minutes. Cover while cooking to avoid water loss. Add the remaining ingredients and simmer until tender, about 1 hour.

———

ANALYSIS FOR 1 SERVING: 1 CUP

Calories: 158, Fat: 1.4 g, Total carbohydrates: 27.5 g, Protein: 10.9 g, Dietary fiber: 9.9 g, Sodium: 274 mg, Net carbs: 17.6 g, Carb choice: 1

———

Saturday

MEAL	PORTION SIZE	CARB CHOICES (number)
Breakfast		
7-Grain Cereal Plus	1 c	1⅓
Strawberries	1 c	½
Toasted chopped walnuts	½ oz (7 halves)	free
Breakfast Beans	½ c	1
Milk, unsweetened soy or almond	½ c	free
Whole Ground Flaxseed	1–2 Tbsp	free
Lunch		
Baked Falafels	2 balls	1
with **Garlic Tahini Sauce**	2 Tbsp	free
served in Ezekiel 4:9 pita pocket	1 half pocket	½
with shredded lettuce and chopped tomato	2–4 Tbsp	free
Smoky Lentils with Caramelized Onions	½ c	1
Brilliant Kale with Red Peppers & Onions	1 c	1
Tossed garden salad	2 c	free
Salad dressing	2 Tbsp	free
Dinner		
Summer Vegetable Soup	2 c	1⅓
Ezekiel 4:9 toast	1 slice	1
Smart Balance Light Buttery Spread	1 tsp	free
Salad of leafy greens and raw vegetables	2 c	free
Salad dressing	2 Tbsp	free
Peach	1 medium	½
Total Carb Choices		9

7-Grain Cereal Plus

YIELD: 3¼ CUPS

3 c water

½ tsp salt

1 c dry Arrowhead Mills Seven Grain Hot Cereal

3 Tbsp whole flaxseed

IN a medium saucepan, bring the water and salt to a boil. Add the cereal and flaxseed and stir briefly. Reduce the heat, cover, and cook until thick, 12 to 15 minutes.

———

ANALYSIS FOR 1 SERVING: ½ CUP

Calories: 91, Fat: 2.5 g, Total carbohydrates: 14.7 g, Protein: 4.0 g, Dietary fiber: 4.2 g, Sodium: 185 mg, Net carbs: 10.5 g, Carb choice: ⅔

———

Baked Falafels

YIELD: 11 SERVINGS

Vegetable cooking spray

4 c canned chickpeas (garbanzos), drained

2 c water-packed extra-firm tofu

3 garlic cloves, minced

½ c onion, finely chopped

2 Tbsp fresh parsley, chopped

2 Tbsp fresh cilantro, chopped

⅓ c Bragg's Liquid Aminos, or low-sodium soy sauce

2 tsp ground cumin

½ tsp ground coriander

1 slice Ezekiel 4:9 sprouted grain bread

Ezekiel 4:9 Prophet's Pocket Bread, or other whole grain pita bread

Garlic Tahini Sauce (recipe follows)

PREHEAT the oven to 350°F and spray a cookie sheet with cooking spray. Place the chickpeas in a food processor and pulse to mash, or mash by hand. Transfer the beans to a large mixing bowl. Rinse the tofu in a colander, drain, and mash; add to the chickpeas. Add the garlic, onion, parsley, and cilantro to the chickpeas along with the liquid aminos (or soy sauce) and seasonings. Mix together well. Break the bread into 4 pieces, place in a blender, and blend to make crumbs. Transfer to a small bowl.

To make falafels, form balls using 2 tablespoons of the chickpea mixture for each one. Roll each ball in the bread crumbs and place on the cookie sheet. Bake 25 to 30 minutes, until golden brown and firm. Meanwhile, make the Garlic Tahini Sauce.

Serving suggestion: Put one serving of Baked Falafels (2 balls) into half of an Ezekiel 4:9 pita pocket, and top with 1 tablespoon Garlic Tahini Sauce, fresh chopped lettuce, and tomatoes.

———

ANALYSIS FOR 1 SERVING: 2 BALLS WITH LOW-SODIUM SOY SAUCE
Calories: 154, Fat: 4.3 g, Total carbohydrates: 20.4 g, Protein: 10.5 g, Dietary fiber: 5.1 g, Sodium: 354 mg, Net carbs: 15.3 g, Carb choice: 1

ANALYSIS FOR 1 SERVING: 2 BALLS WITH BRAGG LIQUID AMINOS
Calories: 154, Fat: 4.7 g, Total carbohydrates: 20.3 g, Protein: 10.9 g, Dietary fiber: 5.4 g, Sodium: 418 mg, Net carbs: 14.9 g, Carb choice: 1

▶ *Garlic Tahini Sauce*

YIELD: ¾ CUPS

3 garlic cloves, minced

½ c tahini (sesame seed butter)

¼ c lemon juice, freshly squeezed

2 Tbsp light soy sauce

In a small bowl, combine all the ingredients and stir together well.
Keep refrigerated in a covered container.

Smoky Lentils with Caramelized Onions

YIELD: 6 CUPS

2 c dry brown lentils

4 c water

1 c yellow onion, chopped

1 Tbsp McKay's Beef Style
Seasoning, vegan

½ tsp liquid smoke

½ tsp salt

2 c onions, sliced

1½ tsp canola oil

COOK the lentils in water, in a medium pot with tilted lid on medium heat until tender, about 30 minutes. No need to stir. Add the chopped onions and seasonings and continue cooking. While lentils are cooking, prepare the caramelized onions by sautéing the sliced onions in the canola oil, about 8 minutes, until dark brown with a syrupy juice. When the lentils are done, top with the caramelized onions.

———

ANALYSIS FOR 1 SERVING: ½ CUP

Calories: 130, Fat: 1.0 g, Total carbohydrates: 22.8 g, Protein: 8.7 g, Dietary fiber: 7.7 g, Sodium: 149 mg, Net carbs: 15.1 g, Carb choice: 1

———

Brilliant Kale
with Red Peppers and Onions

YIELD: 2 CUPS

8 c fresh kale

5 c water

1 tsp garlic, crushed

½ c onion, sliced into half
moons

¼ c red bell pepper, sliced

1 tsp McKay's Chicken Style
Seasoning, vegan

1½ tsp nutritional yeast flakes

½ tsp olive oil

WASH the kale well. If leaves are small, do not chop. If leaves are larger, remove the coarsest part of stem and stack 6 to 8 leaves on top of one another. Cut crosswise into 1-inch strips. Bring kale and water to a boil until the kale turns bright green and shrinks. Drain and set aside. In a saucepan, briefly sauté the garlic, onion, bell pepper, seasoning, and yeast flakes in the olive oil over medium heat until clear, 4 to 5 minutes. Add the kale and raise the heat to medium-high. Sauté another 5 to 10 minutes.

Variation: Try this with other greens, such as collard, turnip, or beet greens in place of kale.

———

ANALYSIS FOR 1 SERVING: 1 CUP

Calories: 127, Fat: 2.7 g, Total carbohydrates: 21.2 g, Protein: 10.3 g, Dietary fiber:
7.2 g, Sodium: 65 mg, Net carbs: 14 g, Carb choice: 1

———

Summer Vegetable Soup

YIELD: 12 CUPS

6 c water

2 c red potatoes, cubed

1½ c zucchini, sliced

1½ c yellow squash, sliced

1 c fresh tomatoes, chopped

1 c celery, sliced

2 c carrots, sliced

1 c onion, chopped

½ c frozen green beans

½ c fresh spinach

1 bay leaf

¾ tsp garlic powder

1½ tsp ground savory

½ tsp dried thyme

1 Tbsp nutritional yeast flakes

½ tsp salt

½ c frozen peas

2 Tbsp fresh parsley, chopped

IN a large pot, place all ingredients, except the peas and parsley, and bring to a boil. Reduce the heat, cover, and simmer until the vegetables are tender. When the soup is ready, add the peas and parsley. Cook several more minutes.

———

ANALYSIS FOR 1 SERVING: 1 CUP

Calories: 55, Fat: 0.3 g, Total carbohydrates: 12.1 g, Protein: 2.2 g, Dietary fiber: 2.9 g, Sodium: 133 mg, Net carbs: 9.2 g, Carb choice: ⅔

———

8

Physical Activity Is Medicine!

THIS CHAPTER INTRODUCES you to Lifestyle Center of America's (LCA) unique physical activity program tailored for weight loss, insulin sensitivity, and blood sugar control. There are four aspects of LCA's plan, all working together with a plant-based diet (PBD) to maximize health in people with diabetes:

- Strolling
- Stretching
- Strength training
- Intermittent training

We stroll, especially after meals, to control our blood sugar and combat insulin resistance; we stretch to increase our flexibility, balance, and range of motion; we do strength training to increase our metabolism, build or tone our muscles, and strengthen our bones; and we practice intermittent training to increase our endurance and get aerobically fit.

Intermittent training should be of particular interest to people with diabetes who have gotten sedentary, because it's based on the idea of "The rest that works." We reject much popular exercise philosophy, especially the pervasive myth of "No pain, no gain" and the idea that a more intense workout equals more weight loss and better conditioning. Instead we present a way to get more physically active at home that's rational, evidence based,[1] and more fun and sustainable. We offer various modes, frequencies, intensities, and durations, depending on your desired results. You'll be happy to know that even modest weight loss (5 to 10 percent of body weight) can result in better glycemic control, improved insulin sensitivity, and decreased cardiovascular risk factors in people with type-2 diabetes.[2] Among people with type-1 diabetes, breaking that insulin resistance will lead to weight loss and less dependence on insulin.

As many of our patients discover, exercise is medicine. And the best medicine is easy to swallow. We'll teach you to *work smarter, not harder.*

ACTIVITY'S THE TICKET

AFTER ALL WE'VE said so far, you might think that it will be enough just to start eating right. However, we consider an increase in activity to be a cornerstone of diabetes care that's as important as a good diet. For people with diabetes, the beneficial effects of an active lifestyle have been known since ancient times.[3] Since the discovery of insulin in the 1920s, researchers have been studying how activity affects insulin and blood glucose levels and overall diabetes care.[4] If you don't have full-blown diabetes, you should know that increasing and maintaining your physical activity can actually slow the progression of prediabetes and even *prevent* type-2 diabetes. Epidemiological studies have proven it.[5] Those with impaired glucose tolerance (impaired ability to deal with blood sugar), gestational diabetes (see Chapter 3), or a family history of type-2 diabetes can especially benefit from a regular program of aerobic activity, as can anyone with some weight to lose.

If you already have diabetes, it's not too late to get on the physical activity train! Even small changes in your activity level can really help.[6] Getting physically active can provide the following major benefits:[7]

Improvement in Blood Glucose Control

Activity, along with a healthful, PBD (and the right amount of the appropriate medicine when absolutely necessary) should be the foundation of diabetes therapy, because it improves blood glucose control naturally.[8] In the short term, the activity causes more glucose to be used by busy cells in need of energy, and causes less insulin to be secreted. This lowers blood sugar without the need for more insulin.[9]

Improved Insulin Sensitivity, Lower Medication Requirement

Physical activity results in improved insulin sensitivity, the measure of how well insulin works to usher glucose energy into cells (how much the Paul Revere Hormone has to shout, "*The Energy's Coming!*").[10] For many people with diabetes, this translates into a reduction in their insulin or oral diabetes medicine dose. Regular activity works in the long term through a process called *improved glucose tolerance*, a measure of how well your body can metabolize blood sugar. The more active you get, the better you train your body to deal with sugar. The key to this process is glycogen, the storage form of glucose, found mostly in the liver and the muscles. Physical activity slows insulin secretion from the pancreas, which causes the liver and muscles to use their stored glycogen to maintain the balance of glucose in the blood. After the physical activity, the glycogen stores in the liver and muscles have to be replenished, which means more glucose from the blood will be absorbed by those busy cells. This process can go on for 24 to 48 hours, until the glycogen is fully restored. During this period of increased insulin sensitivity, insulin ushers more glucose into the cells.[11]

Reduction in Body Fat

Physical activity coupled with moderate caloric intake is considered the most effective way to lose weight. And with weight loss comes increases in insulin sensitivity, which allows many with diabetes to reduce the amount of insulin or oral diabetes agents needed. Remember, insulin's a growth hormone, so the less of it in your system the fewer pounds you will gain. It's breaking this cycle of insulin-chasing-blood-sugar-chasing-insulin that's the real key to diabetes control and lasting weight loss.

Cardiovascular Benefits

Regular activity decreases the risk of cardiovascular disease. This is important to people with diabetes, because they are so much more likely to have cardiovascular problems owing to excess weight, high blood sugar, and high insulin levels. Physical activity can improve your strength and your work capacity; control hypertension (high blood pressure); reduce overall cholesterol, low-density lipoproteins (LDL; the "bad" cholesterol), and triglycerides; and raise high-density lipoproteins (HDL; the "good" cholesterol). It's no wonder the Centers for Disease Control and Prevention (CDC) reports that living a couch-potato lifestyle is the equivalent of being a smoker in terms of cardiac risk.[12]

Stress Reduction

Ahh . . . here's a nice extra benefit to exercise: stress reduction. Stress can disrupt diabetes control by increasing adrenaline, ketones (acidic substances produced when the body uses fat instead of sugar for energy), free fatty acids (fat in the blood), and urine output. Chronic stress increases the risk of heart attack, high blood pressure, obesity, and hardening of the arteries.[13] Stress reduction is an important part of diabetes care. For more on stress and diabetes, see Chapter 9.

Depression Relief

A physical activity program you stick to can even help you overcome depression. Some studies show that getting active can be just as beneficial as antidepressant medication.[14] If you're not depressed, physical activity can still improve your mood. It can even improve your time management skills and your productivity at the office![15] For more on depression and diabetes, see Chapter 9.

Other Benefits

If that's not enough for you, a physical activity program can also do the following:[16]

- Boost your immune system.
- Stave off or improve symptoms of osteoporosis.
- Reduce the risk of bone fractures.
- Ease arthritis pain.
- Diminish insomnia.
- Improve your oral health.[17]

- Improve your memory, keep your mind sharp, and prevent Alzheimer's disease.[18]
- Protect you against some forms of cancer.[19]

ARE YOU OVERWEIGHT?
Using the Body Mass Index

THE BODY MASS index (BMI) is used to assess weight relative to height. Simply put, it gives you an idea of how fat you are. The BMI is calculated by dividing your body weight in kilograms by your height in meters squared (kg/m^2). You can consult the chart on this page or use the following formula, which uses standard American measures:

$$BMI = \frac{\text{Weight (pounds)}}{[\text{Height (inches)} \times \text{Height (inches)}]} \times 703$$

Body Mass Index (BMI) Chart

BMI																	
Height in inches	19	20	21	22	23	24	25	26	27	28	29	30	31	32	33	34	35
58	91	95	100	105	110	115	119	124	129	134	138	143	148	153	158	162	167
59	94	99	104	109	114	119	124	128	133	138	143	148	153	158	163	168	173
60	97	102	107	112	118	123	128	133	138	143	148	153	158	164	169	174	179
61	100	106	111	116	121	127	132	137	143	148	153	158	164	169	174	180	185
62	104	109	115	120	125	131	136	142	147	153	158	164	169	175	180	186	191
63	107	113	118	124	130	135	141	146	152	158	163	169	175	180	186	192	197
64	110	116	122	128	134	140	145	151	157	163	169	174	180	186	192	198	203
65	114	120	126	132	138	144	150	156	162	168	174	180	186	192	198	204	210
66	117	124	130	136	142	148	155	161	167	173	179	185	192	198	204	210	216
67	121	127	134	140	147	153	159	166	172	178	185	191	198	204	210	217	223
68	125	131	138	144	151	158	164	171	177	184	190	197	203	210	217	223	230
69	128	135	142	149	155	162	169	176	182	189	196	203	209	216	223	230	237
70	132	139	146	153	160	167	174	181	188	195	202	209	216	223	230	236	243
71	136	143	150	157	165	172	179	186	193	200	207	215	222	229	236	243	250
72	140	147	155	162	169	177	184	191	199	206	213	221	228	235	243	250	258
73	144	151	159	166	174	182	189	197	204	212	219	227	234	242	250	257	265
74	148	155	163	171	179	187	194	202	210	218	225	233	241	249	256	264	272
75	152	160	168	176	184	192	200	208	216	224	232	240	247	255	263	271	279
76	156	164	172	180	189	197	205	213	221	230	238	246	254	262	271	279	287

A healthy range is 19 to 25 BMI. Between 25 and 29.9 is considered overweight, and a BMI of 30 or above is obese. Weight-related health problems increase beyond a BMI of 25 for most people.[20] The BMI is a useful tool for the general population. It is not as useful or accurate for well-conditioned athletes with large amounts of muscle relative to fat.

The table on p. 171 has already done the math and metric conversions for you. To use the table, find your height in the left-hand column. Move across the row to find your weight. The number at the top of the column is the BMI for your height and weight.

COMMONSENSE CAUTIONS FOR GETTING PHYSICALLY ACTIVE WITH DIABETES

THERE ARE A few important pieces of advice you need to keep in mind before starting the LCA activity plan.[21]

Ask Your Doctor

No one with diabetes should embark on a major new regimen of activity without the guidance of a good healthcare professional. Many people with diabetes are dealing with other challenges, too.[22] Your doctor might suggest a treadmill stress test (if not, ask for one).

Test Your Blood Sugar

Test your blood sugar level before and after your activity. We also recommend breaking for a bit to test your sugar level during the activity, if it lasts more than 30 minutes.

First Things First

If you don't have your blood sugar under control, you should not begin a program of physical activity. In the person with uncontrolled diabetes (blood sugar level less than 70 or more than 250), vigorous physical activity can lead to a state called ketosis, which can lead to problems in the kidneys and liver[23] and can even cause coma or death. We suggest you work on getting off the standard American diet (SAD) first, then start strolling and stretching daily, as described in later sections. When your blood sugar is more under control (above 90 and less than 250), and with your doctor's blessing, you can start your program of increased physical activity. On any given day, if your blood sugar levels are below 90 or above 250, it's not a good idea to do extra physical activity.[24]

Be Patient

Time is required for both musculoskeletal and cardiovascular adaptation. If you attempt to hurry training progress, injuries and "wheel spinning" might result, and this can be discouraging. It takes some time to put on weight, lose your energy and strength, and it will take time to get fitness back, too. The benefits of physical activity diminish quickly if you stop and revert to a sedentary lifestyle. Experts believe it takes at least four weeks to start noticing positive changes from physical activity— possibly longer if you've been inactive for a long time.[25] Though we've seen positive results on the very first day—and very often within a week or two—it's important to remember that good fitness through the LCA activity plan is a lifestyle commitment, not a one-day rarity.

Pain Means You're Overdoing It

Remember above all that the phrase "No pain, no gain" has no room in the sensible, healthful, and fun LCA activity plan. It's not a competition. It's about *you* and *your health*. Remember it takes time to adapt to an activity plan, especially if you've been inactive for a while.

- If you find yourself not recovering from your activity within 2 hours, decrease the intensity or length of time of subsequent workouts. Your physical activity should leave you with a sense of pleasant relaxation and pleasant fatigue—not exhaustion and grief.
- Some shortness of breath is normal when you get active, but it shouldn't be extreme. It should subside soon when you lower the intensity of your activity. Trust the messages your body's sending you. Serious shortness of breath on exertion could be caused by lung disease or heart strain, which is aggravated by exertion. If severe shortness of breath persists or occurs suddenly, stop your activity and alert your physician.
- Headache and faintness during physical activity can be the

result of a variety of causes. They may simply be due to caffeine withdrawal or dehydration. Be sure to drink 8 to 10 glasses of water per day, more on days you are active, especially if the weather is warm. More serious causes include heart irregularity, inner ear problems, heat stress, blood vessel abnormalities, or high blood pressure. If you experience frequent headaches or faintness you need to consult your physician before continuing the activity program.

- *If chest pain develops during your activity, stop immediately!* Rest. If the problem persists longer than 15 minutes (or less if your instincts tell you something's wrong), you need to call 911. If your pain goes away but comes back whenever you are physically active, you need to see a doctor.

Drink Plenty of Fluids

The very best fluid replacement is water. Remember that Gatorade and other sports drinks are loaded with simple sugars. They will raise your blood sugar—that's their whole point. Sweating during your activity will happen, even though you may not detect it, so don't use perceived sweating to determine how much water you're losing. Similarly, *don't wait until you're thirsty* to drink. Thirst is the body's last-ditch effort to get some water. If possible, drink at least 1 pint (2 cups) of water 2 hours before your activity. During your activity, try to drink about 8 fluid ounces (1 cup) every 15 minutes or so.

Keep Track of Effects

Getting active will affect everyone differently—especially when it comes to blood sugar. Log your workouts (see Appendix 1 for sample logs) and look for patterns in your sugar levels. For many people, when their blood sugars are high, strenuous activity will raise it further, but when it's low, the same activity will tend to lower it further.

Watch Your Shots

If you inject rapid-acting insulin, you may want to avoid injecting it into a part of the body that will be exerted (such as the leg if you are going to bike). This may increase absorption of the insulin and cause low blood sugar[26] (though this doesn't appear to happen with slow-acting insulin, such as Lantus[27]).

Time It Right

If you inject or inhale insulin, avoid strenuous physical activity at the peak of the insulin's action. We recommend you take your insulin about 1 hour before starting activity. Watch for symptoms of low blood sugar during your activity—feeling shaky, nervous, clammy, or confused. Check your blood sugar every 30 minutes during your activity, especially if you're doing a new activity or starting a new intensity level. *Stop if your blood sugar is less than 70.*

Remember Drug Effects

Avoid beta-blocker drugs around the time of your activity, because they make it difficult to tell if you're hypoglycemic. Same goes for alcohol. If you're on blood pressure medicine, talk to your healthcare professional before starting physical activities.

Eat Properly When You're Active

In general, 1 hour of activity requires an extra 15 grams (g) of carbohydrates either before or after the activity. It's best to not use glucose tablets to prevent hypoglycemia; try eating something with more fat, protein, and fiber.[28] For example, a slice of whole grain bread with a light smear of nut butter contains 15 g of carbohydrates (1 carb choice). The fat, protein, and fiber cause the carbohydrates to be absorbed gradually during your physical activity.

Treat Low Blood Sugar

If you're actually experiencing a bout of hypoglycemia (blood sugar less than 60 to 70, with symptoms of shakiness, nervousness, clamminess, or confusion), you can take glucose tablets. Keep glucose tablets or other fast-acting carbs (fruit juice, hard candy) available. The usual treatment is three glucose tablets, three pieces of hard candy, or 4 fluid ounces of fruit juice. Don't overdo it! The tendency when you're low is to gorge on sugar. Start with a little, sit tight, test your blood after 15 minutes, and take more carbs only if necessary. Though it's not very common, you should watch for signs of hypoglycemia (low blood sugar) *up to 15 hours after your activity.* For this reason, we don't recommend strenuous activities shortly before bedtime. If you have type-1 diabetes, you should concentrate on reaping the overall health benefits of physical activity—not just lowering your immediate blood sugars. In fact, if you have type-1, you don't really want physical activity to cause precipitous drops in your blood sugar, as they can lead to hypoglycemia.

Keep ID Handy and Buddy Up

If you're getting active outside your own home, always carry identification (such as a MedicAlert bracelet or wallet card listing your medical conditions and the medications you use. Remember to update this information regularly, especially as your medication doses change). If you work out outside or at the gym, let somebody know where you will be in case of an emergency. Whenever possible, do your activity with a partner who knows your condition.

When to See Your Doctor

If you experience pain in your chest, heart palpitations, or severe shortness of breath during your activity, stop immediately and consult your doctor. If you have severe retinopathy or a retinal hemorrhage, you shouldn't get physically active without talking to your healthcare professional first. If you're ill or have an infection, you likewise shouldn't get active. If you experience nausea, this could be a sign of something serious, or it could just mean you need a little less, or more, in your belly before getting active.

Practice Good Foot Care

Wear proper shoes. This is a very good investment in which you usually do get what you pay for. Get some supportive, cotton socks that wick away sweat, too. When you're done with your activity, take your shoes and socks off right away and thoroughly check your feet for blisters, lesions, or other signs of injury.

Mind the Sun

Be careful doing strenuous physical activities in the heat or strong sun. If you have neuropathy (nerve pain or numbness) caused by diabetes, you are prone to heat-related injuries. You might not even notice you're getting a severe sunburn.

Don't Spin Your Wheels

It is possible to overtrain and show what's called *stale* progress. You'll know if this is happening by excessive fatigue, loss of enthusiasm, and lack of results. Be careful about becoming so enthusiastic about being on an activity plan that you place too much emphasis on your *fitness* goals (Gotta run 5 miles today!) and not enough on your *health* goals (I want more energy), which require the other components of good health: a good PBD, proper hydration, adequate rest and sleep, fresh air, sunlight, moderation, and balance. See Chapter 9 for more on these health tenets.

PERSISTENT MYTHS ABOUT FITNESS

TO PARAPHRASE THE recovery community again, "If you keep doing what you've been doing, you're going to keep getting what you've got." This is true when it comes to reaping the benefits of an activity program—or not. First, let's dispel some pervasive myths that prevent so many people from getting the optimal benefits from physical activity.

MYTH
No Pain, No Gain!

When it comes to weight loss, cardiovascular improvements, blood sugar control, and overall health, harder work does not mean better results. In fact, the opposite is true. Much of the pain of vigorous physical activity comes after the body begins to burn glycogen stored in the muscles, and stops burning fat. Again, *you should not feel pain during your activity because that means you're working too hard and are no longer burning fat.* If you define *gain* as keeping your diabetes in check, losing weight, building muscles, increasing metabolism, and increasing endurance, then you must reject the concept of "No pain, no gain."

MYTH
20 Minutes to Benefits

What about the belief that you have to work out for at least 20 minutes before you start gaining any real health benefits? What's the point in walking for 15 minutes or playing a quick round of handball if it won't help you anyway? And what's the point in just strolling around, even it's for 1 hour, if you can't feel the burn? These notions are completely false. When you get active, you burn calories. Period. One of our lecturers, Dr. John Goley, says: *You burn the same number of calories walking a mile as you do running the same mile.* It's true. Of course it *takes longer* to burn those calories walking, but it takes the same amount of energy to get to the end of that mile whether you're walking, jogging, running (or crawling). There's simply no denying the science of it: Calories don't care *how* they're burned, as long as they're burned.

And keep in mind that physical activity is *cumulative* each day. If you do 20 minutes here, 10 minutes there, another ½ hour there, you've been active for 1 hour. So, during your day, calories don't care *when* they're burned, either. Just start burning them.

Remember, though, that fitness is *not* stored from day to day. It must be continually replenished. The benefits of physical activity cannot be crowded into 1 or 2 days a week; the Weekend Warrior is prone to soreness and injuries.

MYTH
Too Late Now

If you're overweight or have pain, that doesn't mean it's too late to start a physical activity plan. In fact, if you're overweight, *you will burn more calories* doing the same activity as a person who is at his or her target weight. A 120-pound person will burn 6.5 calories per minute walking, but a 180-pound person will burn 9.7 calories.[29] You can imagine that it takes more energy to get 300 pounds up a flight of stairs than it takes to get 150 up. Once you start to lose weight, even a few pounds, you will start to experience more energy and less strain on your body.

What about peripheral neuropathy, which affects about 15 percent of all people in the United States who have diabetes? This nerve damage in the feet and legs, caused primarily by persistent high blood sugar, may in some cases be irreversible, but some of it can be alleviated by improvements in glucose control, weight loss, and increased activity. We see this all the time. Physical activity can increase blood flow to the lower extremities and even slow down neuropathy.[30] We surveyed all our patients with diabetes who stayed at LCA for 18 days between January and August 2007. These individuals reported an average of 73 percent improvement in pain and 81 percent improvement in mobility and flexibility. Perhaps as a result of this, they also reported an average 84.5 percent improvement in their attitude and hope for the future. These results are not atypical. Gwen from Texas, who is 66 years old and attended the LCA program in 2006, told us: "I thought my sugar was just going to keep getting higher and then I would eventually die. I used to lose sleep because my legs would hurt and I couldn't stand the blankets on my feet at all. It felt like I was walking on stones, and now it is almost 100 percent better in these few days."

Those who stick with the LCA activity plan over the long haul continue to see improvement. Richard, a 79-year-old with type-2 diabetes from Missouri, was on 75 units of insulin a day when he came to LCA. "I could not climb our stairs or put my socks on," he says. On the LCA plan he started walking and eating right, which allowed us to drastically reduce his insulin. By 3 years after he started the program, he was walking 4 miles a day and had lost more than 70 pounds. "Now," he says, "I can run up the stairs and I can mow the lawn with no help . . . and guess what? My primary-care physician was able to take me off insulin. Wow!"[31]

You will find the right pace for your own limitations—it's never too late to get moving, even if it's just a little bit.

MYTH
There's No Point in Getting Active When There Are So Many Easier Shortcuts

In our quick-fix culture, many people are still looking for the magic bullet. Just look at the number of people getting bariatric surgery, including the invasive, traumatic, and not exactly supersafe[32] gastric bypass operation. Between 1990 and 2000, the number of such procedures increased ninefold.[33] And now, after decades of prescriptions for weight loss, the U.S. Food and Drug Administration (FDA) has made an antifat pill, Glaxo SmithKline's Orlistat, available over the counter. All the experts, even Glaxo officials, are saying it's "not a magic bullet" and it "will not be effective without a weight-loss plan."[34]

The real "magic" comes from healthful, natural, whole foods, and a good dose of sensible physical activity. Eating whole grains, fruits, and vegetables can lower your overall mortality risk.[35] And research has shown that moderate physical activity can add up to 3.7 years to the average person's life—including people with diabetes.[36]

MYTH
If You Feel You Can't Get Active Regularly, There's No Point in Starting

You *can* experience the benefits of getting physically active after just one session. Even if the activity is just walking, you can see reductions in blood pressure, blood sugar, and other health factors. Many people feel overwhelmed by the thought of starting an activity program. Others become overactive too quickly. The best approach is to begin gradually and enjoy the activity you are involved in. Soon it will become easy and enjoyable, and with time it will become a habit you cannot do without.

MYTH
If You Get Active, You Can Eat Anything You Want

You've probably heard that if you exercise, you don't have to watch your diet. But remember the "energy in, energy out" dynamic we discussed in Chapter 3? Increasing your activity *and* consuming the proper amount of calories is the only healthful, natural, and safe way to lose weight.

MYTH
You Can Spot-Reduce Fat

Can you melt away your abdominal fat, just by working that area aggressively? No. You *can* increase the muscle mass in your belly and tone the muscles *under* the fat by doing crunches or other abdominal exercises, but the only way to lose the fat over those muscles is to burn off calories through aerobic activity. Even strolling can help you lose your gut, as long as you reduce your caloric intake.[37]

MYTH
It's Best to Get Active in the Morning

Is the morning really the best time to be physically active? The very *best* time of day for *you* to get active is the time that works for you. If having a morning routine is important to you, and this helps you be consistent with your activity program, then go for it! But some may prefer to do their activity later in the day, after their bodies have had time to "warm up" for a while. Remember: You can break up your activity into more than one session throughout the day. Activity is cumulative. If you have a choice, though, we do recommend doing your physical activity in the morning, as we've found our patients who do so are more likey to stick to their physical-activity routine.

THE FOUR PILLARS

WHENEVER YOU DO even moderate physical activity, like walking, you will probably be able to lower your blood sugar and thus be able to reduce the amount of insulin or oral diabetes medicine you take. You're working at the heart of the diabetes process—on insulin resistance. So the LCA activity plan starts with moderate physical activity and builds to more rigorous activity. The four pillars of this plan—strolling, stretching, strength training, and intermittent training—are discussed in the following sections.

Strolling

The LCA activity plan starts with something most everyone can do: a simple stroll after meals. We don't want you to go on a full-tilt run or even on a particularly brisk walk. In fact, it's important that you *don't* do anything too strenuous right after a meal. After eating, your body needs to devote energy to the process of digestion. A light stroll after meals can facilitate this process—but a heavy workout can rob the digestive system of the energy it needs to do its job. Light strolling can also aid the blood circulation, which is important for good digestion. You don't get good circulation if you nap or sit in front of the TV after eating.[38]

A light stroll can also help keep your blood sugar level down, as testing 2 hours after your meal will show. This is what finally convinced one of our guests, Jim from Oklahoma City, that we were onto something with this active lifestyle stuff. Jim was used to his blood sugar soaring after supper, until he took a walk with his wife one night after eating. He came to the conclusion that lifestyle medicine advocates love to hear: "Hey! Exercise *is* medicine!" If you're interested in the science behind this, look up the references cited in the endnotes to this chapter, but here's a simple way of thinking about this: A light stroll after a meal means that your muscles will demand some of the energy you've just consumed and use some of that sugar, even in the presence of only small amounts of insulin. So if you're taking insulin or oral diabetes medicine, a regular routine of walking can reduce your dose.

The other great benefit of strolling after meals is that you burn off some of the *calories* you just consumed. You're therefore lowering your net caloric intake, which is helpful if weight loss is a goal. Weight loss will lessen your diabetes, and now you're part of a . . . what's the opposite of a vicious cycle? We'll call it a *beneficial cycle.*

In this country, only 20 percent of the population are regularly active, 25 percent are completely sedentary, and 50 percent who start an activity program drop out within the first 6 months.[39] We think a little stroll is the perfect way to start moving you toward good health and fitness, especially if you have diabetes. Go ahead and start today.

If you don't live where outdoor walking is feasible, consider buying a treadmill, or walk the mall (just make sure you keep walking past the Mrs. Fields cookie kiosk!). We also recommend you "park your car where the RVs are." We mean that when you go shopping at superstores or shopping malls, instead of driving around searching for the closest spot to the doors, deliberately park as far away as possible. That way, you'll be forced to take a little stroll.

Stretching

Why Stretch

Stretching nurtures the body and eases the mind. Pete Byrd, a trainer in our fitness center, puts it simply when he says, "Just look at your average tomcat or hound dog: He seems to understand that stretching first thing in the morning, and throughout the day—especially after being sedentary for long periods—is just what the doctor ordered." People have picked up on this wisdom, too: Yogis in the East have been stretching for 5,000 years. You will find, as they do, that regular stretching provides the following benefits:[40]

- Reduces muscle tension, alleviates mental and physical stress, and makes you feel more relaxed in both mind and body
- Increases coordination by allowing for freer and easier movement
- Increases range of motion
- Increases balance
- Helps prevent injuries, such as muscle strains
- Signals the muscles that they are going to be used and prepares your body for more brisk activities
- Increases flexibility and improves posture, so as time passes, you don't get progressively stiffer and more stooped
- Increases circulation and blood flow to the stretched area, which can improve pain and neuropathy (nerve pain and numbness)
- Reduces anxiety and fatigue
- Develops body awareness (as you stretch various parts of the body, you focus on them and get in touch with them)
- Makes getting active much easier (stretching is probably the easiest, least stressful, most enjoyable way to get off the couch and start moving; and if you don't want to get off the couch, you can stretch there, too)

- Can reduce your chances of annoying daily blahs like stomachache, headaches, and nausea as well as more serious, chronic diseases like obesity, diabetes, and cardiovascular disease (all of which are linked to stress and tension)[41]
- Can even help you learn better and be more efficient and productive during the day by calming your mind[42]

When and Where to Stretch

There's no optimal time to stretch, and you don't have to set aside a specific time. You can even stretch while doing other activities. Consider stretching in bed before getting up, during a regular routine before or after breakfast; on the subway, bus, or in your car (at the traffic lights, not on the highway!); on the way to work, at your desk when you start feeling stiff, during lunch hour, in front of the TV, while waiting in line, before bedtime, while you're on the phone, or before and after strenuous activities.

How to Stretch

The granddaddy of stretching in America is Bob Anderson. In his books, DVDs, and software, Anderson says the right way to stretch "is a relaxed, sustained stretch with your attention focused on the muscles being stretched. The wrong way (unfortunately practiced by many people) is to bounce up and down or to stretch to the point of pain: these methods can actually do more harm than good."[43] People have a tendency to push themselves too far when it comes to stretching. Remember, "No pain, no gain" is a harmful fabrication—even when it comes to stretching. Start off easy, stretching just to the point of feeling the muscle tightness, but not pain. After a while, you can push—or is that *pull?*—the stretch a little farther (we're talking about a fraction of an inch here) to develop the muscles and increase your flexibility and range of motion.

Obviously, if you've recently had an injury or surgery, you should be very careful before doing any stretches. Likewise, if you have lost some sensation in your feet owing to peripheral neuropathy or if you have foot ulcers, you should do stretches that don't put too much pressure on your feet and weight-bearing joints. Good upper body stretches and stretches done while sitting or lying on the floor might be best.

Be conscious of your spine. Try to keep the natural curvature of the back in place as you stretch.

LCA'S TOP TEN STRETCHING TIPS

1. For optimal benefits, you should stretch daily to increase joint mobility. Increasing joint mobility increases your range of motion, so performing daily duties will become easier. You can take one day off a week, a kind of "stretching Sabbath," but consistency is the key to long-term benefits.

2. You should stretch all your major muscle groups 6 days a week. Be sure to include stretches for your neck, shoulders, arms, back, abs, and legs. Use the routine in this chapter as a home-stretch program. Or get yourself a DVD or tape, and follow along.

3. Spend extra time stretching those areas that you find are less flexible than others, but don't forget to stretch your entire body.

4. Ideally, you should stretch your muscles when they're already somewhat warm. So take some time to warm up the muscles with a brisk walk or march in place for 5 minutes before stretching. You can do this in front of the morning news shows or while walking your dog, playing with your kids, even while you blow-dry your hair.

5. Hold each stretch for 10 to 30 seconds. As your flexibility increases, you can gradually increase the time that you hold each stretch to 30 seconds or more.

6. Stretching should be static, not bouncy. Gently hold each stretch for the entire duration of the stretch. Bouncing through a stretch can be harmful to the muscle by increasing tightness; and it can cause muscle strain.

7. If it hurts, don't do it. In fact, overstretching can cause injury and even tighten the muscles you're trying to relax.

8. When stretching after a workout, cool down first. Putting your head below the level of your heart, which some stretches require, immediately after a workout can cause dizziness, faintness, and nausea.

9. Breathe deeply while you stretch. Breathe in through your nose and out through your mouth. *Don't hold your breath.*

10. Use stretching time as "me time"; relax and enjoy it. Or stretch with a partner and get some bonding done, too.

The Stretching Exercises

Warm up your muscles before stretching by taking a brisk walk or marching in place for 5 minutes. Do the stretches in the sequence presented here. Hold each stretch for 20 to 30 seconds, and take extra time for areas of your body that feel tight. You should slowly extend your range of stretch—never use a bouncing movement. If you feel pain, you are stretching too vigorously. Breathe in deeply through your nose and out through the mouth. Use your stretching time to relax fully.

NECK, ARMS, AND SHOULDERS

▶ *Neck Stretch*

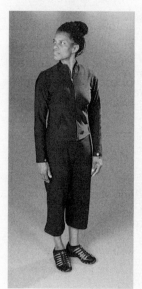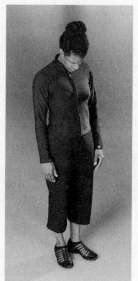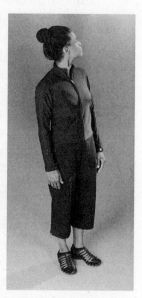

In a standing position with your back straight, slowly look up and over your right shoulder then bring your chin down to your chest. Repeat this on your left side.

▶ *Shoulder Roll*

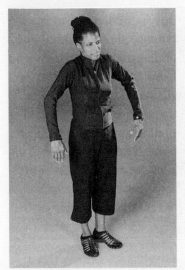 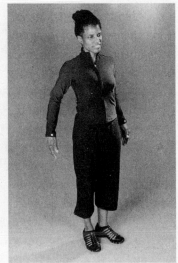

Roll your shoulders forward, making large circles. Then roll your shoulders backward in circles.

▶ *Shoulder Stretch*

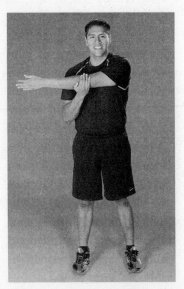

Pull your arm across your chest and lightly press in until a stretch is felt in shoulder. Repeat with the other arm.

▶ *Triceps Stretch*

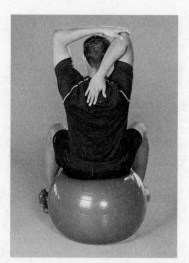

Place your right hand between your shoulder blades. Use your left hand to lightly press up and back on your right elbow until you feel the stretch in the back of your right arm. Keep your back in proper alignment. Repeat, placing the left hand between the shoulder blades.

▶ *Forearm Stretch*

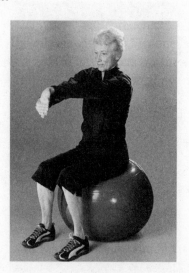

Stretch your arm out in front with the elbow straight and palm facing away. With your other hand, lightly pull the fingers backward until a stretch is felt in the forearm. Repeat with the other arm.

▶ *Rotate Wrists*

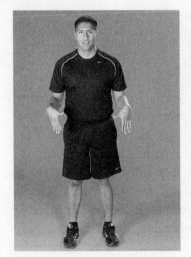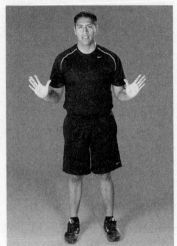

Rotate your wrists in full circles. Rotate clockwise and then counterclockwise.

BACK AND CHEST

▶ *Chest Stretch*

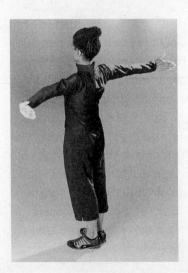

With your arms parallel to the floor, press your arms back and squeeze your shoulder blades together to feel the stretch in the chest.

▶ *Standing Cat Stretch*

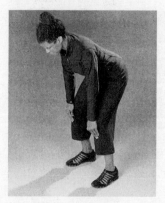 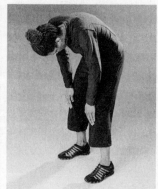

From a standing position, round your back up, then straighten your back to the natural curvature of your spine.

▶ *Single Knee to Chest*

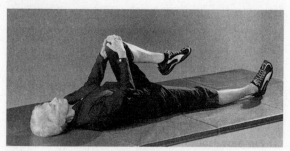

Bring your knee to your chest and hold. Feel the stretch in your back. Repeat with the other leg.

▶ *Both Knees to Chest*

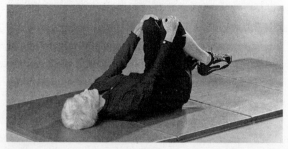

Bring both knees to your chest and hold to feel the stretch in your back.

▶ Low Back

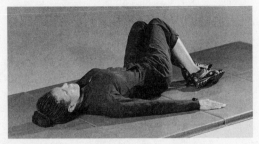

Keeping your back flat and feet together, rotate your knees to one side. Keep your shoulders on the floor. You do not have to touch your legs to the floor. Repeat on the other side.

LOWER BODY: LEGS AND HIPS

▶ Standing Hamstring Stretch

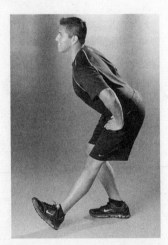

Put one leg straight out with your heel down and toes up. Slightly bend the other knee and sit back into the stretch. You should feel this in the hamstrings (back of leg). Repeat with the other leg.

▶ *Seated Hamstring Stretch*

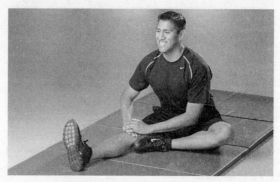

Sit with one leg straight and the other leg bent. Keep your chest lifted and shoulders down to maintain the natural curvature of your spine. Lean forward slightly until you feel the stretch in the hamstrings (back of leg). Repeat with the other leg.

▶ *Standing Inner Thigh Stretch*

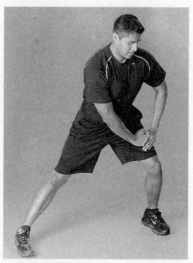

With feet wide apart, slowly shift your weight to one side until a stretch is felt in the inner thigh. Do not let your knee go past your toes. Repeat on the opposite side.

▶ *Sitting Inner Thigh Stretch*

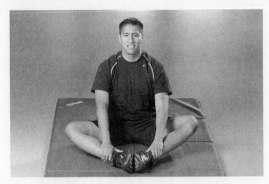

Sit up straight while gently pushing your knees to the floor to feel the stretch.

▶ *Calf (Chair or Wall) Stretch*

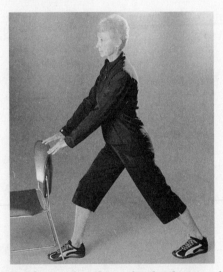

Stand with one leg forward and one leg back. Your back leg should be straight, with the heel on the floor and both feet pointing forward. Lightly press against the chair or wall until a stretch is felt in the calf. Repeat with the other leg.

▶ *Quadriceps Stretch*

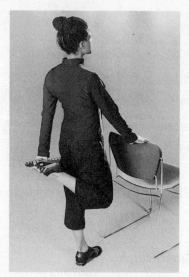

With your left hand, grasp your right ankle and gently pull the heel toward your buttocks until a stretch is felt. Repeat on the opposite side.

▶ *Quadriceps Stretch (Modified)*

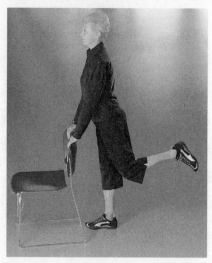

Keeping your knee bent and foot flexed, extend your leg backward, just moving at the hip joint, until a stretch is felt in the front of your upper leg. Repeat on the opposite side.

▶ *Rotate Ankles*

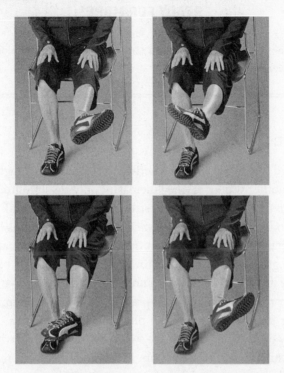

Rotate your ankles clockwise. Repeat going counterclockwise.

▶ *Hip Stretch*

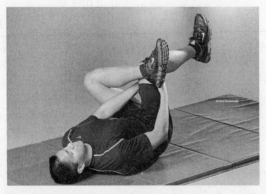

Rest your left ankle on your right knee. Hold your right leg and pull it in toward you until you feel the stretch in your left hip. Repeat on the opposite side.

> ### READY FOR MORE?
>
> ●
>
> FOR examples of more advanced stretching routines, go to our website (www.diabetesmiracle.org).

Strength Training

The third pillar of the LCA activity program is strength training, which is another way of saying "increasing muscle strength." There are two kinds of muscle development: strength training and bulk building. If you want to look like Arnold Schwarzenegger looked in his heyday, you want bulk building. That's not what the LCA activity plan is all about. It's about strength training, which provides the best health benefit. And don't worry if you're a woman with no interest in looking like Popeye the Sailor: Your mix of hormones will prevent this from happening.

Strength training works by the phenomenon known as *the overload principle.* By overloading the muscle system with more than what it is normally accustomed to, muscle fibers increase in size and number in a process called *hypertrophy.* As the muscle gets bigger, it gets stronger because of an increase in the contraction ability per square inch of muscle.

The primary focus of the LCA activity plan is overall health for people with diabetes. For this reason, we recommend you start a light strength training program, because it will help you perform simple activities of daily living (what the fitness industry calls *functional* fitness), such as opening jars, mowing the lawn, vacuuming a carpet, and playing with your grandchildren: It's not about dead lifting 500-pound barbells. We just need to develop our muscular strength a little, because nowadays, most of us work in jobs that don't require too much strength—unless you think pushing pencils is tiresome. Building strength also improves stamina and energy. You'll find you'll be more prepared to deal with the mental and social stresses of life when you're more physically fit. In short, good muscular fitness can help you work longer and harder before you tire out.

Strength training, sometimes called resistance training, has also been shown to improve glycemic control and even protect against the metabolic syndrome (the constellation of health challenges that can include

impaired fasting glucose, high blood pressure, obesity, and high cholesterol and triglycerides). One recent study of a group of men in their late
60s with type-2 diabetes found that two weekly sessions of strength
training improved their insulin sensitivity and blood sugar levels.[44]

A Simple Strength Training Plan

Strength training can be done with dumbbells or household "weights"
like soup cans, water bottles, and detergent jugs. You can also use resistance tubes, which are lightweight, flexible rubber bands of various thick-
nesses that approximate weight lifting (the thicker the tube, the greater
the resistance). The strength training routine laid out in this chapter
presents strength training with free weights and resistance tubes.

Here's what we recommend to start:

- Prepare your muscles for strength training with a brief warm-
  up. Take a brisk walk or do another form of aerobic activity for
  5 minutes. You can also do your strength training after your
  intermittent training session (discussed later in the chapter),
  when your muscles will already be warmed up.
- Test the maximal weight (or resistance) that you can comfortably lift one time, without overstraining or hurting yourself.
  Settle on 50 to 70 percent of that weight for your routine.
- Begin by doing one set of 10 repetitions (reps) for each activity.
  The last 1 or 2 reps should be comfortably hard but not agoniz-
  ing. If you can do one set very easily and could do more reps,
  the weight (or resistance, if you're using tubes) is too light. If
  you can't get through 10 reps, the weight or resistance is too
  heavy. Adjust accordingly.
- As you progress, add sets. Try two sets of 10 reps, then three
  sets. Once you're at three sets and the activity becomes easier,
  start increasing the weight or resistance incrementally.
- Lift with as full a range of movement as possible, starting at full
  contraction (the effort) and going to full relaxation (bringing
  the muscle back to its starting position).
- *How* you lift is much more important than *how much* you lift.
  Faster is not better. When you do strength training too quickly,
  you wind up using momentum, and you do not properly isolate

and work the muscle to get the full benefit. It should take 2 seconds to lift a weight (or resistance tube) and 2 seconds to lower it. Try it: You'll find it's much harder than the quick, jerky, bouncy, or pendulum-swinging movements many people do.

- Use intermittent training. *Rest* the muscles you're working for 30 to 60 seconds between *sets* (not between reps). You'll find that it's easier to do 100 sit-ups if you do a set of 10, then rest for a 10-count, then do another set, and so on, up to a count of 100.

- Workouts should begin with the largest muscle groups and proceed to the smaller muscle structures (for example, legs, then back, then abdominals, then arms).

- Increases in muscle strength come easiest when you do *brief* and *infrequent* training, so aim for strength training two to three times per week, not to exceed 30 minutes per session. Don't overdo it.

- You must let your muscles recuperate after strength training. *There should be at least 48 hours between workouts,* but not more than 96 hours.

- Because of these last two facts, it's best to do strength training every other day. Another option is to alternate upper and lower body training sessions, whereby you work a major muscle group every other day. If your goal is to *maintain* strength, 2 to 3 days per week is sufficient. If your goal is *build and tone,* 4 days a week is recommended—but remember to alternate upper and lower body muscle groups.

- Stay focused. Concentrate on the muscle doing the work. This will help you maintain the proper form, which will provide maximum benefits and reduce the chance of injury. Don't just go through the motions. Picture the effort your muscle is going through, and even tell your muscle to lift the weight; that's what professional athletes do.

- Correct breathing is important when strength training. *Don't hold your breath!* Breathe out during the contraction phase (the effort) and breathe in during the extension phase (returning the muscle to the starting position). (See "Breathe!" on p. 199.)

- Cool down after strength training. Walk slowly or do any other light activity for 5 minutes or more, stretching the muscles you've worked (this will reduce soreness).

> ## BREATHE!
>
> ●
>
> TEMPTING as it is, *don't hold your breath when lifting weights or using resistance tubes.* Correct breathing technique will help maintain a low blood pressure during training and will help prevent strains and injuries. Holding your breath while straining to perform a lift causes a decrease in the amount of blood returning to the heart, which means that blood cannot be pumped as easily to the brain. Doing this can cause dizziness and fainting: Not good when you're holding a heavy weight.
>
> The simple principle is to breathe out when you are exerting the most. In general, you exert the most at the beginning of your lift, so this is the time to breathe out. For example, if you are working on your biceps muscle (upper arm) by curling a weight, the first motion is lifting the weight up toward your shoulder. This is the time to breathe out. Then, breathe in when you return the weight to the starting position down at your hip.

Proper Strength Training Form: Oh, My Aching Back!

Back injuries are among the serious mishaps that can happen when you do strength training incorrectly. They can be prevented if you follow some basic principles of lifting:

- Keep the weight or resistance tubing as close to your body as possible. The farther out you hold a weight from your body, the more strain on your back.
- When picking up a weight from the ground, keep your back straight and your head level or up. Bending at your waist with straight legs places tremendous strain on the lower back muscles and spinal disks of the lower back. Do most of your lifting with your legs. The large muscles of the thighs and buttocks are much stronger than those of the back, which are better suited to maintaining an erect posture. Keep your hips and buttocks tucked in.
- Don't twist your body while lifting. Twisting places an uneven load on back muscles, causing strain.
- Lift the weight smoothly, not with a jerky, rapid motion. Sudden motions place more stress on the back muscles and disks.

- Allow for adequate rest between lifts. Fatigue is a prime cause of back strain.
- Don't lift beyond the limits of your strength. Listen to your body. There's no competition here. Strength training is not about being macho, it's about getting healthy.
- When using a weight machine, make sure it's properly adjusted to your body. Get help from someone at the gym (or, if you use a machine or weight equipment at home, make sure you read and understand the directions). Improper settings can cause you to use a muscle group that is not supposed to be targeted by the equipment. Uncomfortable, twisted positions may place unnecessary stress on vulnerable back muscles and nerves.
- Stretch before and after strength training.

STRENGTH TRAINING CAN INCREASE	STRENGTH TRAINING CAN DECREASE
Motor skill performance	Fat weight
Size and strength of connective tissue	Percent body fat
Insulin sensitivity	Risk of falling and the need for custodial care[45]
Bone mass and bone density	Insulin resistance
Lean body weight	Fatigue from life's activities
Speed, power, balance, agility, flexibility	

DO I HAVE TO WARM UP?

WARMING up is always a good idea. Athletes wouldn't think about performing before warming up. Warming up raises your body temperature gradually and slowly increases the demands put on your cardiovascular system. It gives your body—especially your heart—adequate time to prepare for a more vigorous activity. Oxygen delivery to the exercising muscles occurs more easily at higher muscle temperature. This means that a warm-up increases blood flow to the working muscles. They are then better prepared to work aerobically, so your workout feels easier. Without a proper warm-up, you could experience abnormal heart rhythms, muscle injury, and joint pains, and your workout will feel noticeably more difficult.

The Strength Training Exercises

Many of the activities illustrated here can be done from a sitting position. Beginners should use a chair and then advance to an exercise ball. Always keep a light but firm hold on the dumbbells or tubing you are using. Also, watch your wrists when doing each activity and make sure they stay flat and in line with your arm. Keep your abdominal muscles tight to stabilize the trunk during these activities to minimize back pain or injury. Follow the sequence of activities as presented. You may do all of them in one session, with a day off between sessions. Or you may do daily sessions and focus on the lower body and abdominals one day and the upper body on the next, in an alternating fashion.

LOWER BODY

▶ **Squat (with Chair)**

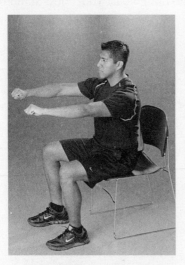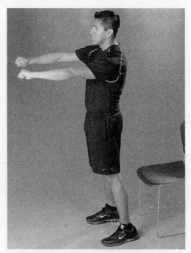

Sit on the edge of a chair, with good posture and with your feet apart. Stand up without leaning forward. Keep your arms out to assist with balance. Sit back down and repeat.

► *Squat*

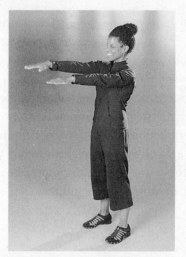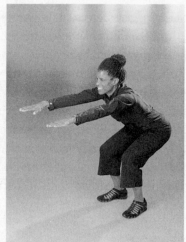

Stand with the feet apart, good posture, and the head up. Bend at the knees and extend your buttocks back until your thighs are parallel to the floor. Make sure your knees do not go past your toes. Stand back up and repeat.

► *Single Step*

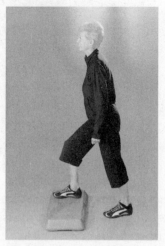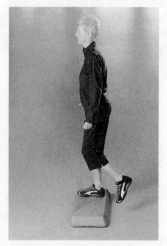

Step up with your right foot followed by the left until both feet are on the step. Step back down beginning with the right foot followed by the left. Repeat, starting with the left foot. Keep alternating feet with each cycle.

▶ *Calf Raise*

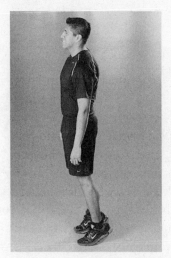

Stand with the feet apart, good posture, and the head up. Slowly raise up on your toes, then lower your heels to the floor and repeat.

▶ *Leg Extension*

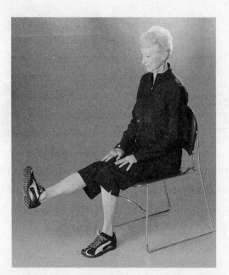

In a sitting position with good posture, extend one leg out. Return the foot to the floor and repeat with the other leg.

ABDOMINALS

▶ *Crunch*

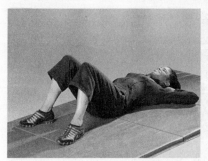
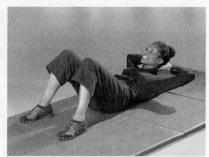

Place your hands behind your head. Tighten your abdomen and raise your shoulders and upper back off the floor. Keep your head and neck in line with your spine. Keep the same space between your chin and chest. Lower back down and repeat.

▶ *Reverse Crunch*

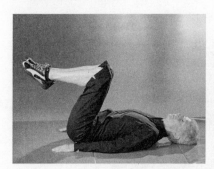
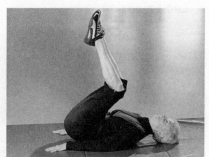

With your knees bent about 90 degrees, tighten your abdominals and curl your hips up until the lower back is off the floor. Use the abdominal muscles to lift, not momentum or your body weight. Return to the starting position and repeat.

▶ *Oblique Crunch*

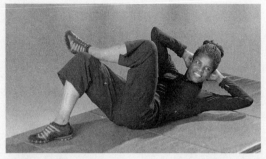

Place your hands behind your head. Put your left ankle across your right knee. Tighten the abdomen and twist your right shoulder toward the left knee. The goal is not to touch your elbow to the opposite knee. Keep good form and think about the abdominal muscles contracting. Repeat on the other side.

UPPER BODY

▶ *Biceps Curl (Dumbbells)*

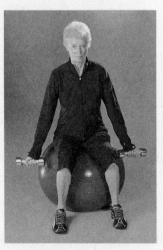 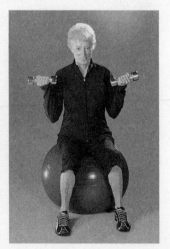

Hold the weights at your sides with your palms forward. Curl your arms toward your shoulders. Keep your elbows at your side and bend just at the elbow joint.

▶ *Biceps Curl (Resistance Tube)*

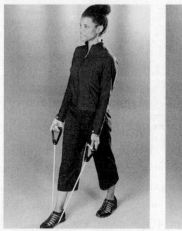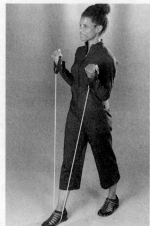

Anchor the resistance tube under your front foot in a stride stance. With palms forward, curl your arms toward your shoulders. Keep your elbows in at your side and move just at the elbow joint.

▶ *Triceps Extension (Dumbbells)*

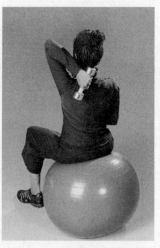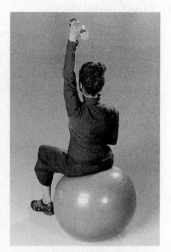

Extend one arm up above your head. Slowly lower the weight behind your head to the upper back. Repeat with the other arm.

▶ Triceps Extension (Resistance Tube)

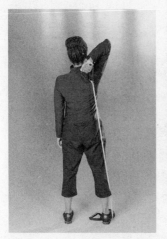 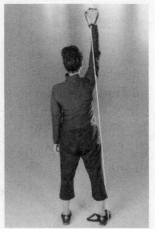

Place your feet shoulder width apart, with one foot on the end of the tube. Raise the tube up behind you until your hand is near your shoulder blade, your elbow is up, and your arm is by your ear. Straighten the arm up, keeping the arm by the ear and bending only at the elbow joint. Do not press out in front of you. Repeat with the other arm.

▶ Shoulder Shrugs (Dumbbells)

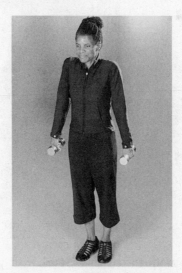

Assume a comfortable stance with your knees slightly bent, and the arms straight, raise your shoulders as high as possible. Repeat.

▶ *Shoulder Shrugs (Resistance Tube)*

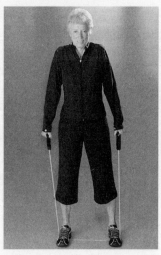

Place the tube under both feet with your legs shoulder width apart, the knees slightly bent, and the arms straight. Raise your shoulders as high as possible and repeat.

▶ *Overhead Press (Dumbbells)*

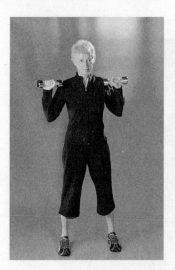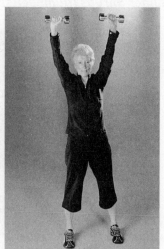

Bring the weights up to shoulder level with your palms forward. Press the weights straight up to extend your arms. Repeat.

▶ *Overhead Press (Resistance Tube)*

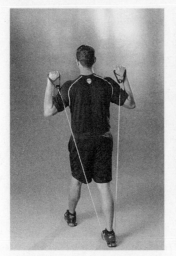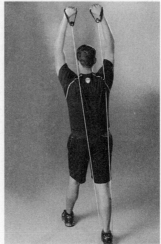

In a stride stance, place the tube under your back foot. Distribute your weight evenly on both feet. Bring the tube behind your body and up to your shoulders for the starting position. Lift your arms straight up overhead, keeping them in line with the body. Repeat.

▶ *Side Raise (Dumbbells)*

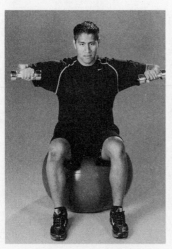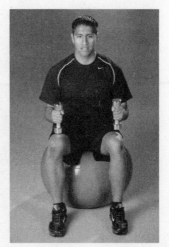

Hold your elbows at a 90 degree angle. Raise the hands and elbows level to your shoulder and parallel to the floor. Return to the 90 degree angle and repeat.

▶ *Side Raise (Resistance Tube)*

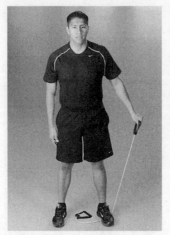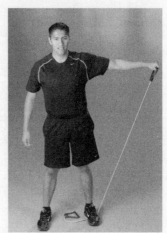

Place your feet shoulder width apart, with one foot on the end of the tube. Face your palm toward the body and lift the tube out to the side. Raise the arm only until it is parallel to floor. If you cannot lift the tube up to parallel, go to where you are comfortable and work up from there. Repeat with the other arm.

▶ *Front Raise (Dumbbells)*

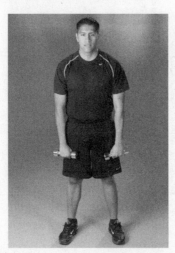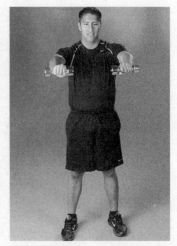

Put your feet shoulder width apart with the knees slightly bent. Place the arms in front of the body with palms facing down. Keep the elbows straight and slowly raise the weights parallel to the floor. Return to the starting position and repeat.

▶ *Front Raise (Resistance Tube)*

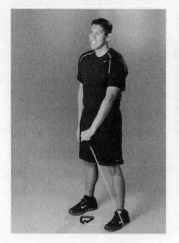 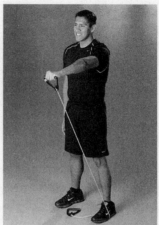

Place your feet shoulder width apart with one foot on the end of the tube. Face the palm toward the body and lift the tube out in front of the body. Raise the arm only until parallel to floor. If you cannot lift the tube up to parallel, go to where you are comfortable and work up from there. Repeat with the other arm.

▶ *Push-Up (Standing with Chair or Wall)*

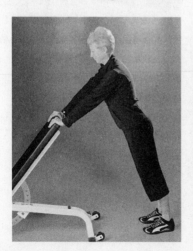 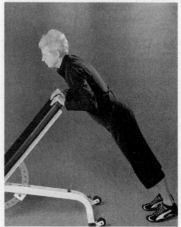

Using a wall or chair, keep your back straight and slowly lower your body down, then push your weight back up. Repeat.

▶ *Push-Up (Modified)*

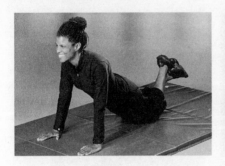 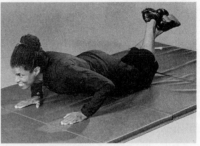

Start with your knees on the floor, back straight, and arms fully extended. Now lower your body toward the floor, and then press back up. Repeat.

▶ *Push-Up*

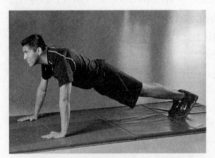 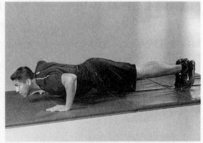

Keeping your back straight, fully extend your arms and lower your body to the floor, then press back up. Repeat.

▶ *Upright Row (Dumbbells)*

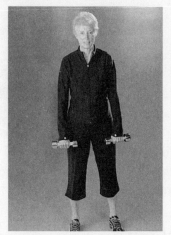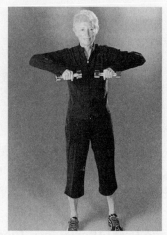

Stand with your feet shoulder width apart and the knees slightly bent. Place your arms in front of the body with the palms facing down and weights close together. Lift the weights to chest level, leading with your elbows. Repeat.

▶ *Upright Row (Resistance Tube)*

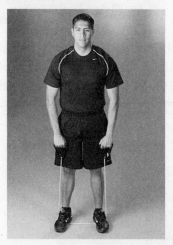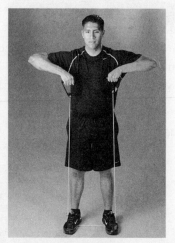

Stand on the tube with the feet shoulder width apart and knees slightly bent. Place your arms in front of the body with the palms facing down and shoulder width apart. Raise your hands to chest level, leading with your elbows. Repeat.

▶ *Bench Press (Dumbbells)*

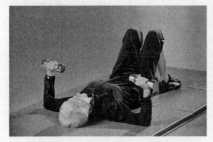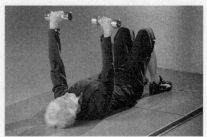

Lie on the floor or a weight bench with the arms forming a 90 degree angle at the elbows. Straighten the elbows as you lift the weights up. Return to the 90 degree angle and repeat.

▶ *Bench Press (Resistance Tube)*

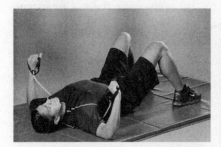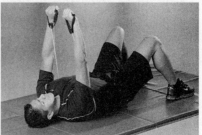

Lie on the floor or a weight bench with the tube under the back and arms forming a 90 degree angle at the elbows. Straighten the elbows as you lift the tube up. Return to the 90 degree angle and repeat.

▶ *Back Extension*

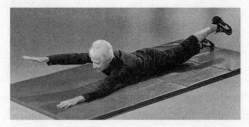

While lying on your stomach, place your arms and legs out as straight as possible. Lift the opposite arm and leg. Alternate sides.

READY FOR MORE?

●

FOR more examples of strength training routines, go to our website (www.diabetesmiracle.org).

Intermittent Training

The last of the four pillars of the LCA activity plan is intermittent training (IT). The basic premise of IT is simple: Your heart is a muscle, and IT is the best way to "weight-lift your heart," to make it stronger.

We're going to make a bold claim here: We believe that IT is *the* key to increasing physical activity among sedentary Americans. IT is a *non-continuous* activity that incorporates an active-rest period for a fraction of every minute of moderate activity.[46] Benefits from IT come after only moderate intensity[47] and short intervals of physical activity with rest.[48] You make your body work a little, then you let it rest a little, then you make it work again, and so on. You do this by exerting to five heartbeats above your target heart rate and then rest to five heartbeats below your target heart rate. *Active rest* means you don't stop your activity completely; you just slow it down enough to rest. For example, you jog, then you walk (you don't *stop*), then you jog again.

You might assume that during those rest periods, you'll be pretty much wasting your time. But our own research and the research of others support what we've experienced clinically and what people who practice IT report: You get equivalent aerobic benefits if you *rest* for part of each minute as do those who practice the old-fashioned continuous aerobic exercise.

You get the same health benefits if you rest during your activity as those who don't rest.

And you get *added benefits*, too—big ones: Dr. Harold Mayer and Dr. David DeRose, former colleagues at LCA, determined that with IT you get *greater* weight loss and *greater* body fat loss, too.[49] And it's been proven that IT activities are more appealing, more rewarding, and easier to maintain for most people than continuous "No pain, no gain" exercise.[50]

It's important to consider how people *feel* about the physical activity that doctors, the government, and health organizations recommend they do. It's also very important to consider the *disease-specific effects* of physical activity:[51] People with diabetes are different from people with other challenges or with no challenges at all. The research we've done in the medical, fitness, and behavioral health departments of LCA has shown that attitudes significantly change toward physical activity when *rest* is interposed with exercise. This is especially true of people who've been sedentary, people with diabetes, people who are overweight, and the elderly.[52] Those who do IT aerobic activities report that they like it better, find it easier, and are more likely to maintain it, as contrasted to those who do more traditional activities, such as continuous aerobic exercise. Again, physiological measures demonstrate significant and equivalent fitness improvement for both groups, *even though exercise quantity was significantly less for the IT exercise technique.* Just one example: People who do IT activities demonstrate a significant drop in resting heart rate after their 18 days with us.[53]

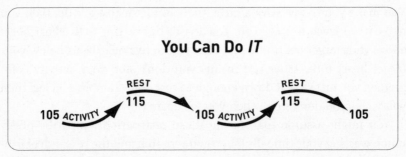

You Can Do *IT*

Intermittent training (IT) means that you work within a heart rate range of 10 beats per minute (bpm). For example, if your target heart rate is 110 bpm, you would work in a range of 105 to 115 bpm. You work until you reach the top of the range, then rest (slow down but don't stop) until you reach the bottom of the range, then start working again. This is called the active-rest *method.*

Why IT Works

Energy for activity comes from two basic metabolic sources: oxygen metabolism (aerobic) and muscle metabolism (anaerobic).[54] Anaerobic fitness requires large bursts of energy in very short periods of time: Sprinting or heavy-lifting would qualify. The intensity of the activity exceeds the ability of the heart and lungs to get oxygen (O_2) to the muscles being worked. Anaerobic activity builds strength. But it's how fit your body is *aerobically* that's the gold standard of health, fitness, and well-being. This is where IT comes in, because practicing IT, with its periods of rest after working at a high intensity, prevents the body from metabolizing anaerobically. Intermittent training keeps the workout in the aerobic zone. That means any oxygen debt accumulated during the hard parts of the activity is paid back during the rest intervals.

Why is this important? Well, for one thing, it's *easier* to work aerobically than anaerobically. If we gave you a choice of climbing a mountain with or without the aid of oxygen, you'd go with the oxygen, because a little air onboard would certainly make that activity easier. But aerobic activities are also *less painful*, and, therefore, easier to stick to for the long run. Here's why.

Anaerobic activities use glycogen, the form of sugar stored within muscle cells. Using glycogen generates a syrupy, liquid byproduct called *lactic acid*, or lactate, which in simple terms is the stuff that causes burning muscles during strenuous physical activity, decreases fat metabolism, and even contributes to lack of motivation.[55] When your workout is too intense (too hard or too long) your body bypasses the aerobic phase, in which it burns fat, and burns glycogen instead, producing lactic acid. The less fat you burn, the less weight you lose. Again, intense physical exertion produces large amounts of lactate, especially in previously sedentary people. The more inactive you've been, the more it will hurt or burn your muscles if you suddenly start a vigorous activity. Researchers have found that inactive people accumulate lactate (indicating anaerobic metabolism) even when they're only moderately active.[56] We believe that increased amounts of lactate—in addition to causing bad physical sensations—negatively influences people's *attitude* toward physical exertion. So, slow down, and forget that "No pain, no gain" myth. Yes, you're eventually going to have to raise the intensity level of your activity to get good cardiovascular benefits and meaningful weight loss, but with IT, you'll always get to rest as soon as that burn is about to occur. The experience of IT will give you a desire to keep active.[57] Over time, we want you to increase your aerobic capacity. But if you always stay in the aerobic range, without tipping over into the anaerobic zone, you will get the best results for weight loss and diabetes moderation.

Before You Begin IT

Before you get going on this part of the activity plan, you're going to need to do some easy prep work to set your IT *target heart rate* (THR) zone.

STEP 1: LEARNING HOW TO TAKE YOUR PULSE

The pulse rate indicates the frequency at which your heart is pumping. Learning to count your own pulse is a very positive step toward becoming active in your own healthcare. Pulse monitoring is especially important when performing physical activities or undertaking any new activity, so that you do not overtax your heart. It's also a good way to periodically check your progress: In general, the slower your pulse rate during complete rest (first thing in the morning, for example), the better shape you're in.

Count your pulse at regular intervals to determine the intensity of your activity. Find your pulse quickly to get a fair representation of your working heart rate. Count your pulse for 10 seconds and multiply this number by 6 (when you count, remember that first beat is 0, a "reference beat").

Two common places where you can probably feel your pulse easily are at the:

- Wrist (radial artery), located at the base of either thumb and best felt by the pads (not tips) of two or three fingers of the opposite hand. Pressing the artery too hard may cut off the pulse, whereas a light but firm pressure should allow you to feel it well.
- Neck (carotid artery), found on either side of the windpipe. It's one of the largest arteries in the body and one of the most easily felt. It's probably easiest to feel this artery by placing both the index and middle fingers just to the side of the windpipe. Don't press both carotid arteries at the same time—or press either one too hard—as this can cause you to faint. Feel only one carotid artery in the middle of the neck for accurate pulse counts. Use your finger, not your thumb. Don't press the carotid near the jawbone, as this can stimulate nerves that slow the heart rate.

The "techno-pulse" is the one you get after purchasing a heart rate monitor, a fairly cheap transmitter device you strap around your chest. You read your heart rate on a watch that continuously picks up the signal.

STEP 2: FINDING YOUR TARGET HEART RATE AND IT TRAINING ZONE

There are complicated methods and mathematical formulas available to determine your target heart rate (THR) and IT training zone. For those who want to use these more scientific and complex methods, you'll find instructions on our website (www.diabetesmiracle.org).

But we want you to just get moving—right now. So we have a very simple way to do that, beginning at a target heart rate we think nearly all can safely use. To get your personal THR, subtract your age in years from 220. Then take that number and multiply it by 0.65. This is your target heart rate. Your IT training zone will be between 5 beats lower and 5 beats higher than your target heart rate. Use the following table to find your target heart rate and IT training zone based on your age (round off your age to the closest 5-year level).

YOUR TARGET HEART RATE AND IT TRAINING ZONE

AGE	TARGET HEART RATE	IT TRAINING ZONE
30	124	119–129
35	120	115–125
40	117	112–122
45	114	109–119
50	111	106–116
55	107	102–112
60	104	99–109
65	101	96–106
70	98	93–103

Because this is such a simple method of determining your target heart rate and training zone, it may not work ideally for some people. For example, if your resting heart rate is quite high (85 or above, for example), you may get into your calculated training zone with very minimal exertion. However, as you become more conditioned, even by doing small amounts of exertion, your resting heart rate will go down, and it will take you longer to reach your training zone. Also, certain medications, such as beta blockers (propranolol, metoprolol, and most medications that end in *-olol*) can slow your heart rate response to activity, and you will achieve your training zone only with larger levels of physical exertion. We recommend you consult your physician to determine your initial THR zone if you are taking beta-blocker medication or if you are older than age 70.

RATE OF PERCEIVED EXERTION

The rate of perceived exertion (RPE) is another method to determine how hard you feel you're working during your activity—and with no math! It's a simple scale from 0 to 10, with each number corresponding to a rating of how you feel about your *total* physical stress, effort, and fatigue: from "nothing at all" (0) to "extremely strong" (10). It turns out that the RPE, although it's subjective, correlates pretty well to your actual heart rate, rate of oxygen consumption, and lactic acid accumulation—in other words, you pretty much know the intensity of your workout.[58]

Rating of Perceived Exertion (RPE)

```
0 . . . . . . . . . . Nothing at all
0.3
0.5 . . . . . . . . . . Extremely weak
0.7
1 . . . . . . . . . . . . Very weak
1.5
2 . . . . . . . . . . . . . .Weak
2.5
3 . . . . . . . . . . . . . . . . .Moderate
4
5 . . . . . . . . . . . . . . . . . . . Strong
6
7 . . . . . . . . . . . . . . . . . . . . . Very strong
8
9
10 . . . . . . . . . . . . . . . . . . . . . . .Extremely strong
11 . . . . . . . . . . . . . . . . . . . . . . . . . . Absolute maximal
```

You can do intermittent training using the RPE by working within a zone from about number 3 on the scale to about number 5. Go up to 5, then down to 3, then up again.

ADJUSTING YOUR TRAINING INTENSITY

●

TO work out at the right intensity, we recommend updating your training level periodically. Performing your activity at the right intensity will help you progress safely and efficiently, with maximal results. Documenting your progress will motivate you to continue on a regular activity plan. When you find you've become too comfortable at your training intensity, it's probably time to upgrade your workout plan.

- Set a goal to work out 5 or 6 days a week.
- Gradually increase the amount of time you're working out each day, up to 60 minutes a day.
- Once you are working for 1 hour, 5 to 6 days a week, raise your training zone 5 beats per minute. Use the RPE to assess whether the new range is too much or too little, and make adjustments accordingly. (Instructions for a more accurate and scientific method of increasing your training intensity, which takes your age and resting heart rate into account, are available on our website, www.diabetesmiracle.org.)
- Spend at least 2 weeks at each 5 percent increase. You will eventually want to work up to 60 to 75 percent. Any more than that, you'll risk going anaerobic and losing some benefits.

Putting Your Training Zone to Work

Once you know your training zone, you can start your activity. IT is designed for use with cardiovascular (aerobic) activities that are rhythmic and repetitive and use large muscle groups: walking, jogging, running, swimming, cross-country skiing, rowing, stair-stepping, elliptical training, and so on. Warm up for a few minutes, then begin building up to your zone. If you get tired, slow down, then increase your intensity again until you get to 5 beats per minute above your THR. Slow down again (don't stop completely, just work at about half the intensity) until you get down to the low number again, 5 beats below your THR. Until your endurance builds, you will get to your THR rather quickly. Depending on your age and physical condition, it might take 30 seconds to a couple of minutes to get your heart rate back down to the low end of the 10-beat range. When doing IT properly, it should take 30 to 60 seconds to get your heart rate back up to the high end of the 10-beat range. Don't let your heart rate go back up more quickly than this. As you practice IT, you'll start to get fitter fast.

After a while you'll notice that it's taking longer to get up to the high end of the zone and shorter for your heart rate to drop to the low end of the zone. Don't get discouraged. This means you're getting healthier! Your heart muscle is stronger and better able to cope with the activity. Eventually, you may find it's just too easy to get up to the high end of your training zone; then it's time to bump up your zone by 5 points. In other words, if you're working in a heart rate training zone of 100 to 110, you should move up to 105 to 115.

How Often Should You Do IT?

The fact is, any good physical activity if done consistently begins to train your metabolism to burn energy better, all the time—even when you're resting. The fitter you are, the fitter you tend to stay, as long as you keep up with it. We recommend you practice IT at least three times a week to start, for 30 to 60 minutes a day. This time doesn't count strolling, stretching, or strength training, either: just your IT workout. Remember you can break that time up throughout the day, though, and accumulate the same benefits.[59]

Every bit of calorie-burning activity can help; but if weight loss is your goal, we're certainly not convinced that everyday living or even doing IT three times a week will be sufficient for you to see real results. Assuming you don't change your diet much, doing your IT activity only three times a week is likely to merely *maintain* your current health and weight (and keep your blood sugars moderately down during and briefly after your workout). That's a start, but don't expect to lose any weight or gain meaningful cardiovascular improvements or drops in cholesterol unless you can get active five to six times a week for up to 60 minutes. If you have diabetes and if you've been a couch potato (or "mouse" potato if the computer's your poison) you should endeavor to build up to a 5- to 6-day activity regimen. After you're at your ideal weight and fitness level, you can ease up and do a maintenance program three to four times a week.

If that seems exhausting, consider putting your stair stepper, treadmill, or elliptical trainer machine in front of the TV. There are several studies out there showing that the more you watch TV, the less you get physically active (and the fatter you get),[61] but this is a great way to buck that trend: You burn calories, and you don't have to give up your favorite show. It's much easier to work out for 60 minutes when you're watching a good show or movie.

BONUS ENERGY BURNERS!
●

NONEXERCISE activity thermogenesis (NEAT) is the energy used by everything you do except eating, sleeping, and dedicated exercise. This includes your job, relaxation activities, and everything else you do during everyday living: talking, walking, standing, sitting, shopping, stair climbing, even the energy required for fidgeting. NEAT energy actually accounts for more energy expenditure than dedicated exercise, even for exercise junkies.[60] It's important, therefore, that you choose more active ways of living your daily life. Take the stairs rather than the elevator; park farther away and walk into the restaurant even if there's a drive-through window (better yet, don't eat anywhere that has a drive-through); use a push mower and don't buy a lawn tractor; shovel snow by hand and leave the snow blower in the garage; wash dishes by hand instead of using the dishwasher. The burning of these little bits of energy will add up.

MIXING IT UP A BIT

IT'S AMAZING HOW creative we can get when it comes to excuses for slowing down or stopping our physical activity. Getting active can at first be very invigorating. But after a while, you might find it difficult to get jazzed about your morning walk or your visit to the gym after work. Even the most dedicated fitness fiends occasionally get bored with their routine. If you find your enthusiasm waning or if you find yourself cutting your workouts short, your activity plan is probably getting stale. Here are a few ideas to help you get reinvigorated about getting active.

The Quick Fix

Evaluate your current routine to determine what really bores you. A new variation on your favorite activity—such as kickboxing instead of step aerobics or hoisting free weights instead of working on machines—may be enough to reinvigorate your monotonous routine. If you've been logging miles on a treadmill, stair climber, or stationary bike, you could try to move your workout outside for a welcome change of scenery. Run, hike, or bike on trails; swim in a lake or the ocean.

Bigger Changes

When tweaking your routine isn't enough, try taking up an entirely new activity, especially something you never thought you'd do. If you've always stuck to solitary pursuits, why not sign up for a team sport, such as volleyball, basketball, or doubles tennis? Or tackle something you've always shied away from: Indulge your thirst for adventure with a rock-climbing class (start on an indoor wall, then move to the real thing as your skills improve). What about the trampoline? You're never too old! New activities have the dual benefit of keeping you excited and providing slightly different health advantages. For example, some recent research[62] on Alpine hikers made the intriguing discovery that the different physiology involved in the distinct phases of hiking had different effects on fats and sugars in the blood. In particular, going uphill cleared fats from the blood faster, but going *downhill* reduced blood sugar more.

Good Company

Working out alone can be an oasis of solitude during an otherwise busy, stressful day, but some people find they need company to stay motivated. Activity companions add a social element to any routine. Ask a friend to be your workout partner—you'll be less likely to skip a workout if someone is waiting for you. Or consider a four-legged friend. If you consistently make your dog part of your activity plan, it will become a habit that's good for both of you.

Just about every sport or activity has a club, too. To find one, ask around at gyms or community centers. Remember, it's not about competition; but having said that, keeping up with the crowd also means you'll be challenged to improve your skills, as any marathon runner can attest.

Goal Setting

Many people work out simply to stay in shape, and most of the time that's just fine. But sometimes it helps to have a specific goal to work toward. Maybe you want to complete a rough-water swim or climb your state's highest mountain. A goal like this can give your daily workouts more meaning. You can start by incorporating bursts of speed into your workouts. After a gentle warm-up, alternate a fast pace with a slower one for recovery. This can be as simple as sprinting to the next tree, or as structured as running intervals on a track or sprinting laps in the pool, both IT activities.

Add Variety

Elite triathletes pioneered the popular cross-training concept, and it works for the rest of us, too. If you usually focus on one activity, substitute another a few days a week. Ideally, any activity plan includes elements of cardiovascular activity, weight training, and flexibility.

New Toys

Exercise gadgets aren't necessary, but they can make your workouts more fun and challenging. Heart-rate monitors, aquatic toys, music, and safety equipment are just a few items to consider. Find out which new training doodads are available for your favorite activity.

Innovate

Don't use your creativity to come up with novel excuses—use it for novel solutions. Dr. James Levine, an obesity researcher at the Mayo Clinic in Rochester, Minnesota, rigged his desk so he could walk on a treadmill while reading his e-mail, taking calls, and working on his computer. Soon, 10 other employees got the modified workstation, too.[63] The staff walks 1 mile per hour on their treadmills, burning about 100 calories each mile, which adds up to 30 or 40 pounds a year!

PUTTING IT ALL TOGETHER

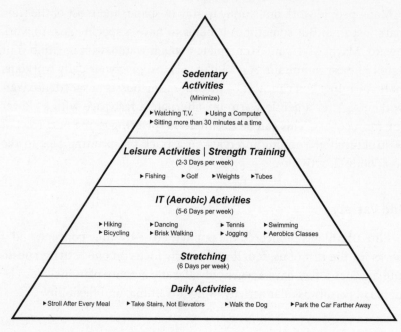

Lifestyle Center of America's activity plan

The activity pyramid shown in the figure here can serve as a reminder of when and how often to practice each of the four pillars of the LCA activity plan:

- Strolling: every day
- Stretching: 6 days a week
- Strength training: every other day
- Intermittent training: 5 to 6 days a week

Keeping Track of Your Progress

And finally, but certainly no less important, we suggest you create and maintain a regular log to track your progress. See Appendix 1 for examples and how you can get ready-made log sheets.

9

Secrets to Long-Term Success

LONNIE CARBAUGH, BEHAVIOR health director at Lifestyle Center of America (LCA), fights daily alongside our patients on the front lines of the emotional battle that is life with diabetes. About half of the patients with diabetes who come to LCA are suffering some form of depression or other emotional challenge related to their disease—and *suffering* really is the right word. This statistic correlates well with other studies that show high rates of depressive symptoms in people with diabetes, across ethnic lines:[1] Depression rates among people with diabetes are about double that of the general population. Lifestyle medicine is perfectly suited to deal with these issues; and in the last decade, we've honed an approach that we believe can set people with diabetes free from many of the mental and spiritual problems commonly associated with diabetes.

In this chapter, we'll present simple, everyday self-help tools for maximizing your potential for following and sticking to the 30-Day Diabetes Miracle program and for achieving great overall health by overcoming the most common mental obstacles, such as food addictions, inertia, and defeatist ("victim") thinking about disease. We'll also review common threads among our patients who've maintained their tight blood sugar control and weight loss and stayed on a plant-based diet (PBD) and intermittent training (IT) regimen for the long term. The secrets to endurance lie in understanding our choices and their likely consequences, in an awareness of our natural rhythms, in an ownership spirit, in a support network, in an attitude of gratitude, and in the mastery of the motivational triad—a life-altering principle we'll explain in detail right off the bat. We've found that people with diabetes who learn strategies for reducing anxiety, anger, fear, and emotional and physical fatigue tend to do much better, so we'll outline how you can start on that positive path today. As peak performance consultant, and dedicated vegetarian, Anthony Robbins says, "The road to success is always under construction."[2]

THE MOTIVATIONAL TRIAD

AS YOU KNOW, there's a lot more to living with diabetes than blood sugar levels and insulin. Much of your success in conquering your disease will take place not in your pancreas, but in your brain. Preventing or treating insulin resistance through weight loss and physical activity certainly does improve cognitive function.[3] But another critical component to achieving the miracle in the 30-Day Diabetes Miracle program is learning to deal with the emotional, spiritual, and cognitive aspects of diabetes self-healing.

Let's start with some valuable questions:

- Why do we do the things we do?
- Why do we eat the way we do when we know that it's often not good for us?
- Why don't we get more active when we know it will improve our health?
- Why do we seek magic-bullet solutions to problems that we intuitively know require time and energy to resolve?
- Why do we often ignore serious health issues?

Would you be surprised to learn that there actually *are* answers to these painful questions? And those answers are so simple and practical that they can change your life profoundly if you put them into practice? And you can start today—right now! The answers are based on a fascinating concept called the motivational triad, described brilliantly by Douglas Lisle and Alan Goldhamer in their book *The Pleasure Trap*.[4] The motivational triad is a key to human (and animal!) behavior and human emotions that we've found indispensable in helping people with diabetes live to the utmost. It helps us understand the very basics of what leads us to do the things we do. The motivational triad concept of human behavior is as simple as one, two, three:

1. We seek pleasure.
2. We avoid pain.
3. We conserve energy.

This system is embedded into the genetic design of all humans, indeed all complex animals that ever lived. Everything we want, and don't want, is motivated by these three factors: pleasure seeking, pain avoidance, and conservation of energy. Lisle and Goldhamer put it this way: Why does the shark eat? He eats because of the pleasure of eating and to avoid the pain of hunger. And he eats efficiently. He's hard-wired to respond to the smell of blood because an injured fish (or unfortunate surfer) is relatively easy to hunt and kill for food. Why go through all the trouble of chasing healthy, vigorous prey?

That's all well and good for the beasts of the sea or the Serengeti, but what about the rest of us who are more highly developed? It's true that humans are complex, multidimensional beings. But though it seems like an oversimplification, it really is true: The motivational triad works for us, too, all the time:

- *Someone goes to work.* The bottom line is he believes that more money will provide the spoils that will give him a more *pleasurable* life and help him *avoid the pain* of feeling impoverished.
- *Someone strives to be healthy.* She doesn't want to live the next 50 to 75 years suffering from chronic illness. What she really wants is to live a long time, and feel good along the way, so she can be with her family, see her kids and grandkids grow up, travel the world, and bring her fondest dreams to fruition. These are all things that would bring her *pleasure* and help her *avoid pain.*
- *Someone gets married.* He wants the *pleasure* of loving and being loved, companionship, intimacy, comfort, and security. Plus he believes marriage will help him *avoid the pain* of being lonely. Nobody wants to get into a bad, loveless marriage. People want to live happily ever after.
- *Someone goes on a diet.* She may say it's because she wants to

feel and look better. That means she's experiencing *pain* (either physical, emotional, or both) she'd rather avoid, and she wants to get more *pleasure* out of her life—pleasure she believes will come with weight loss.

Simple, but true. All of us will pursue pleasure and run from pain. And we will do so in an energy-efficient manner, nearly every time. Everyone's heard of "love at first sight." Does anyone talk about "love at one-hundredth sight?" That's not a very energy-efficient way of achieving the pleasure of a long-term relationship. Does anyone advertise "get rich slowly" schemes? Rarely. The most sought-after ways to achieve the supposed pleasure of wealth are by winning the lottery, inheriting money, or otherwise jumping the queue. Same again with weight loss. Can you imagine a TV commercial marketing a weight-loss solution that promises—guarantees!—that you'll lose 1 pound a month? Nobody would buy. That would take too much effort, too much time, *too much energy*. The irony of this mentality is that time will pass anyway, one month after another. If you had a choice to be the same weight in 2 years or 24 pounds lighter, wouldn't you choose the latter?

The motivational triad makes sense: In the natural world, those things that *feel* good usually bring about good results. We're designed in such a way that sex feels good, and that's a good thing, because it's good for us to "be fruitful and multiply." Eating feels good, too, and it's good to get energy to live another day (another day to be fruitful!). Both food and sex are biological imperatives: They're fundamentally necessary for us to continue as a species, so they both feel good to get and lousy to forgo. Good plan, right? Sure, as long as you don't confuse the system with something like a chocolate cannoli. Or cocaine. These things, and other addictive substances, including caffeine, alcohol, and nicotine, are so alluring to us because of a trick they play on the motivational triad:

- *They give us pleasure.* They feel good, so our brains think they are good, and we seek more.
- *They help us avoid pain.* They give us a temporary stay against the feeling of deprivation or they mask other painful feelings we may be experiencing. At the worst, they drug us into stupefaction—an unawareness of our real feelings—or give us a high from an artificial feeling of well-being.

■ *They provide these benefits with very little effort* (a bite, a toke, a swig, a shot) so the energy-conservation feature of the motivational triad is also at play.

Obtaining gratification and pleasure quickly and easily can fool the brain into thinking we have succeeded biologically, and we seek out more of whatever it was that gave us that pleasure "high." These deceptively good feelings short-circuit our normal neurochemical reaction, disrupting our normal pleasure-seeking behaviors. Unfortunately, the things in our lives that would normally give us pleasure no longer do so. This is the reason why it might still seem to you that a chocolate bar or a slab of cake will always give you more pleasure than even the perfect salad.

Sometimes, we must learn not to trust our instincts about what we want, what feels good, what we think we need. There's startling evidence for how easy it is to deceive the motivational triad: If you get male pigeons hooked on cocaine, they will start preferring the good feelings of cocaine to the good feelings of sex (which, of course, means they'll stop reproducing and the species would die out, surely a bad decision). Similarly, when you give lab rats access to both cocaine and food, they consume the coke ravenously, ignoring the food entirely, because the good feelings are much more intense with coke. But without food, the animals die.[5]

Putting the Motivational Triad to Work

Once we realize that our basic motivation for what we do involves just three factors, we can then begin to use the motivational triad to intelligently make good things happen for us and achieve long-term success. For example, let's start with the realization that there are at least three ways we can look at finding pleasure in our lives:

■ We can look for *immediate gratification*. We seem to be hardwired to do this, and our energy-conservation circuits love to take over all other motivators. Just look at drug, food, or sex addiction. We enjoy the immediate pleasure of a cigarette or feel the near-instantaneous rush of indulging our appetite for a highfat, high-sugar food (make no mistake about it, that doughnut alerts the same brain chemicals—dopamine, endorphins, serotonin—that make you feel good as do heroin and sex).[6]

■ Alternatively, we can learn to delay gratification so that we enjoy even more and more meaningful pleasure and avoid a whole lot more pain down the road. So, for instance, if we quit smoking, we will enjoy a longer life with greater health (and much more money! You could go on a very nice cruise eventually by saving that cigarette money). Or if we eat healthfully, with a thought toward tomorrow—or at least modify our eating habits so that we still enjoy our food and maintain good health—we will have more pleasure and less pain in our lives. It is interesting that eating a health-promoting diet and making progress at a worthwhile task (like changing to a PBD) can also affect some of our brain's neurotransmitters (chemicals that transfer information from one neuron to another), specifically serotonin, in a positive way,[7] giving us the same feelings of pleasure that the quick hit of sugar and fat give, with none of the negative consequences,[8] only a strong feeling of success and satisfaction.

■ We don't necessarily have to substitute short-term hedonisms for long-term gain. You just have to stick with a few new healthful behaviors long enough to experience the new kind of pleasure you'll feel, and soon this powerful pleasure will outweigh the alternative. Look at it this way: If you went down a few waist sizes or dress sizes or if you were able to walk a mile again or if you could go to bed one night knowing your blood sugar was totally under control that day, wouldn't that give you pleasure? Wouldn't that help you avoid pain? And that newfound pleasure-seeking, pain-avoidance mechanism would kick in to the point that indulging in that ice cream cone would actually seem like it might *cause* pain. People on a regular physical activity plan, like the one described in Chapter 8, know this all too well. If you start your day burning 300 calories on a stair-stepping machine, you tend to look at a 300 calorie piece of cake differently: It no longer seems like it will give you as much pleasure. Instead, you sense the pain it will cause you (it will undo that good feeling of accomplishment you had when burning the calories). It is interesting, though, that you're actually less likely to crave that junk food anyway, because your brain will have gotten a similarly satisfying high from your workout.

STRESS AND BURNOUT CAN INFLUENCE DIABETES

EVERYONE EXPERIENCES STRESS in their lives—emotional, physical, and occupational. One recent poll found that almost one fourth of all people are chronically "angry or somewhat angry" at work.[9] Day in and day out, life and our reactions to it cause physiological stress on our bodies, which can trigger the onset of disease, including diabetes.

A study done in Israel examined job burnout, which is characterized by emotional exhaustion, physical fatigue, and something called "cognitive weariness" from work; we all get that from time to time! It looked at the risk such burnout might pose for healthy workers in developing type-2 diabetes. The researchers concluded that chronic burnout was associated with a 1.84-fold increased risk of developing diabetes.[10]

Not only does work-related stress increase your risk for diabetes but emotional stress does as well. Researchers in Amsterdam did a study suggesting that better blood sugar control is associated with a better mood and better overall well-being.[11]

Remember, too, that stress often comes from the change it implies, be it positive or negative. Getting married, having a baby, even embarking on a new lifestyle can bring about a certain amount of stress if you let it.[12]

So how and why does stress cause an increased risk in diabetes? Stress results in overproduction of cortisol, a hormone that counteracts the effect of insulin and results in elevated blood sugar.[13] Over time, chronic stress affects the body's normal fat and protein processing, and reduces the body's sensitivity to insulin. Cortisol, as an insulin antagonist, makes it harder for glucose to enter cells and, therefore, raises blood sugar. Cortisol also has the nasty habit of increasing abdominal fat, which contributes to the cycle of insulin resistance. People with metabolic syndrome, a risk factor for type-2 diabetes characterized by abdominal obesity, insulin resistance, increased triglycerides, and high blood pressure, have an even greater output of cortisol.[14] If you already have diabetes, you cannot adequately metabolize the increase in blood glucose owing to lack of adequate insulin. Consequently, stress can potentially lead to chronic elevated blood sugar.

People with diabetes may be additionally stressed from coping with the disease. Daily stress can interfere with the management of diabetes and make it difficult to control. Therefore, stress management is critical to overall health—for people with diabetes to maintain glycemic control and for others to decrease the risk of developing diabetes.

The good news is that simple stress management strategies and coping-skills training work—and they can save your life. Middle-aged adults with explosive tempers are more likely than mellow people the same age to suffer from coronary heart disease–related events, such as heart attack and death.[15] Practice what Australian motivational speaker and author Matthew Kelly calls the art of slowing down: "Slow down. Breathe deeply. Reflect deeply. Pray deeply. Live deeply. Otherwise you will spend your life feeling like a bulldozer chasing butterflies or a sparrow in a hurricane."[16]

Such techniques will help you both emotionally and physically. Studies show that a group stress management program resulted in lower long-term blood sugar levels in people with type-2 diabetes.[17] Another study showed that patients with type-1 diabetes displayed improved coping techniques and lower long-term blood sugar levels after 3 months of stress management training classes.[18] Stress management along with a regimen of physical activity and regular use of relaxation techniques can help reduce stress, decrease the risk for disease, and improve overall health. Now there's even more reason to take a vacation!

Some simple ideas to relieve stress:

- Breathe deeply, hold your breath, then slowly release.
- Listen to classical music.
- Walk or pet your dog.
- Take a stroll in nature.
- Read a book.
- Meditate or pray.
- Learn and practice yoga.
- Give yourself positive affirmations ("I'm at peace, I'm balanced, I'm calm") and repeat them, visualize them, and really believe them. Inspirational radio host, publisher, and human behavior expert Earl Nightingale said, "Whatever we plant in our subconscious mind and nourish with repetition and emotion will one day become a reality."[19]
- Do IT, which will spur surges in stress-relieving endorphins, speed the release of toxins, and get more oxygen in the blood, all of which will de-stress your system.

- Avoid mood-altering substances, including caffeine, nicotine, alcohol, and sugar.
- Gently but firmly say "Stop" as soon as you start feeling stressed; then focus on the parts of your body where you're holding stress, and try to release it.[20]
- Find your own way to bring yourself peace, balance, and calm, and take time often to practice it.

If you have uncontrolled diabetes or other chronic health problems, the best way to relieve stress is to focus on bettering your health and well-being. When you begin to experience improvement, especially blood sugar control, you're naturally going to feel better.

DIABETES AND DEPRESSION

YOU MIGHT HAVE noticed that blood glucose instability can cause depression, mood swings, irritability, weariness, and fear. A recent University of California, San Francisco study showed that people who were having a grumpy day were more likely than people in a good mood to report higher than normal blood sugar levels the next morning.[21] There are a few recent studies that question the direct relationship between depression and diabetes.[22] But for centuries, research and clinical experience have shown such a link exists. More than 300 years ago, British physician Thomas Willis, the first person to recognize that glucose in the urine was a sign of diabetes, noted that there is a close relationship between depression and diabetes. In fact, Willis believed that diabetes was caused by depression.[23] It's still not clear which comes first, but the relationship between the two problems makes intuitive sense to physicians: It isn't surprising that depression would be associated with a life-changing disease such as diabetes.

But there is evidence that depression worsens chronic illness, too—and this does surprise many doctors[24] who are not prepared to deal with the whole patient instead of the disease process alone. But deal that way doctors must: Did you know people with diabetes who are also depressed have worse glycemic control?[25] They also have higher rates of chronic complications.[26] Preexisting depression can even increase the risk of subsequent development of diabetes.[27] In fact, if you have diabetes, your chances of also having depression are twice as likely as someone who does not have diabetes. Recent research by Patrick Lustman, professor of medical psychology at Washington University School of Medicine in St. Louis, notes that having depression, independent of weight gain and other factors, doubles your risk of later developing diabetes.[28]

Now, what does depression have to do with the *outcomes* of diabetes? On the surface it seems deceptively simple: Depression reduces patients' adherence to their diet, activity, and medicine regimens. This might be true for some patients, but research reveals a more complex answer. Depression can directly influence specific physiological body processes that can make diabetes worse. These include immune responses,[29] inflammation,[30] and even insulin resistance.[31] Whatever comes first, diabetes and depression are related. There is a mind-body connection that can't be denied. "Low risk of depression in diabetes? Would that it were so," writes a leading endocrinologist at Massachusetts General Hospital.[32] It seems obvious: Once diabetes complications occur, the prevalence and risk of depression increase. On the other hand, depressed people are "more prone to illness than happy people." Unhappiness "shuts down the immune system."[33]

How do you know if you're one of the 30-plus million Americans with depression?[34] If you have five or more of the following symptoms present more days than not for at least 2 weeks, and they interfere with routine daily activities such as work, self-care, childcare, or social life, then seek an evaluation for depression:[35]

- Persistent sadness or feeling empty
- Feelings of hopelessness
- Feelings of guilt, worthlessness, or helplessness
- Loss of interest or pleasure in hobbies and activities that you once enjoyed
- Decreased energy, fatigue
- Difficulty concentrating and making decisions
- Insomnia or oversleeping
- Appetite and/or weight changes
- Restlessness, irritability
- Thoughts of death or suicide (if you have this one, even if it's the *only* symptom, please get help immediately)

Don't allow depression and diabetes to defeat you. Use our easy-to-learn way to overcome depression (as well as anger, anxiety, and other "stinkin' thinkin'"). You can begin working with this plan at home, using the instructions that follow.[36]

Rational Emotive Behavior Therapy: Gateway Through Stinkin' Thinkin'

While more research might be needed to establish the exact nature of the murky relationship between the physical and mental aspects of diabetes, one thing *is* perfectly clear: In both the treatment and the prevention of diabetes, depression and the other emotional challenges associated with the condition need to be taken seriously. When it comes to depression, the news is good; it's a very treatable disorder. According to the National Institute of Mental Health, the various therapies available alleviate symptoms in more than 80 percent of those treated. Unfortunately, less than half of those who have depression get the help they need.[37]

One of the most effective treatments for depression, anxiety, and anger among people with diabetes, is a form of therapy known as cognitive behavior therapy (CBT).[38] At LCA, we've adapted and applied one of CBT's earliest and most useful forms, called rational emotive behavior therapy (REBT), which was originated in 1955 by Dr. Albert Ellis in New York. REBT starts with a very simple premise: When people are depressed or otherwise emotionally upset, they think and behave differently from when they are not depressed or emotionally upset. REBT helps people change their thinking and behavior patterns to help them overcome their mental trouble. REBT can also be used educationally to help in the prevention of depression, anger, fear, and anxiety.

RATIONAL EMOTIVE BEHAVIOR THERAPY

●

Rational = the way we *think* and reason
Emotive = the way we *feel*
Behavior = the way we *act*
Therapy = the way we *heal* ourselves and get better

We find REBT works particularly well for easing depression. When we include REBT as part of the program for our LCA patients with mild to severe depression, the vast majority show significant improvement by the time they leave.

The best part is that this sort of miraculous success doesn't require massive time or intensive therapy. After you learn a few basic principles, you can do REBT on your own, at home, a little bit every day. It doesn't work overnight. It's not a cure-all. But it is remarkably simple, adaptable, and effectual.

The 10 Principles of Successful Thinking

Here are 10 principles of successful thinking that we've adapted from expert teachings on REBT and from our experience helping thousands of patients deal with depression and diabetes.

1
It's All in Your Head

To feel better and to be mentally healthier, better able to cope, and happier, you have to grasp that past traumas and disappointments don't much matter. In fact, even the specific sources of your present stress, anxiety, fear, and depression are not very important. It doesn't really matter what kind of relationship you had with your mother when you were a child, whether your boss is mean to you, or if people cut you off on the highway. Instead, what matters in REBT is how you think about these and other things, how you respond to these and other things.

Frankly, it's all in your head—and you have a choice in most cases about how you organize, judge, and act according to that which is in your head. After all, it is your head. No matter how or when you got into the habit of thinking and believing the things you do, it is up to you whether or not you choose to continue thinking in that manner.

Please be assured that we don't say "it's all in your head" to blame you for unhealthy thinking. REBT is more concerned with whether your thinking is helping you achieve what you want in life (the pursuit of pleasure, the avoidance of pain, and the conservation of energy) or whether your thinking is holding you back or otherwise causing you suffering.

And, of course, we recognize that if you have just had your legs amputated, your bad feelings are in both your head and your legs. The important thing to know is that only one of those things can be changed. You can't bring your legs back. But you *can* change what's in your head, so you should focus there. You can choose to feel victimized and worthless based on your situation—or you can accept the reality of the circumstances and move on. Consider the famous Serenity Prayer, written by theologian Reinhold Niebuhr and adopted in the 1940s by Alcoholics Anonymous: "God, grant me the serenity to accept things I cannot change, the courage to change the things I can, and the wisdom to know the difference." It's become a cliché, but there's a lot of truth in that.

The idea of the power of positive thinking, as posited by Norman Vincent Peale in the 1970s,[39] has been very appealing to millions of people. And while it's true that a positive attitude and emotional state can strengthen the body's immune system and help fight disease just as assuredly as a good diet, activity, and avoidance of drugs and alcohol,[40] positive thinking alone has its limitations. You can't bring your legs back once they've been amputated. You can't change your difficult boss (or loud kids or the obnoxious guy who cut you off on the freeway). Instead, dealing with such unpleasant things requires good, old-fashioned serenity. But you can change your reply to your cranky boss, your reaction to your feisty children, and your response to the rude driver.

We are response-able (required and able to respond) only for our part of these exchanges. We're responsible for what goes on in our own heads. It is up to you whether or not you choose to think negatively about upsetting events in your life, and as a result feel emotionally down.

2

Mind the Gap

Realize it's not your boss, your kids, that other driver, or even the tragedy of your amputated legs that are making you feel bad. Between stimulus and response, there lies a gap.[41] Human productivity expert Dr. Denis Deaton explains it elegantly in his helpful little book *The Ownership Spirit Handbook.*

Seeing a gooey piece of pie makes you want to eat it. Or noticing your blood sugar is high one evening makes you angry and disappointed in yourself for being such a failure. Your husband's snide comment about what's on your plate causes you to get sullen and have a bad time at the party. It would seem that these things are mere cause and effect. What's wrong with this interpretation? It is incorrect to assume that our environment forces us into responding in a specific way. Humans have the ability to think and to choose, and therefore we can select how we will respond to a set of circumstances.

This choosing happens in the gap between stimulus and response. That's where (or rather, when—in a fraction of a second) we can consider, select, and act, rather than simply react to the stimulus. Something happens—you see a bag of candy in your cupboard (or you just think about it). It's your favorite candy, the one you've savored since you were a toddler. What are you going to do? It might feel as if you are a slave to sweets. It might feel as though you don't really have a choice. But deep down, you know you do. There is a voice echoing out of that gap. It's just that we usually don't like to listen. All we ask is that before you reach immediately for the candy—pause, just for a second, in that gap. This will prevent you from simply reacting mindlessly. It will encourage you to listen to your voice of choice. It's choice that separates humans from other creatures: You think, therefore you are.

If in the end you take the candy, just make sure it's a real decision.

3
Activation–Belief–Consequence

Going a little deeper, realize what usually happens in that gap between stimulus and response. What happens has to do with what we believe and what we say to ourselves. We call this the *ABCs of Our Emotions*.[42] Developed by Ellis, the ABCs are a mainstay of REBT and all forms of CBT.

- A = *activating event*: A stressor, bad memory, or other unpleasant situation we encounter (it could also be a good memory or pleasant experience).
- B = *our belief system*: What we tell ourselves silently about what the activating event "means"; this has to do with how we judge the activating event (as good, bad, or something else).
- C = *consequences*: The emotional and behavioral response to the activating event, filtered through our belief system; for example, anxiety, anger, depression, fear, serenity, gratitude, or joy.

The key here is that it's our beliefs, along with what we tell ourselves based on those beliefs, that really cause the feelings we have. This all happens in the gap between the activating event (the stimulus) and the consequence (response). It's not your spouse. It's not your lawn mower. It's not the war, the economy, or the world making you feel the way you do. It's all in your head. If you understand what we have just said, you won't be offended. If you are offended by our assertion, please read this section again: It is all in your head.

At this point we find it's helpful to work on our toxic self-talk. The first step is to understand that many challenges can be overcome by not focusing on our feelings and emotions (the consequences) so much as focusing on the messages we give ourselves—the self-talk connected to our beliefs—that fuel the feelings and emotions. Can you see in the examples that follow how our beliefs go hand in hand with our self-talk and lead to negative consequences, like emotional upset?

UNHEALTHY, IRRATIONAL, COUNTERPRODUCTIVE SELF-TALK	HEALTHY, RATIONAL, PRODUCTIVE SELF-TALK
There I go again, eating like a pig. I'm so disgusting.	I overdid it, but I'm going to stop right now, go for a stroll, and get right back on my program.
Why am I so weak willed that I can't get up and stroll after dinner?	Who says I have to feel like going for a stroll in order to do it? I can do just about anything for 5 or 10 minutes (and if I walk 5 or 10 minutes from here I'll have to walk it back as well)!
She's making me feel dumb again by using all those fancy doctor words. I'll never get control of this disease.	I don't understand what's being explained to me. I'm not a doctor, of course. I'd better ask some questions for clarification. After all, no one is an expert in everything, but I'd better learn as much as I can about my condition, because I really want to get it, and get better.
So, I'm on insulin now. Guess that means it's just a matter of time before I go blind and die.	I don't like the fact that I'm on insulin. It would behoove me to learn as much about my condition as possible and take care of myself so that I don't become more dependent on this than I have to. You know, this is a helpful wake-up call.
Well, I had that first Pop-Tart, so I might as well eat the other one now that I've ruined my diet today.	That Pop-Tart wasn't the best thing for me to eat right now, but one is better than two. I'll go for an extra stroll and be careful what I eat the rest of the day.

One more idea about combating toxic self-talk, and this one's not rocket science. Just start to say nice things to yourself, even if doesn't feel natural at first.[43] Just make sure the nice things you say to yourself motivate you to take constructive action. Such as, "I've made many really neat new choices lately. The results look great. I'm going to keep doing that." You don't want to demotivate yourself with niceties such as, "I deserve a break today, so I'm going to eat a dozen Krispy Kremes."

4

Unconditional Self-Acceptance

Stop judging yourself: Stop judging your *self*. In other words, you can look at your behaviors critically (and make necessary changes accordingly). But you should not judge your whole self (either negatively or positively). Ellis calls this *unconditional self-acceptance*, or USA. You're not a bad person because you ate a jelly doughnut. You've just behaved in a way that did not further your goal of eating healthful foods. It doesn't call into question your worth as a human being. Nor does it make the guy who cuts you off on the way home a bad person—he or she is just someone driving badly at that moment. You know it's funny; if we ever talked to our friends the way we talk to ourselves—"You fat pig!" "You lazy slob!" "You loser!"—we wouldn't have many friends left, would we? Yet we continue to go on berating ourselves with these ongoing, mean-spirited, self-defeating scripts.

Ellis puts it this way: "Accepting yourself involves acknowledging that you are a complex, ongoing, ever-changing process that defies being rated by yourself or others."[44]

USA does not come easy, especially after a lifetime of negative self-talk. You have to keep working on it, every day, for the rest of your life. "There is no magical way for you to change your personality and your strong tendencies to upset yourself," writes Ellis. "You really change with *work* and *practice*."[45] Think of it as mental fitness. It will get easier as you get mentally fitter; but if you stop practicing, you'll get flabby again and probably resort to that old stinkin' thinkin'. Remember, if you struggle with any of these principles at first, don't berate yourself for it ("I'm so stupid I can't even accept myself unconditionally"). Obviously, that would miss the point entirely!

Keep track of your progress with USA. For some more help, see Appendix 1.

5
Recognize Irrational Beliefs

Now, pause in the gap between the activating event (the stimulus) and the consequence (the response); and during that very brief time, be conscious of what you say to yourself, what self-talk scripts (beliefs) come up. We say scripts, because often we tend to repeat self-defeating talk, which continually reinvigorates unhealthy beliefs and perpetuates bad feelings: Your father yelled at you for eating too much as a child. Because it was in front of your friends, you were thinking he should never do such a thing to you. Whenever you think about that scene, you replay those feelings, tell yourself the same things, and engage in still more unhealthy thinking—such as "My father was right. I am a glutton" and "Nobody ever understands me. It started with my father, and now it's hopeless."

The secret, again, is to pause in the gap when the feelings and self-talk first come up. Listen to your mind. Try to hear what you say to yourself and figure out what triggered the thoughts. This gets to the heart of REBT, which posits that some thoughts are rational and some are irrational. Irrational beliefs are simply those that block you from achieving your goals. They fuel extreme emotions like road rage, stinging humiliation, bitter disappointment, and hopelessness. They also lead to behaviors that harm you and/or others. Irrational beliefs also tend to distort reality—they contain exaggerated or otherwise illogical ways of evaluating oneself, others, and the world. In the following irrational beliefs and toxic self-talk scripts, look for exaggerations and distortions and look for what we call *demandments* (extreme and impossible demands we place on ourselves, others, and the world):

- "You just can't run a restaurant without serving meals for vegetarians. I demand you change your menu!"
- "I must always work out 1 hour every day, or I'm a complete failure."
- "He should eat as well as I do lately. He's making all the wrong choices."
- "It's not fair that I have diabetes!"
- "This pain in my feet is just awful! The worst! I can't stand it!"[46]
- "I never get to eat what I want."

6
Substitute Rational Beliefs

Realize that you can replace your typical irrational beliefs and toxic self-talk with more rational, healthy ways of believing, thinking, and talking to yourself. You have to dispute and replace irrational beliefs to do this.

Use what Ellis calls rational analysis.[47] Actively seek out and destroy all the *shoulds*, *oughts*, and *musts* in your thinking. Be rational about it. There's no law that says anything really must be a certain way. Is it bad that you have diabetes? Probably. But can you rationally argue that there's some law of the universe that says you absolutely ought not to have gotten diabetes? Should your friends and family always be patient with you when you explain your new lifestyle? It would be nice—but there's no law. In fact, if there's any absolute, it's that the world and its people should, ought to, and must always be . . . totally unpredictable! This is mental fitness, so you have to do it every day, many times, before it really starts to take hold.

Use a "catastrophe scale" to put things in perspective. When you start thinking, "I can't stand this high blood sugar again. This is the absolute worst thing that could ever happen. It's literally unbearable," slow down, breathe, mind the gap, and think rationally:

- Can you stand it? Yes, you can. You could probably stand a whole lot worse if you had to. In fact, it might be a universal law (or a great gift in how we're made) that the worse things get, the better we seem able to cope.
- Is it the absolute worst thing that could ever happen? No, there are far worse things that could happen, and even those could still be worse into infinity. We're not asking you to think of yourself as some sort of martyr capable of enduring worse and worse deprivation and suffering—just the opposite. Realize that whatever you're going through is very often not that bad. It's just unpleasant, not unendurable. If you tell yourself that, you will feel a whole lot better.
- Is it unbearable? No, there have been plenty of people who used their rational thinking to keep hope alive in very dire circumstances far worse than high blood sugar.[48]

Replace irrational overgeneralizations, magnifications, and all-or nothing thinking.[49] You don't "always" gorge on junk food. You don't have the "world's worst blood sugar control." You haven't "blown your diet completely" if you have a handful of M&M's—just don't go on to eat the rest of the bag! Don't forget that thinking is self-perpetuating and self-fulfilling. "The mind moves in the direction of our currently dominant thoughts," said Nightingale: "You become what you think about."[50]

7
Prefer Not To

You don't need to quash real feelings and emotions, or ignore or avoid strong, appropriate consequences of truly challenging stimuli. Say you have stubbornly refused to get your blood sugars under control, and now you find out that the blurriness in your eyes is retinopathy that will prevent you from driving. This is tough news. But it's not the end of the world. Can you just brush it off, though? That would take someone superhuman. And it wouldn't be healthy or normal. You can and should still experience the natural response to difficulties in your life—just don't blow them out of proportion.

Choose the way you respond (mind the gap) and change your toxic self-talk. Instead of saying, "This is a catastrophe, terrible, horrible, tragically devastating," say, "I'd prefer to keep driving. I'd prefer to see better. But it's not like I must keep my license. There's no law that says my eyes can't go bad." The key is in the word *prefer*. You can tell yourself what you'd prefer—even strongly prefer—as long as you don't get caught in the irrational belief that things must be a certain way as though some cosmic law ordained it. "I'd prefer it if my coworkers brought less tempting snacks into work." You can see how that's different from, "You *have* to stop bringing in cookies! It's killing me!" The former will keep you centered and strong-willed; the latter will drive you nuts, because your coworkers and the rest of the world will not magically come into line with your thinking—ever.

The key to emotional health is to keep our desires as preferences, even strong preferences, without turning them into absolute demands. When our preferences are violated, we experience only appropriate, and often constructive, negative emotions (like regret, sadness, or annoyance). When demands are violated, however, we experience unhealthy, destructive, negative emotions. When you experience unhealthy negative emotions, don't get down on yourself. Instead, accept yourself unconditionally while you forcefully and vigorously challenge your demands until they become mere preferences.

8

Plant-Based Diet

Nutritional counseling is almost never offered to people suffering depression or other mental illness, and this is a huge mistake. At LCA, we start by putting people with depression on a PBD, a treatment based on good nutritional science with no ill health effects. Here are a few reasons why the PBD works to fight depression.

A PBD is high in tryptophan, an essential amino acid (see Chapters 5 and 6) absolutely necessary for the production of serotonin, a neurotransmitter in the brain associated with depression. Serotonin must be boosted in people with depression and to do so naturally requires tryptophan. Tofu is perhaps the best source of tryptophan, with nearly 750 milligrams (mg) per 100 grams (g). Other good sources include ground flaxseed (644 mg/100 g), roasted pumpkin seeds (578 mg/100 g), and gluten flour (510 mg/100 g). You can mix fresh ground flaxseed in your oatmeal or your chili beans. Milk, which many people assume is a good source of tryptophan (part of the warm milk at bedtime old wives' tale), is actually quite low in the amino acid. Because some people with depression are hypersensitive to small adjustments to tryptophan, this natural and tasty treatment can have a rapid and profound effect.

A PBD diet is high in omega-3 fatty acids. Omega-3 is one of only two absolutely essential fats (the other is omega-6, which is much more abundant in food). They are termed essential because humans cannot manufacture them from simpler nutritional building blocks; therefore, it is essential that we get them in our diet. Omega-3 is necessary for proper brain functioning, and deficiencies are associated with numerous brain glitches. This is why many experts recommend eating fish or taking fish oil supplements, which contain a lot of omega-3 fatty acids. However, there are many potential problems with getting your omega-3 from fish—not the least of which is all the cholesterol and toxins fish have onboard.

It is interesting that fish do not manufacture omega-3 fatty acids either; they get them from a plant source: algae. We can get them from plants also. We recommend some plant-based sources of omega-3, which come via a healthful plant fat called alpha linolenic acid (ALA), which the body converts to omega-3. Again, the best source is flaxseed (linseed) oil.[51] It has a whopping 7,520 mg of ALA per tablespoon, which, when converted, is about equivalent to the omega-3 content of a can of tuna packed in water (930 mg). Another great source of omega-3 is English walnuts (2,043 mg per ¼ cup); canola oil, black walnuts, wheat germ oil, soybean oil, and dark green, leafy vegetables are other good sources. One dietary caution: If you consume trans-fat, ALA will not be efficiently converted into the omega-3s that are crucial for brain health.

A PBD is high in folic acid (sometimes called folate). Folic acid deficiency can cause depression. Dr. Neal Nedley, lifestyle medicine colleague and author, has found this deficiency is a relatively common cause of depression among meat eaters. "Patients who are depressed due to folate deficiency *tend not to improve at all with standard antidepressants.*"[52] The real treatment is simple—foods high in folate. Good sources of folate include chickpeas, black-eyed peas, lentils, red kidney beans, okra pods, navy beans, spinach, and mustard greens. Animal products are very low in folate.

9

Other Lifestyle Treatments

GET OUTSIDE

Lots of natural light or light therapy provides vitamin D, which is produced in the skin when ultraviolet (UV) light (found in sunlight) strikes the skin. Recent research shows that low levels of vitamin D are related to wintertime depression, or seasonal affective disorder. Supplementation of vitamin D in the wintertime alleviates the symptoms of seasonal affective disorder.[53] Furthermore, vitamin D appears to increase serotonin levels in the brain (which is what combats seasonal depression). Regular exposure to bright light will increase the brain's levels of serotonin (separate from, and in addition to, the effects of vitamin D), and this alleviates feelings of depression.[54] This type of light exposure should be to the eyes—but not directly, only indirectly. We feel the best light source is sunlight, especially in the early morning soon after awakening. An alternative is to use a light box that emits at least 6,000 lux of light. Use it for 30 minutes in the morning soon after you get up.

It's interesting to note that obesity is a well-known risk factor for vitamin D deficiency,[55] so getting out and walking in the morning sun can have a dual benefit on depression. Regular physical activity is essential to overall health and well-being, including coping with emotional challenges associated with chronic disease. Please see Chapter 8 for a complete discussion of the benefits and techniques of a regular physical activity program.

GET MORE SLEEP

Those who suffer from insomnia and sleep deprivation are at increased risk for developing depression.[56] As it turns out, there is a hormone partially responsible for ensuring you have a good night's sleep: melatonin. Melatonin is produced in the pineal gland. When we are in a bright-light environment, the eye sends information to the brain that shuts off the formation of melatonin. As the light in our environment decreases, the eyes send this information to the brain, and the brain, in turn, tells the pineal gland to start making melatonin. The pineal gland uses serotonin as a building block for melatonin; this is the same hormone that is produced by our exposure to light during the day! It makes sense, then, that you will experience that relaxed and restful sleep on the nights when you have been outdoors and exposed to a lot of sunlight. Your serotonin levels are soaring (be sure to eat a diet rich in tryptophan because this is what serotonin is made from); and as the day turns into darkness, your melatonin levels will soar, too. You'll sleep like a baby. For maximal melatonin production, it's important for you to sleep in a totally dark room and to get sunlight exposure—especially in the morning hours. Remember that the serotonin your body makes today will not last until tomorrow, so you need outdoor sunlight exposure every day.[57]

SLEEP WELL WITH DIABETES

●

GOOD sleep helps ease the diabetes process.[58] Dr. K. Spiegel of the University of Chicago[59] found that healthy young men had 40 percent lower blood sugar uptake by their tissues (meaning their blood sugar was higher) when they got only 4 hours of sleep for 6 consecutive nights compared to the 6 nights before, during which they got enough rest. Further, insulin released from the pancreas was 30 percent lower after sleep deprivation than after nearly 1 week of adequate rest. The ability of blood sugar to enter body cells without help from insulin dropped 30 percent, to a level usually seen in type-2 diabetes. In other words, sleep deprivation left healthy young men with an ability to handle blood sugar comparable to an elderly person with diabetes! One explanation for this is that loss of sleep appears to raise stress hormone levels, which in turn might increase insulin resistance.[60]

GIVE UP SMOKING

Everyone knows smokers get chronic lung diseases like bronchitis and emphysema—about 85,000 smokers a year die of such pulmonary diseases, and another 100,000 die of lung cancer caused by smoking. But did you know that smokers also tend to have the following:[61]

- A much shorter life span—by some government estimates up to 21 years lower
- More heart attacks—smoking causes 30 to 40 percent of all coronary disease deaths in the United States each year
- More cancers, in addition to lung cancer, such as lip, mouth, throat, larynx, trachea, esophagus, stomach, cervix, skin, colon, breast, and penis
- Reduced bone strength and more fractures
- Greater risk of back pain and injury
- Hormonal abnormalities
- More rapid loss of agility, balance, and endurance
- Accelerated skin wrinkling, hair loss, and graying
- Accelerated vision loss
- Difficulty sleeping

- Heartburn
- Stomach ulcers

Even so, many people still smoke,[62] and a large number of them have diabetes. Among patients with diabetes in the United States and in some western European countries, about 25 percent are smokers.[63] Diabetes already increases the risk for cardiovascular disease, retinopathy, and nephropathy—and smoking increases the risk even higher.[64] It's like putting two bullets in a gun and playing Russian roulette. Several studies have shown that smoking has negative effects on metabolic control in people with diabetes and increases their risk for complications.[65] Furthermore, smokers who do not have diabetes have a 1.5- to 3.0-fold increased risk of developing type-2 diabetes. In addition to creating an unhealthy lifestyle, nicotine from smoking negatively influences insulin sensitivity and, therefore, worsens glucose metabolism.[66] Smoking worsens insulin resistance, a problem that individuals with type-2 diabetes are already fighting. This causes the pancreas to secrete large amounts of insulin, which accelerates the development of large blood vessel disease (coronary and carotid arteries, aorta, etc.).[67] Smokers who have type-1 diabetes experience higher average blood sugar levels.[68]

CAN SMOKING CAUSE DIABETES?

●

A British study showed that infants of mothers who smoked 10 or more cigarettes during pregnancy had a four times greater risk of developing early type-2 diabetes. The same study showed a 1.35 times greater risk for developing adult obesity (there was also a 3.62 times greater risk of developing diabetes in teenagers who were themselves smoking 30 or more cigarettes per week).[73] What about secondhand smoke? In 2005, for the first time, researchers determined that exposure to tobacco smoke raises the risk among teens of the metabolic syndrome, the disorder associated with excess belly fat that increases the chances of diabetes, heart disease, and stroke. Teens have a 1 percent chance of developing the metabolic syndrome if they're not exposed to tobacco smoke, a 6 percent chance (or more, depending on exposure level) if they are exposed, and a 9 percent chance if they're active smokers.[74]

For proper glycemic control and decreased risk of complications as well as several other health benefits, cessation of smoking should be a critical part of lifestyle intervention for diabetes. If smoking is terminated and there is no subsequent weight gain, insulin sensitivity should progressively return to normal.[69]

If you're worried about weight gain after quitting smoking, you should know that this is usually caused by increased energy intake (more food), decreased metabolism, decreased physical activity, and enzyme changes that contribute to extra pounds.[70] However, if a healthy diet, rich in plant-based foods and whole grains, and a regular physical activity program are followed, weight gain can be prevented.[71]

Don't give up the fight against nicotine. Most ex-smokers "re-decided" to quit several times before they succeeded. In fact, most ex-smokers finally quit on their *eighth* serious attempt.[72]

10
Believe in Something

Religious people get over their depression more quickly than nonbelievers. More than 850 studies have now examined the relationship between religious involvement and mental health,[75] and three-quarters or more of them show people experience better mental health and adapt more successfully to stress if they're religious.[76] But it doesn't have to be an organized religion you believe in—just believe in something. At your core, in your heart and soul, in your bones, believe in something. Believe you're here on earth to teach junior high school math to reluctant students. Believe in the bond between you and your horses. Believe in your country, in the work you do, the art you create, your parenting, or your partnership with your spouse. Know and truly believe your own answer to the question, "Good health—for what?"

ONE FINAL WORD on successful thinking. For REBT to work, you have to make getting over your misery one of your most important goals in life, "something you are *utterly determined to achieve*."[77] Make the restoration of your health a very strong preference—and believe you can do it. Remember, whether you believe you will succeed or fail, you're right.

IS FAITH HEALING?

WHEN DIAGNOSED WITH a chronic illness such as diabetes, it can be difficult to remain positive. Hope and faith are sometimes in short order when you're coping with a serious disease, but they can make all the difference. Many studies have shown that negative emotions have negative influences on our bodies. Science has proved that consciously selected thoughts can immediately and directly alter states of body.[78] A positive outlook, therefore, can improve overall health and the body's physical condition. Psychosomatic medicine long ago proved that our stomachs, liver, heart, and sensory organs all function better when we're happy.[79]

Many people rely on religion or spirituality for their positive outlook: More than two-thirds of U.S. citizens belong to a church or synagogue, and even more incorporate some form of spirituality into their lives.[80] There is direct evidence that shows an association between religious involvement (organized religion) and spirituality (values and mission) and better health outcomes.[81] This could be because religious and spiritual practices evoke positive emotions, such as love, hope, contentment, and forgiveness. These values tend to reduce negative emotions. It could also be more technical than that. Positive emotions can increase activation of the sympathetic branch of the autonomic nervous system and decrease the release of stress hormones, such as cortisol and norepinephrine. This response has effects on the mind and the body, such as oxygen consumption, decreased anxiety, blood pressure, and heart rate—all of which can enhance overall health.

People with a spiritual or religious practice actually have better immune function, which can help fight off infection. In addition, they have more optimism and expect a better health outcome, which suggests they may be more likely to achieve their goals.[82]

Believe it or not, religious involvement and/or spirituality is associated with lower mortality rates, too. It appears that a belief in God can actually help you live longer, which might be another reason why "There are no atheists in foxholes." Believing in God is also correlated to less cardiovascular disease and lower blood pressure. One reason for this is that spiritual and religious people are more likely to engage in other health-promoting behaviors, such as physical activity, smoking cessation, and a healthful diet. Furthermore, religious involvement and spirituality are linked to lower rates of new depression as well as recovery from existing depression, which is a common occurrence in those suffering from chronic disease.

Religious or spiritual people may also be more effective at coping with their condition. Quality of life is improved with religious involvement and spiritual well-being. People involved in a religious community often have strong social support systems, which are known to have physical and mental health benefits.[83] Don't get too excited before you consider this, though. Just engaging in religious activities does not equal good health. Some important facts are often ignored when looking at the effects of religion on health.[84] The bottom line is, whether or not a person is religious, health needs to be a core value to be experienced. Spiritual needs may be increased during disease, and engaging in religious or spiritual practices may promote healing and result in overall better health.[85] Doctors would be wise to remember this and to practice the mantra, "Our calling as physicians is to cure sometimes, relieve often, comfort always."[86]

Many Look Up—and Some Look In—for Essential Help

Whether you believe unwaveringly in God, sense there might be some higher power out there, or are still searching for meaning that makes sense to you, you might find yourself in need of a few words once in a while from the world of faith.

The Bible says, "Be still and know that I am God."[87] Many successful people find strength to reach for their grandest vision in setting aside time for thoughtful, meditative, contemplative appreciation of a higher power. It is all too easy to get unconsciously caught up in the rush of mundane daily thoughts, words, feelings, and actions, only later to deny they are related to what we experience in life. That's why we believe it's so important to be still and allow the truth to sink in—that is to recognize the connection between our thoughts and feelings and their outcomes.

Many thousands of years ago, wise King Solomon said, "A merry heart doeth good like a medicine: but a broken spirit drieth the bones."[88] Perhaps this is why most of the major religions in the world, including Judaism and Christianity, prescribe joy, rejoicing, thankfulness, and cheerfulness as a means to the good life.[89]

Often people rely on a power outside of themselves to help them deal with unhealthful practices, such as smoking, alcohol, and food addictions. It is faith that allows believers to look away from self to an all-powerful, all-loving God who is able to accomplish what they cannot accomplish for themselves: "Beloved, I wish above all things that thou mayest prosper and be in health, even as thy soul prospereth."[90] "For I will restore health unto thee, and I will heal thee of thy wounds, saith the Lord."[91] "And the prayer of faith shall save the sick, and the Lord shall raise him up."[92]

On the other hand, you needn't necessarily give up self entirely or give in to some force greater than yourself to find freedom from your challenges. The will is within each of us, and we have a responsibility to look after ourselves, even when we believe firmly in God.

MODERN HUMANITY IN SEARCH OF A SOUL?

IN 1933, Carl Jung, a monumental figure in the founding of the science of psychology, wrote something so profoundly rooted in a spiritual understanding of humanity that you might not expect from a distinguished 20th-century psychologist:

> During the past thirty years, people from all civilized countries of the earth have consulted me. I have treated many hundreds of patients. Among all my patients in the second half of life—that is to say, over thirty-five—there has not been one whose problem in the last resort was not that of finding a religious outlook on life. It is safe to say that every one of them fell ill because they had lost that which the living religions of every age have given to their followers, and none of them has been really healed who did not regain his religious outlook.[93]

Jung hit on an essential truth. We are soul and body linked together intricately and mysteriously; and as the young inspirational Christian writer Matthew Kelly puts it, "Maximum health and well-being can be reached only when we attend to each of the elements of our being. Ignoring the spiritual component of our being necessarily reduces our health, effectiveness, well-being, and efficiency."[94]

THREE QUICK KEYS TO
SUCCESSFUL LIFESTYLE CHANGE

DR. A. J. PALMER and associates recently studied the impact of metformin, a popular diabetes drug (see Chapter 3), compared to lifestyle
intervention with no medicine in people with prediabetes (fasting
blood sugars between 100 and 126). The results were not surprising to
us: The group that got the standard lifestyle advice, such as that given
by the American Diabetes Association, along with the drug metformin
saw a 31 percent reduced risk of developing full-blown type-2 diabetes.
But the group that made intensive lifestyle changes such as those we
recommend reduced their risk by twice as much—a full 58 percent—
with no medicine at all! Considered over a lifetime, the lifestyle modification group could expect nearly three times the improvement in
mortality risk than the drug group.[95]

So, what do you need to be successful in making such lifestyle
changes? There are a lot of different ways to answer this question, but
here are our top tips based on our conversations with LCA alumni who
have successfully implemented the principles of lifestyle change that
they learned from our program:

- *Be clear about your goals.* Let's say you are traveling south on I-
  35 from Sulphur, Oklahoma, and you stop and ask someone, "Is
  this a good way to go?" The response will be, "Depends on
  where you're going!" Those who are successful know where
  they are going, and they stay focused on going in the right
  direction, mastering incremental steps (one meal or mile
  marker at a time), ultimately leading to their goal. A good goal
  might be working on overcoming your insulin resistance to live
  longer and healthier without diabetes complications.
- *Set specific target behaviors* designed to help you achieve your
  goals. For example, your specific target behaviors might include
  eating a plant-based diet, strolling after meals, starting an intermittent training activity, and cutting out evening snacks.
- *Make the time to reach the goals.* Even when you know where
  you want to go and how to get there, you still need to establish
  time and prepare to devote resources (like your energy and
  focus) on actually engaging in your target behaviors. In this

case, you have to put yourself first. If health is not at the top of your list of values—even above family and work—you won't be around as long as you can be to satisfy your commitment to all your other values.

Coping with the Uncertainty of Diabetes

Life is uncertain, whether you have diabetes or not. None of us can say with any certainty what's going to happen to us tomorrow, let alone next week, next month, or next year. We all live in this constant state of uncertainty. But when we use words like *anguish* and *turmoil* when we think about and describe this reality of our existence, all we do is increase our level of psychic pain. If we link inevitable uncertainly to anguish and turmoil, then this perfectly natural uncertainty becomes such an awful, terrible experience that we believe we can't possibly cope with it. But if we accept it as a routine part of our experience, then we can go about our lives and creatively work on the problems we face, despite life's uncertainties. It's possible you might be surprised one day at an unusually high or low blood sugar level, despite your earnest efforts to change your lifestyle. It's possible that some other health crisis might befall you. It's possible that your type-2 diabetes will begin to reverse after a short period of following our recommendations, and some day might vanish completely. All of these things are possible in our world of uncertainty.

Remember the tenets of REBT: We get ourselves into trouble when we hold to a belief that does not fit the natural laws of the world we live in. If we believe that outcomes in life should be certain, we're in trouble: "My blood sugar should not be so high!" If we accept uncertainty, then each day we make the best decisions that we can (accepting that they will be imperfect in some way or another) and adjust those decisions as new evidence emerges. In doing so, we learn that we actually have much control over many factors, and we can tweak the way we do things to stack the odds more in our favor. In other words, the key to living in an uncertain world is to be flexible—not flexible with our character or our values or our mission in life, but flexible with the things we cannot control.[96]

To refuse uncertainty is to disturb ourselves emotionally. People who demand that life should be certain will go through life disappointed and might even become angry at life or at God. They might turn to alcohol or drugs (to mask the pain of life not being the way they think it should be); they might give up on pursuing a healthy lifestyle; or they might become depressed, anxious, or afraid. We can see the results of people demanding that life be certain whenever a person sues McDonald's for making them fat. In this case, the unspoken demand seems to be, "I should be able to eat anything I choose, any time I choose to eat it, and expect to remain slim and healthy." That's like believing, "I should be able to defy gravity as I sail my body off this cliff."

In this world of uncertainty, it can be incredibly empowering when we take responsibility for our beliefs and our actions—and let go of demanding the consequences be exactly as we demand.

BREAKING THE RULES

AT LCA WE encourage each patient toward the end of his or her stay to design an individual plan. We encourage you to do the same. We recognize that you are always free to choose: *Lifestyle* and *choice* are synonymous. Remember that it's okay that you're not perfect. Nobody is.

The secret to following, or not following, the 30-Day Diabetes Miracle program is threefold:

- Simply do the very best you can today, then start again tomorrow. Don't let a lapse turn into a relapse. Had junk food for lunch? Have a light, healthful, plant-based supper. Been slothful for the past few days? Get up and take a hike today.
- Accept the consequences of your behaviors and move on. Can you eat the occasional piece of fish on the LCA plan? Can you splurge a little on your birthday? Can you skip a few days of your IT physical activity? Of course you can. We're not recommending it. But it's your own goals that will determine how much of our lifestyle prescription you want to put into practice. If you find you're not getting the results that you want, you might have to put more into practice. From an emotional standpoint, we get screwed up by doing 50 percent and expecting 100 percent results. So, for example, if your goal is to lose 30 pounds, conquer your insulin resistance, and get your blood sugar levels under control, then eating chocolate bars and never getting active is probably not going to work. Again: Let your own goals be your guide.

- Know thyself. Thus saith Socrates. Then plan accordingly, we say. In other words, if you know that you can't eat just one tiny square of chocolate, don't keep huge chocolate bars in the house. The myth of moderation[97] has been the bane of many people who've attempted change: Can most alcoholics have just one drink without major consequences?

10

30-Day Prescription for a
Personal Diabetes Miracle

CONGRATULATIONS! YOU'RE NEARLY at the end of this book, and well into your own journey toward a healthful, diabetes-busting lifestyle. If you want to join a growing number of people who've overcome their diabetes challenges, this chapter is for you. It's where the rubber meets the road—the practical application of our entire book. It's about changing your habits, transforming your lifestyle, and vastly improving your diabetes condition and overall health. There are some important tips and recommendations in this chapter: If you put the 30-Day Diabetes Miracle prescription to work, your transition to health will be faster and easier, and you'll obtain the best possible results. Remember that it all comes down to choice. You just have to decide you're really going for it, then . . . go for it!

When they arrive at Lifestyle Center of America (LCA), many patients have the notion they are about to enter a world of restriction, a world where "You can't do that!" is far more common than "Yes, you can!" They soon find this isn't true. It's all about perception and attitude. If, for example, all you ever eat for dinner is a burger and fries, then it's likely you *will* at first feel restricted by our diet. You can choose to look on this change negatively or you can realize that by not confining yourself to the same unhealthy way of eating, you are actually opening up a whole new world of endless variety—one you never allowed yourself to experience until now. The feeling of restriction is largely based on how you *choose* to view your circumstances.

LET THE MOOSE RUN

As you begin the lifestyle journey that we feel confident will change your life forever, we want to share a few words from the book *Paddle Whispers* by Douglas Wood, which Dr. Seale has found inspirational in his life:

> *Setting out to do something with your life is like sitting down to eat a moose. Nobody ever did anything successfully with their life. Instead they did something with their day. Each day . . .*
> *Each day is your life.*
> *Let the moose run. Eat some blueberries.*[1]

Don't look at the changes you're about to make as if they are as big as a moose you're sitting down to eat. Let the moose run (in this case, literally as well as figuratively!), and eat some blueberries instead. Take things one day at a time and, for that matter, one *meal* at a time. When you do this, the changes we recommend won't seem like such a big deal. Just take one day, one meal, one step, at a time.

Here are some tried-and-true tips to help you avoid feeling deprived as you undergo change. We want you to follow our recommendations, starting today. Give it 30 days. It will get easier the longer you do it, and we bet that within a few days or weeks, you'll feel better—and you'll *be* better, physically, emotionally, and spiritually.

REJECT THE SAD AND EMBRACE A PBD TODAY

Here are our *Super Seven Tips* for getting off the standard American diet (SAD) and getting on a plant-based diet (PBD) with minimal distress:

- **Make a clean break from eating addictive foods.** "Betcha can't eat just one" is more than a clever slogan. It's a reflection of human nature and a testament to the power certain substances have over us. It's best to simply avoid these foods completely, just like an alcoholic needs to avoid alcohol completely to recover. Be honest with yourself and identify the foods that are addictive for you. If you try to just cut back on the substances that have a hold on you, you'll always feel deprived, *and* you'll continue to fuel your addictive cravings. When you take these trouble foods out of your diet completely, your cravings will soon disappear. You'll no longer feel restricted.

■ *Don't just choose to eat healthfully, choose to enjoy eating healthfully.* You likely have taste buds that have become used to a diet high in salt, sugar, artificial sweeteners and flavors, fats, and refined (processed) carbohydrates. You may have actually developed addictions to these types of foods. It's safe to say that eating a PBD will not initially satisfy your taste buds or your cravings (at least not like the SAD does). However, after 2 or 3 weeks of following our prescription, your taste buds will adjust, and you will be amazed at the enjoyment you get from your diet. You can choose to remain skeptical—or you can trust us and try it.

■ *Evaluate your reluctance.* If you have difficulty following our recommendations, write down the reasons and closely evaluate them. We find that most reasons people come up with for rejecting a healthful lifestyle are really nothing more than elaborate excuses and counterproductive justifications. The message here is, if your motivation is strong enough, most reasons can be dealt with and solutions found.

■ *Make your home a safe house.* When you're tired, stressed, hungry, or bored, it's easy to make bad food choices. If you fill your kitchen and pantry with a variety of healthful food choices and if you keep unhealthful food out, you'll be much safer when you're most vulnerable. Stock up on fruits to satisfy the urge for something sweet. Use an air-popper to make popcorn, instead of buying the microwave variety. Munch on crisp cut vegetables instead of chips—you get the picture. Just keep the stuff you crave out of the house. If there's a huge tub of ice cream in the freezer, it will begin to serenade you sweetly.

■ *Eat wholesome foods the way nature created them.* The processed version will *never* be as good. The closer a food is to the way it came off of the tree, vine, or plant when you eat it, the healthier it is likely to be. Processing, refining, and the addition of artificial flavorings, sugars, and salt degrades our foods. When you shop, read labels. Remember, the healthiest foods will have the shortest ingredient list. If you want to buy beans, for example, you want to see only beans listed.

■ *Try a new fruit, vegetable, or whole grain every week.* The variety is endless. If you don't like something the first time, try it again later prepared differently. Have you ever tried millet, spelt, or quinoa? How about jicama, fennel, or blue potatoes? If possible, find a market that has a large selection of produce. Try all of the fruits and vegetables you have never heard of or eaten before. If you do this, you'll realize how truly *restrictive* the SAD is and how *liberating* a PBD can be.

■ *Make mealtime special.* Don't multitask eating with driving, watching television, paying bills, or other activities. Concentrate on enjoying the foods you've taken the time to prepare. Eat slowly and savor the natural flavors of simple, unprocessed foods. You may be surprised by what you've been missing. Also, break the habit of eating whenever you are being entertained. It's a safe bet there's nothing healthy for you to eat at a movie theater or an amusement park—a veggie dog on a white bun with ketchup and mustard doesn't make the grade!

HOW AND WHAT TO EAT ON THE 30-DAY DIABETES MIRACLE PROGRAM

IN CHAPTERS 5 and 6, we showed you how a PBD is best for battling diabetes. Here's how to put that diet into practice.

Eat a Total Plant-Based Diet for Optimal Health

Eliminate meats, milk, cheese, and eggs. There are milks made from nuts, beans, and grains (almond, soy, rice) that can be used in place of cow's milk (for those with diabetes, plain, unsweetened soy milk is recommended). Meat substitutes can be used as you make your transition. However, we recommend these meat analogs (fake meats) be used sparingly, as they can be high in fat, calories, and sodium. A far better meat substitute is beans. When you're not filling up on meat and dairy, you will naturally eat more vegetables, fruits, and grains.

Eat Breakfast Like a King, Lunch Like a Prince, and Supper Like a Pauper

Eat 50 to 60 percent of all your daily calories at breakfast (3 to 5 carb choices). Breakfast is the most important meal of the day. This is when you should eat *substantial* foods. You can even have foods traditionally served for evening meals. Bean chili on whole wheat toast with a side of steamed Swiss chard is very satisfying on a cold winter morning.

Eat 30 to 40 percent of your calories at lunch (3 to 5 carb choices). You could have vegetable barley stew, a mixed greens salad, and some fruit. Or a great on-the-go meal might be whole wheat pita bread stuffed with hummus; sliced sweet peppers, cucumber, and red onion; sprouts and fresh basil leaves. Use your imagination and the choices become endless.

Eat 10 percent or less of your calories at supper (0 to 3 carb choices). If you choose to eat in the evening, a plate of steamed above-ground vegetables, vegetable soup, a green leafy salad with lemon juice, or a piece of Northern Hemisphere fruit is the best choice. If you can avoid supper altogether, that's probably the best option, so try working toward that as an ultimate goal.

Eat a Sensible Breakfast and Lunch with No Snacking

Eat a sensible, plant-based breakfast and lunch (and possible light supper) at regularly scheduled times, with no snacking in between. Careful—you can gain weight on a PBD if you don't watch calories. For more menu planning ideas, recipes, and a pantry list, go to our website (www.diabetesmiracle.org).

Eat 8 to 10 Servings of Fruits and Vegetables per Day

Eat mostly above-the-ground vegetables like cucumbers, peppers, squash, and celery. These are typically low glycemic. Limit below-the-ground, or root, vegetables to ½ cup or so per day. These include potatoes and carrots. Have 1 or 2 cups of dark green, leafy vegetables like spinach, kale, and chard daily. Choose mostly northern fruits, or those grown in the Northern Hemisphere, such as apples, pears, berries, peaches, apricots, and cherries because these are typically low glycemic. Citrus is fine, too, especially grapefruit. Maximize dark, colorful fruits and vegetables that have strong flavors and smells (blueberries, cherries, blackberries, onions, garlic). Limit southern, or tropical, fruits such as bananas, pineapples, mangos, and papayas as well as melons because these typically have a higher glycemic index and will raise blood sugar rapidly. Don't drink fruit juices; eat the whole fruit instead. Limit vegetable juices made from root vegetables and those that contain high levels of sodium (more than 500 milligrams per serving).

Eat 2 to 3 Servings of Beans Every Day

Try pinto, black, red, and kidney beans, soybeans (tofu products), and lentils. Include ½ cup of beans at breakfast and lunch daily. Be creative with beans. Try hummus (garbanzo bean spread) one day, black bean soup the next, and scrambled tofu (soybeans) the day after that.

Eat 6 to 9 Servings of Whole Grains Daily

Grains that have not been ground are preferred. For hot cereals try whole wheat berries or oat groats; for bread look for sprouted grain breads (Ezekiel 4:9 bread is our favorite; you can find it in the frozen food section). Limit foods made from flour. *Ground grains will raise the blood sugar rapidly, even if whole grain.* Avoid all enriched, unbleached, bromated, or other flours made from grains not preceded by the word *whole*.

Eat 1 Ounce of Unsalted Tree Nuts Each Day

Eat a small, cupped handful of almonds, walnuts, or pecans. Cashews, too, are remarkably versatile and can be used in many recipes. Nuts are great, but don't go nuts with your serving size.

Eat 1 Tablespoon of Whole, Freshly Ground Flaxseed Daily

Flaxseed is an excellent source of essential omega-3 fatty acids. Buy a mini-coffee grinder and grind up flaxseed each morning; add it to your oatmeal, beans, or salad.

Take Vitamin B₁₂ Daily for the Rest of Your Life on a PBD

Bacteria manufacture vitamin B_{12} in the large intestines of most animals, including humans, but animals cannot absorb it from that location. When animals are slaughtered and processed, the meat is often contaminated with the intestinal bacteria, which then becomes the main source of B_{12} for most meat-eating humans. Vitamin B_{12} can also be manufactured in soil, which used to be a rich source until modern industrialized agricultural methods essentially sterilized soil of this vital nutrient. Therefore, those on a PBD should take a B_{12} supplement. We recommend 1,000 micrograms (µg) daily.

Limit Fat Intake

Add as little oil as possible to your foods, and limit your intake of foods that are visibly oily. Eat only plant fats—the best are olive oil and canola oil. Avoid saturated fats, which are found mainly in animal oils but are also present in coconut and palm oils. Eliminate all trans-fats— they're prevalent in snack foods, fast foods, and restaurant foods. Don't eat any products that have the words *hydrogenated, partially hydrogenated, interesterified, margarine,* or *shortening* as ingredients.

Avoid Refined and Processed Foods of All Kinds

Remember, the best foods have only one ingredient, such as whole wheat, brown rice, black-eyed peas, or Jonagold apples.

Limit Salt Intake

Your daily salt intake should be about ½ teaspoon (approximately 1,000 milligrams) per day. Don't use added (table) salt at all. The best place for your salt shaker is buried deep in the cupboard; take it off of the table!

Avoid Food and Drinks That Are Sweetened

Train your taste buds to enjoy foods that are naturally sweet, without additives such as preservatives, refined sugars, or artificial sweeteners.

Eliminate Caffeine

Caffeine can cause dehydration, affect blood sugar control, and increase blood pressure while at the same time decreasing the body's ability to boost blood flow to the heart during physical activity.[2]

Eliminate Alcohol

Alcohol is high in calories and can cause dehydration and severe hypoglycemia if you are taking diabetes medication or insulin.

Drink 8 to 10 Glasses of Water per Day

The best way to tell if you're drinking enough water is to observe the color of your urine—it should be clear or pale yellow. If it is dark yellow, you need to drink more! If you have trouble drinking water, try adding an herbal (decaffeinated!) tea bag. Begin the day by drinking 16 to 24 ounces of room temperature or slightly warm water. If this is difficult, try adding a slice of fresh orange, lemon, or cucumber to your glass. Stop drinking ½ hour before meals and don't resume drinking for 1 hour after meals. Stop drinking all liquids in the early evening.

THE LCA ACTIVITY PLAN

START YOUR PHYSICAL activity regimen as soon as you can, because it's just as important to a healthy lifestyle as your new diet.

- Do gentle stretching for 30 minutes each morning, 6 days a week. Use an instructional video or DVD if this helps. You should also stretch before intermittent training (IT) and strength-training sessions.
- Be physically active 60 minutes daily, 5 to 6 days per week. The time does not need to be done in one session and can be accumulated daily.
- Use IT, and increase your intensity level by 5 beats per minute approximately every 2 to 3 weeks, or as tolerated, until you are at 75 percent intensity. You should not feel muscle burning if you're doing IT correctly.

- Choose pleasant, invigorating physical activities that you enjoy doing. If you choose walking, use a pedometer and try to build up to 10,000 steps per day.
- A heart monitor will help you stay in your target zone and help you progress more efficiently.
- Slow walk (stroll) after each meal for 15 to 20 minutes.
- Avoid vigorous physical activity for 1 to 2 hours after meals.
- Do resistance (weight) training exercises 3 times per week. A small amount of muscle soreness the day after a workout is acceptable, but joint pain should not be present. If it is, cut back on the intensity of your workout or skip a session completely. Remember, do not do strength training 2 days in a row.
- Get physically active outdoors in the sunshine whenever possible. Try to avoid areas with high levels of automobile exhaust fumes.

THESE SHOES ARE MADE FOR WALKING

●

ALONG with a PBD, increased physical activity is a major component of the 30-Day Diabetes Miracle program. You'll gradually start increasing your activity during the 30-day program, but before you begin, you'll need a few items we feel are important:

- *Quality walking shoes.* Go to a good sporting goods, hiking, or outdoor store where they have knowledgeable sales staff and buy the *best pair of walking shoes you can afford.* Don't scrimp here, especially if you're overweight or have some level of peripheral neuropathy (nerve pain or numbness in the feet). If you buy cheap shoes, your feet, legs, knees, and hips will suffer. If you use the shoes as you should, expect to replace them every 3 to 6 months.
- *A heart rate monitor.* Nothing fancy is needed here, but a model that has a programmable heart rate zone is desired. Polar brand monitors are reliable, durable, and work with many aerobic exercise machines you find in fitness centers.
- *A basic pedometer (step counter).* These are helpful in telling you how much you're moving each day. The goal is to walk 10,000

continued . . .

steps per day. Of course, if you do more, that's okay, too! You don't need to calibrate it to measure distance walked. The important thing is to get the 10,000 steps in per day, working up to it gradually if necessary.

- *A set of weights or resistance tubes.* We find tubes are safe, effective, convenient, and easy to use—they're also cheaper than weights and easier to store and tote.

You don't need a membership to a fancy gym or an expensive piece of equipment in your basement or bedroom. Of course, if you have these things, great—use them. But all you really need is a good pair of walking shoes and a place to walk that's safe and fairly level (or hilly if you want to do IT), and you'll be set to go. (You can find more suggestions for the tools that can assist you in your active lifestyle, including the brands we recommend, on our website, www.diabetesmiracle.org.)

SUNLIGHT AND REST

AFTER DIET AND physical activity, there are two more important lifestyle medicine prescriptions for ideal health: sunlight and rest.

- Get early morning light exposure for 30 minutes every day, for optimal rest and rejuvenation that night.
- Get 15 to 20 minutes of sunlight exposure to your arms, face, and hands between the hours of 10 a.m. and 3 p.m., three to four times per week. This is for vitamin D production. Don't exceed these times, to avoid burns!
- Go outside daily, even on cloudy days.
- Sunlight exposure should be increased in the winter. If you live north of the 37th latitude (about even with Oklahoma City), you likely will not make adequate vitamin D in the winter and should take a supplement of 1,000 units per day.
- Avoid lying down for 2 hours after a meal.
- Keep your bedroom neat and clean; it will help you sleep more peacefully.

- Sleep 7 to 9 hours nightly in a completely dark, cool room.
- Sleep 2 to 3 hours before midnight for optimal rest and rejuvenation.

DON'T SETTLE FOR NORMAL WHEN YOU CAN BE OPTIMAL

IN GENERAL, PHYSICIANS, laboratories, and health organizations don't employ optimal values when setting health goals for patients. They base their goals, in part, on what they feel patients will likely achieve—and not what they optimally could achieve. We've compiled a list of important health parameters and corresponding results that are optimal, based on current research as well as our experience with patients at LCA. We know these results are obtainable, usually through lifestyle changes alone (meaning without medicine), because we see it happen daily. When you have the tests on this list done, do not be satisfied with a result because you are told by your laboratory or doctor that it's in the normal range. Being *normal* in this country means you may be overweight or have high cholesterol, prediabetes, or heart disease. We strive for *optimal*, not normal. Be certain you know the actual results of your tests and compare them with the optimal values in the box on p. 270. We suggest you share these ideal health parameters with your doctor.

THE 30-DAY PRESCRIPTION FOR A PERSONAL DIABETES MIRACLE

BEFORE YOU BEGIN the 30-day Diabetes Miracle Prescription found at the end of this chapter, we ask that you make an appointment with your doctor. If you feel your physician would like to have information specifically directed to him or her by Dr. House and Dr. Seale, please go to www.diabetesmiracle.org where you can find a link for physician's guidelines. Print them out and take them with you to your next physician visit. This will give your doctor the information needed to coach and monitor you. We've made recommendations in the physician's guidelines, but it's up to you and your doctor to make the final decisions concerning medication adjustments, frequency of follow-up visits, and so on. Please follow your physician's advice. If you find your doctor does

IDEAL HEALTH PARAMETERS AND OPTIMAL RESULTS

●

HEALTH PARAMETERS	OPTIMAL VALUES
Fasting glucose	60–86 milligrams per deciliter
Serum C peptide	0.6–3.2 nanograms per deciliter
Fasting insulin	less than 6 micro International Units per milliliter
Microalbumin/creatinine	less than 30 micrograms per milligram
Hemoglobin A_{1c} (HgA_{1c})	less than 5.0 percent
Mean blood sugar	less than 90 milligrams per deciliter
Fructosamine	190–270 micromoles per liter
Triglycerides	less than 100 milligrams per deciliter
Total cholesterol	less than 150 milligrams per deciliter
High-density lipoprotein (HDL) cholesterol	more than 50 milligrams per deciliter
Low-density lipoprotein (LDL) cholesterol	less than 70 milligrams per deciliter
Total cholesterol to HDL cholesterol ratio	less than 3.5
Homocysteine	3–7.2 micromoles per liter
Serum B_{12}	about 1100 picograms per milliliter
Serum folate	more than 24 nanograms per milliliter
25-hydroxy vitamin D	30–68 nanograms per milliliter
Thyroid stimulating hormone (TSH)	1–2 micro International Units per liter
γ-Glutamyltransferase (GGT)	2–80 Units per liter
Aspartate transaminase (AST)	2–50 Units per liter
Alanine aminotransferase (ALT)	3–60 Units per liter
Alkaline phosphatase	20–125 Units per liter
Resting blood pressure	less than 115/75 millimeters of mercury
Body mass index (BMI)	18–24

not want you to participate in our program, see "How to Find a Doctor Who Can Be Your Lifestyle Coach," on p. 272.

We recommend you follow the prescription for 30 days before you judge whether or not you're benefiting from it. You should begin to feel better, have better blood sugar control, and take fewer medications if you follow the directions carefully. It's important to understand that lifestyle medicine's potency or power will be determined primarily by *you*. If you make a dramatic change from your current lifestyle, following the prescription to the letter, you can expect dramatic results. If you make adjustments or substitutions, you can expect diminished results corresponding to the amount of substituting you have done. As you continue to live the LCA lifestyle, you will likely see more and more improvements in your health over time. If your diabetes is accompanied by extra pounds, the good news is that you can achieve normal weight as you continue the plan. We feel confident this is a prescription that is like no other ever given to you, and you will likely be amazed by the results you receive from it! We think you'll agree with us that this is one prescription you'll want to refill over and over again, for life.

IS YOUR DOCTOR RIGHT FOR YOU?

WHILE WE BELIEVE in a proactive, patient-centered, patient-guided program, we strongly urge you to find a like-minded, knowledgeable, positive physician to coach you and guide you. It's very important that your doctor knows what you're doing each step of the way. We're certain that if you start acting on our precepts you will see marked improvements in your health as soon as today. Because of that, your medicine needs can change quickly.

We're not setting about to bash doctors. We have enormous empathy for the pressures they face. But it's important to note that much of the problem resides within our current healthcare system. You should ask these questions about your doctor:

- Does your doctor prescribe medicine before other approaches like lifestyle changes?
- Does your doctor explain things to you in a way you can understand?
- Does your doctor rush you or not seem to listen?

- Does your doctor treat only your symptoms—or also their causes?
- Does your doctor look healthy to you; does he or she have healthy habits?
- Does your doctor ever patronize you or seem condescending in his or her attitude?
- Does your doctor communicate regularly with the others on your healthcare team?
- Does your doctor consider the whole you or is the focus primarily on some medication, symptom, diagnosis, or number?

How to Find a Doctor Who Can Be Your Lifestyle Coach

As you begin following our recommendations, we strongly advise you to find a supportive physician who will work with you, monitor your progress, and adjust your medications as the power of lifestyle change kicks in. You should find someone who will encourage your efforts. Here are some suggestions as you seek just the right doctor:

- Talk to your current doctor. Describe what you're going to do, as well as your goals, and find out if your doctor is willing to coach you through the process.
- Ask your doctor for a referral. Your current physician may not feel adequately trained to work with you, or may be in disagreement with the changes we recommend. However, they may be willing to refer you to a colleague who is capable of being your coach.
- Contact the American College of Lifestyle Medicine (www.life stylemedicine.org). Someone there may be able to give you the name of a lifestyle medicine physician near you.
- Contact your local county medical society and ask for a referral to a physician who specializes in adult wellness or preventive medicine.
- Talk to your friends and neighbors. Ask them if they would recommend their doctor.
- Visit a health club and ask if there are any doctors who are frequent users. This will not tell you much about them professionally, but it will help determine their personal view about fitness and health.

Whomever you choose as your doctor(s), tell him or her about the program you're about to begin. Share with the doctor(s) the checklist that appears in the following section, "Working with Your Doctor." Ask if he or she is willing to monitor you in the manner suggested. Continue to assess whether or not your doctor is right for you, using the guidelines given in this book.

Working with Your Doctor

By now, we hope you recognize the crucial role you play in the management of your diabetes. How well you succeed in taking control of your health does not rest solely on the shoulders of your doctor! To help you partner with your physician as he or she coaches you through the transition you're about to make, we have devised a checklist of items you should discuss at your upcoming doctor visits. If you feel your physician would like to have information specifically directed to him or her by Dr. House and Dr. Seale, please go to www.diabetesmiracle.org where you can find a link for physician's guidelines. Print them out and take them with you to your next physician visit.

Laboratory Tests

We recommend you have the following tests done before starting the program and then repeated after 3 months:

- Fasting chemistry panel
- Lipid profile
- Fasting insulin level (if you have type-2 diabetes or are overweight with a BMI greater than 25)
- HgA_{1c} (if you have type-1 or type-2 diabetes)

Medications

As you follow the program recommendations, it's likely that certain medications will need to be reduced. The following are medication adjustments you should discuss with your physician:

- *Insulin.* If you're taking insulin, it's likely your dosage will need to be reduced fairly quickly into the program; this

should be done under physician guidance, based on blood
sugar test results.

- *Oral diabetes medications (pills).* These medications also typically should be reduced or eliminated. We usually discontinue
everything except metformin or Januvia at the beginning of
the program.
- *Blood pressure medication.* After about 2 weeks on the program, blood pressure usually comes down naturally, and medications can be reduced. This should be done only on your
doctor's recommendation.
- *Cholesterol- and triglyceride-lowering medications.* Because
this program also works to lower cholesterol and triglycerides,
it's very likely you may be able to reduce, or even eliminate,
these medications when you have your blood retested after 3
months. Your doctor will be able to help you decide.

Medical Visits

- If you have diabetes, we recommend you be seen at least twice
per week for the first 2 weeks, then weekly until blood sugar
and medication adjustments are stable.
- For those with high blood pressure, we advise weekly visits
until blood pressure and medication adjustments are stable.

All other patients should be seen at intervals recommended by their
physician.

YOU HAVE IN your hands the best available hope for dodging the dire
consequences of uncontrolled diabetes: A proactive program that puts
you in charge of addressing the cause, not just the symptoms, of your
disease. We want you to join the thousands who've embraced our
lifestyle approach and realize that the consequences of diabetes are not
inevitable or irreversible. Are you still skeptical? Ask yourself what *good*
reason you have *not* to try our program for 30 days. Are you afraid it will
be too hard? How hard will it be to deal with blindness, amputations,
and an early death? Or are you afraid of failure? Many of us freeze in
the face of this fear before ever trying to change. Yet isn't what you've
been doing to treat your diabetes failing thus far? Are you simply a
doubter of miracles? Ask yourself, if you lower your blood sugar, insulin

resistance, weight, cholesterol, blood pressure, and risk of heart attacks, strokes, Alzheimer's disease, and cancer—all with good food and less medicine, or none at all—couldn't you call that a miracle? Could you even call it a cure? You decide.

30-DAY DIABETES MIRACLE PRESCRIPTION

Attitude

- Set specific, attainable lifestyle goals, both short and long term.
- Identify behaviors that will allow you to achieve your goals.
- Devote resources (time and money) necessary to engage behaviors needed to reach your goals.
- Keep in mind universal self acceptance (USA). If you fail to attain a goal, just start over again!

Nutrition and Water

- Follow a plant-based diet, eliminating meat, eggs and dairy.

  - Breakfast: 3 to 5 carb choices, including a serving of beans.
  - Lunch: 3 to 5 carb choices, including a serving of beans.
  - Dinner: skip completely, or limit to 3 carb choices.
  - For more meal plans and recipes, go to our website at www.diabetesmiracle.org.

- Eat 8 to 10 servings of colorful fruits and vegetables; 6 to 9 servings of whole grains; 2 to 3 servings of beans; and 1 ounce of nuts and seeds per day.
- Drink 8 to 10 glasses of water per day. Start your day by drinking 2 glasses upon awakening. Don't drink within ½ hour before eating or within 1 hour after eating.

Activity

- Gently stretch for 30 minutes each morning.
- Stroll for 15 to 20 minutes after each meal.
- Use IT and set your heart rate monitor to your initial target

zone; increase your target heart rate by 5 beats per minute every 2 to 3 weeks until you reach a 75 percent intensity workout level. Do 60 minutes of total IT activity, 5 to 6 days per week.

- Do resistance training (with weights or tubes) for 30 minutes, 3 days per week.

Rest

- Get 7 to 8 hours of sleep every night.
- Go to bed early and get up early.
- Sleep in a room that is totally dark.

Sunlight

- Get outdoor light exposure for 30 minutes, within 30 minutes of awakening—preferably before 7 a.m.
- Get 20 to 25 minutes of sunlight exposure between 10 a.m. and 3 p.m., 3 to 4 times per week.

Medical

- If you have diabetes

  - Blood sugar: Check daily upon awakening, immediately before meals, 2 hours after every meal, and at bedtime. If you are on insulin, you may also want to check at 1 a.m. to be sure your sugar does not go too low in the middle of the night. Keep a daily log for your doctor.
  - Doctor visits: See your physician twice weekly for blood sugar and medication review until you are stable, then follow the advice of your physician.
  - Medications: Your physician is ultimately in charge of adjustments. General guidelines were given earlier in this chapter, or on our website, www.diabetesmiracle.org, under "Physician's Guide to the 30-day Health Prescription."

■ If you have high blood pressure

  • Check your blood pressure 3 times per day. Report any light headedness, dizziness, or consistent blood pressure readings below 100 (top number) or 60 (bottom number) to your physician. Keep a daily log of your readings.
  • Doctor visits: See your physician weekly for blood pressure and medication review.
  • Medications: Your physician is ultimately in charge of adjustments. General guidelines can be found earlier in this chapter, or on our website, www.diabetesmiracle.org, under "Physician's Guide to the 30-day Health Prescription."

■ Take 1,000 micrograms of vitamin B_{12} per day.

KEEPING TRACK

IT'S ALWAYS A good idea to keep track of your progress and to maintain records that will help you and your healthcare professionals. See a sample daily log in Appendix 1.

APPENDIX 1

Keeping Track of Your Progress

THROUGHOUT THIS BOOK you are encouraged to keep track of activities, nutrition, health markers, and behaviors. Lifestyle Center of America (LCA) has devised logs to make this simple and you can download the log sheets at no charge, or order a whole book, from www.diabetesmiracle.com. If you do not have Internet access call 1-800-685-7310 or write to: Lifestyle Center of America, Free Booklet, Rt. 1, Box 4001, Sulphur, OK 73086. Or you can use the following examples as a guide to create your own logs.

Date **11/18**   Day of the Week **Day 1/Tues.**

	Night	Fast	Brkfst	+ 2-hr
Time		5:45	6:15	8:15
Blood Sugar		190	169	224
Insulin — Lantus			10u	
Insulin — Humalog			6 u	5 u
Blood Pressure	—	123 / 77	117 / 67	
Pulse		79		

Breakfast/Lunch/Dinner	Amount	Total Carb (g)	Fiber (g)	Net Carb (g)	Carb Choice
Homemade biscuits	1	20	2	18	1
Gravy	1/3 cup	6	1	5	1/3
Breakfast beans	1/2 cup	16	6	10	2/3
Multigrain cereal	1/2 cup	10	5	5	1/3
Apple	1				1
Grd flax seed	1 Tbl	4.1	3.3	.8	Free
PB Dinner roast	1 slice	16	1	15	1
Mashed potatoes	1/2 cup	17	1.6	15	1
Country gravy	2 Tbls	2.1	.3	1.8	Free
Peas	1/2 cup	11	4	7	1/2
Broccoli	1 cup	7.8	4.6	3.2	1/3
Kale salad	1 cup	7	2.3	4.7	1/3
3pm Orange juice	1 cup	26	1	25	2
Green salad	1 cup	9	3	6	1/3
	Totals				9

	Lunch	+ 2-hr		Supper	Bedtime
	1 pm	3 pm		6 pm	9 pm
	164	60 oJ.		136	181
		8 oʊ		10 u	
	6 u			8 u	
	121 / 74			152 / 62	
	62				

Aerobic/Exercise Activity	Duration	I.T. HR Zone		RPE 0-10
Treadmill	30 min.	135 — 145		5
Recumbent bike	20 min.	" — "		6
		—		
		—		
		—		
		—		
		—		

I did my LCA Stretching Routine today! ☑
I strolled after meals today! ☑
I did my strength training today!* ☐
*3-4 times a week

Water Intake ☒☒☒☒☐☐☐ Total Water 2 liters

Goal #1 I stuck to the PBD today: Yes ✗ No ___
Goal #2 I practiced USA* today: Yes ✗ No ___
Goal #3 I got enough sleep/rest today: Yes ___ No ✗
Goal #3 I got enough sunshine/light today: Yes ✗ No ___

*Unconditional Self Acceptance

NOTES See Doc. ASAP! My blood sugars will go down soon on this diet.

Carb-Counting Guide

F OLLOWING IS A list of the Carb Counts of some healthy, plant-based foods. For a comprehensive database of other foods, visit our website, www.diabetesmiracle.org.

Key

" = inch
~ = approximately
c = cup
frzn = frozen
g = gram
lb = pound
lg = large
med = medium
oz = ounce
sm = small
Tbsp = tablespoon
tsp = teaspoon
w/ = with
w/o = without

FRUIT

NAME	SERVING SIZE	CALORIES	TOTAL CARBS (g)	FIBER (g)	NET CARBS (g)	NUMBER OF CARB CHOICES	AMOUNT THAT EQUALS ~ 1 CARB CHOICE
Nontropical	1 c or 1 med whole fruit	50–150 (typical)	Varies‡	Varies‡	15 (typical)	1 (typical)	1 c or 1 med whole fruit
Apple	1 med (2¾" diameter), raw w/skin	81	21	3.7	17.3	1	~ 1 med
Blueberries	1 c, raw	81	20.5	3.9	16.6	1	~ 1 c
Grapefruit	½ med (3¾" diameter), pink and red, raw	37	9.4	0	9.4	⅔	¾ med
Kiwifruit	1 med, raw	46	11.3	2.6	8.7	½	1¾ med
Orange	1 med (2⅝" diameter), all varieties, raw	62	15.4	3.1	12.3	⅔	~ 1¼ med
Pear	1 med, raw	98	25.1	4	21.1	1⅓	~ ¾ med
Raspberries	1 c, raw	60	14.2	8.4	5.8	⅓	2½ c
Strawberries	1 c whole, raw	43	10.1	3.3	6.8	½	~ 2¼ c
Tropical*	1 c	100–150	Varies	Varies	30 (typical)	2 (typical)	½ c
Dried fruit†	‡	‡	‡	‡	‡	‡	‡

*For example, banana, papaya, mango, pineapple.
†Much higher in calories and carbs per equivalent volume of fresh fruit.
‡See the website (www.diabetesmiracle.org) for more information.

VEGETABLES, ABOVE-GROUND

NAME	SERVING SIZE	CALORIES	TOTAL CARBS (g)	FIBER (g)	NET CARBS (g)	NUMBER OF CARB CHOICES	AMOUNT THAT EQUALS ~1 CARB CHOICE
All vegetables that grow above the ground*	½ c	5–50 (typical)	Varies†	Varies†	< 5 (typical)	Free	1½ c (for starchy vegetables, such as squash) to 5 c (for leafy vegetables, such as spinach)

*For example, asparagus, broccoli, celery, cabbage, lettuce, bell peppers.
†See the website (www.diabetesmiracle.org) for more information.

VEGETABLES, BELOW-GROUND

NAME	SERVING SIZE	CALORIES	TOTAL CARBS (g)	FIBER (g)	NET CARBS (g)	NUMBER OF CARB CHOICES	AMOUNT THAT EQUALS ~1 CARB CHOICE
Beets	2 whole (2" diameter), cooked	44	10	2	8	½	3¾ whole
	1 c, raw	58.5	13	3.8	9.2	⅔	1⅔ c
Carrots	½ c slices, cooked	35	8.2	2.6	5.6	⅓	1⅓ c
	1 c chopped, raw	55	13	3.8	9.2	⅔	1⅔ c
Onion	1 c chopped, boiled	92	21.3	2.9	18.4	1	~ ¾ c
	1 c, raw	61	13.8	2.9	10.9	⅔	1½ c
Potato, baked	1 med w/ skin	161	36.6	3.8	32.8	2	~ ½ med
Potato, boiled	1 med w/o skin	144	33.4	3	30.4	2	½ med
Sweet potato	1 med, baked w/ skin	117	27.7	3.4	24.3	1⅔	⅔ med
Yam	1 c cubed, baked	158	37.5	5.3	32.2	2	~ ½ c

CEREALS

NAME	SERVING SIZE	CALORIES	TOTAL CARBS (g)	FIBER (g)	NET CARBS (g)	NUMBER OF CARB CHOICES	AMOUNT THAT EQUALS ~ 1 CARB CHOICE
Cooked*	1 c	100–200 (typical)	Varies†	Varies†	Varies†	1 ½–2 (typical)	½ c (typical)
Ready to eat, cold	1 c	50–200 (typical)	Varies	Varies	Varies	1 ½–2 (typical)	½ c (typical)
All-Bran, Kellogg's	½ c	81	22.9	9.9	13	1	~ ½ c
Kashi Go Lean	1 c	140	30	10	20	1⅓	¾ c
Uncle Sam	1 c	190	38	10	28	2	½ c

*For example, barely, oatmeal, rice, and wheat.
†See the website (www.diabetesmiracle.org) for more information.

GRAIN PRODUCTS

NAME	SERVING SIZE	CALORIES	TOTAL CARBS (g)	FIBER (g)	NET CARBS (g)	NUMBER OF CARB CHOICES	AMOUNT THAT EQUALS ~ 1 CARB CHOICE
English muffin, whole wheat	2.3 oz muffin	134	26.7	4.4	22.3	1½	~ ¾ muffin
English muffin, 7-sprouted grains, Ezekiel 4:9	½ muffin	80	16	3	13	1	~ ½ muffin
Sprouted grain burger buns, Ezekiel 4:9	1 bun	170	34	6	28	2	½ bun
Sprouted 100% whole grain flourless bread, Ezekiel 4:9	1 slice, original	80	15	3	12	⅔	1¼ slice
Pita bread, whole wheat	1	170	35.2	4.7	30.5	2	½
Pocket bread, Ezekiel 4:9 Prophet's	1	100	21	4	17	1	~ 1
Taco shells, blue or yellow corn Garden of Eatin'	2	140	17	1	16	1	2 shells
Tortilla, corn	1 med	53	11.2	1.2	10	⅔	1½ med
Tortilla, flourless, Ezekiel 4:9 sprouted 100% whole grain	1	150	24	5	19	1	¾ tortilla
Tortilla chips, baked, Guiltless Gourmet	1 oz (18 chips)	110	22	2	20	11/3	0.75 oz (~14 chips)

NAME	SERVING SIZE	CALORIES	TOTAL CARBS (g)	FIBER (g)	NET CARBS (g)	NUMBER OF CARB CHOICES	AMOUNT THAT EQUALS ~1 CARB CHOICE
Tortilla chips, Garden of Eatin'	1 oz (18 chips)	140	19	2	17	1	1 oz
Pasta products (white, whole grain, or sprouted)	1 c, cooked	175 (typical)	40 (typical)	Varies*	30–35	2	½ c
Popcorn, plain	1 oz (~3½ c), air popped	108	22.1	4.3	17.8	1	0.84 oz (~3 c)
	1 oz (~2⅔ c), oil popped	142	16.2	2.8	13.4	1	~1 oz (~3 c)
Crackers, Ryvita	2 slices, dark rye	70	15	3	12	⅔	2½ slices
	1 slice, pumpkin seeds and oats	60	9	2	7	½	~2 slices
Crackers, Wasa	1 slice, fiber rye	30	7	2	5	⅓	3 slices
	2 slices, light rye	60	13	3	10	⅔	3 slices

*See the website (www.diabetesmiracle.org) for more information.

LEGUMES (BEANS, PEAS, AND LENTILS)

NAME	SERVING SIZE	CALORIES	TOTAL CARBS (g)	FIBER (g)	NET CARBS (g)	NUMBER OF CARB CHOICES	AMOUNT THAT EQUALS ~1 CARB CHOICE
Beans, peas, and lentils	½ c, cooked	100–150 (typical)	Varies*	Varies*	Varies*	1	⅓ c

*See the website (www.diabetesmiracle.org) for more information.

NUTS, NUT BUTTERS, AND SEEDS

NAME	SERVING SIZE	CALORIES	TOTAL CARBS (g)	FIBER (g)	NET CARBS (g)	NUMBER OF CARB CHOICES	AMOUNT THAT EQUALS ~1 CARB CHOICE
Cashews	1 oz	163	9.3	0.9	8.4	½	1.8 oz
Other nuts and peanuts	1 oz	160–200 (typical)	Varies*	Varies*	Varies*	Free	3–12 oz
Nut and peanut butters	1 Tbsp	100	Varies	Varies	Varies	Free	4–7 Tbsp
Seeds	1 oz	150–160	Varies	Varies	Varies	Free	4–6 oz

*See the website (www.diabetesmiracle.org) for more information.

APPENDIX 3

Glycemic Index Guidelines for a Plant-Based Diet

LISTED HERE ARE low-glycemic, plant-based healthy foods. For a comprehensive database of other foods, visit our website (www.diabetesmiracle.org) or see www.glycemicindex.com.

FRUIT, FRESH AND DRIED

Apples, fresh (38)
Apples, dried (29)
Apricots, dried (30)
Bananas, ripe (52)
Bananas, slightly underripe (42)
Blueberries (53)
Grapes (53)
Grapefruit (25)
Kiwifruit (53)

Lemon (0)
Lime (0)
Oranges (42)
Peaches (42)
Pears (38)
Plums (39)
Raspberries (0)
Strawberries (40)

FRUIT JUICES

WE RECOMMEND YOU eat the whole fruit and use juices sparingly.

Apple juice, unsweetened (40)

Carrot juice, fresh (43)

Grapefruit juice, unsweetened
  (48)

Orange juice, unsweetened (53)

Pineapple juice, unsweetened
  (46)

Tomato juice, unsweetened (38)

VEGETABLES

Artichoke, Jerusalem
  (sunchoke) (0)

Bok choy, raw (0)

Broccoli, raw (0)

Cabbage, raw (0)

Carrots, raw (16)

Carrots, cooked (41)

Cauliflower (0)

Celery (0)

Corn, sweet (47)

Cucumber (0)

Green Beens (0)

Lettuce (0)

Mushrooms (0)

Onions (0)

Peas, green (48)

Peppers (0)

Radishes (0)

Spinach (0)

Squash, yellow (0)

Sweet potato (46)

Swiss chard (0)

Tomato (0)

Turnip (0)

Yam (37)

Zucchini (0)

BEANS AND BEAN PRODUCTS

WITH THE EXCEPTION of fava beans, which are high glycemic, all bean varieties are considered low glycemic.

NUTS, SEEDS, AND AVOCADOS

ALL NUTS, SEED, and avocados are considered low glycemic, but because they're all high in fat and calories, we advise you to limit these foods to 1 ounce per day or less.

GRAINS AND CEREALS

PRODUCTS MADE FROM flour will have higher glycemic indices than those made without flour.

All Bran (34)
All Bran Fruit 'n Oats (39)
All Bran Soy 'n Fiber (33)
Barley, pearled (25)
Barley, cracked (50)
Bran Buds w/ psyllium
  (Kellogg's) (47)
Buckwheat groats (54)
Muesli, natural (40)

Muesli, toasted (43)
Oat bran, raw (55)
Oatmeal, steel-cut oats (52)
Quinoa (51)
Rice bran (19)
Rye, whole kernels (34)
Wheat, cracked (bulgur) (48)
Wheat, whole kernels (41)

BREADS, ROLLS, AND FLATBREADS

100% whole grain bread (Natural
Ovens, USA) (51)
9-grain multigrain bread (43)
Chapatti, baisen (Indian) (27)
Corn tortilla, Mexican (52)
Healthy Choice Hearty 7-Grain
  Bread (55)

Muesli bread (54)
Oat bran and honey bread (45)
Pumpernickel bread (50)
Rye bread, seeded (51)
Sourdough rye (48)
Sourdough wheat (54)
Soy/flaxseed bread (55)

PASTA AND NOODLES

Capellini (45)
Fettuccine, egg noodles (40)
Linguine, thick (46)
Linguine, thin (52)
Macaroni (47)
Mung bean noodles (33)
Soba noodles (46)

Spaghetti, white,
  durum wheat (44)
Spaghetti, whole wheat (42)
Split-pea/soy pasta shells (29)
Vermicelli, white,
  durum wheat (35)

DAIRY ALTERNATIVES

Soy milk (40)

Soy milk smoothie, low-fat (30)

Soy yogurt, fruited (50)

Other Conditions

ABOUT 80 PERCENT of the patients who come to Lifestyle Center of America (LCA) for treatment have diabetes. But our program was originally designed as a restoration program for health damaged by any number of disorders. The explosion in obesity and type-2 diabetes in the last two decades changed the demographics of our patients. We noticed early on that more of LCA's patients were obese and had type-2 diabetes, so it was natural for us to focus more intensely on those treatments, and we soon became a specialty center using lifestyle to treat diabetes—the only one of its kind. We got together, doctors and patient, to write this book, to present the amazing power of lifestyle medicine to those who have diabetes or are at risk for developing it.

MORE GOOD NEWS

BUT WHAT ABOUT treatment for the other 20 percent of our patients— those who have heart disease, high blood pressure, high cholesterol, arthritis, or a history of strokes or cancer? How is the LCA program customized to meet the needs of these individuals? As difficult as it may be to believe, the answer is, that we don't have to customize! That's another huge benefit to lifestyle medicine—its ability to effectively treat multiple disorders, without the need to alter the principal recommendations made. Basically, one lifestyle treatment fits all. Research proves that the best treatment and prevention of the leading three killers in the United States (coronary heart disease, cancer, and stroke) is a plant-based diet (PBD) combined with regular physical activity. Although the role of a cancer or heart disease specialist is important, there is much about these diseases that is totally within your control with lifestyle modifications.

There have been some interesting innovations developed by researchers and pharmaceutical companies over the years. As mentioned earlier in the book, a "polypill" has been developed, which consists of a combination of aspirin; three blood pressure–lowering medications, each at half their usually prescribed strength; a statin drug to lower cholesterol; and folic acid. In the minds of the developers, *everyone* over the age of 55 and *everyone* who has diabetes or heart disease (regardless of their age) should take this pill. The claim is that if everyone in these groups took this wonder drug, there would be an average gain of 11 years of life, free from heart attack or stroke. Of course, there would also be adverse side effects in 8 to 15 percent of those who went on the drug.[1] Those of us who practice lifestyle medicine, and daily witness the amazing benefits of lifestyle change in our patients, just shake our heads when we learn of absurdities such as the polypill. Does it make any sense to live a fast-food, sedentary existence that brings about chronic disease and then develop a pill to try and prevent the ill effects of such a misguided lifestyle?

At LCA, we already prescribe a polypill—it's our diet loaded with fiber, antioxidants, phytochemicals, low glycemic index (GI) complex carbohydrates, beneficial fatty acids, minerals, vitamins, and other micronutrients plus a regimen of proper physical activity and a cognitive behavior approach to thinking about ourselves and the world we live in. This prescription is much more potent than any conventional pill that can ever be devised by modern medicine. It costs nothing, and has *no* adverse side effects! And this lifestyle polypill provides a miracle for people with diabetes *and many other disorders.*

HEART DISEASE

HEART ATTACK IS the number one killer of both men and women in this country. Every hour, 135 Americans suffer a heart attack—52 of them will die—nearly one death every minute from this *preventable* disease. Each year there are 664,000 balloon angioplasties and 427,000 coronary artery bypass surgeries performed.[2] Without lifestyle changes like those we recommend, many (if not most) of these procedures will need to be repeated, because the blood vessels will likely block again.

When Dr. House and Dr. Seale were in medical school, they were taught that once arteries became blocked with cholesterol sludge, the only possible remedies were surgery, angioplasty, or medication. We now know this is not true. Research has shown that coronary arteries can be unblocked naturally if a PBD is followed.[3] If you suffer from coronary artery disease, you can now have the same hope of disease reversal as our patients with type-2 diabetes, if you follow the 30-Day Diabetes Miracle program. For patients of our lifestyle medicine colleague Dr. Caldwell Esselstyn, 75 percent had a regression of their artery blockages after 5 years of treatment with a plant-based diet![4]

CANCER

ABOUT 1.5 MILLION Americans will be diagnosed with cancer this year, not counting skin cancer. At least 1,500 people per day (560,000 per year) will die from one of many types of cancer, making this the second leading cause of death in the United States.[5] Even though heart disease kills more people, cancer is probably more feared, likely because of the ravaging nature of the disease.

To fight cancer, our bodies need to neutralize free radicals before they have a chance to damage our cells' DNA. Antioxidants and phytochemicals serve this need, by acting like free-radical sponges. Antioxidants are found almost entirely and phytochemicals are found exclusively in plant foods. The second line of defense is our immune system, which also depends on antioxidants and phytochemicals.

In numerous studies, a diet high in fruits, vegetables, and whole grains is associated with a lower incidence of several types of cancers.[6] In contrast, a diet high in animal protein and refined (processed) grains and low in fruits, vegetables, and whole grains is related to an increased risk of various cancers.[7] Regular physical activity reduces risk of colon, breast, prostate, and possibly lung cancer.[8] The recommendation, then, to reduce your risk of getting most forms of cancer is to eat a plant-based diet and do moderate physical activity at least five times per week. Sound familiar?

STROKE AND HYPERTENSION

STROKE IS THE third leading cause of death in the United States, killing 150,000 people per year.[9] Another 550,000 will suffer from nonfatal stroke,[10] and many of these people will be left with crippling disabilities such as paralysis, speech and swallowing disorders, visual difficulties, or mental incapacity. Research has shown that for every increase of three servings of fruits and vegetables in the diet, stroke risk is reduced by 22 to 31 percent.[11]

High blood pressure is a prime risk factor for stroke. It has been shown that for every 20-point increase in the systolic (top number) blood pressure, the risk of stroke will double.[12] Effective ways to reduce high blood pressure include eating a PBD, losing weight, and doing routine physical activity.[13] The same recommendations we make to stop diabetes.

WAIT, THERE'S EVEN MORE

THERE ARE STILL more conditions for which this lifestyle modification prescription is effective.

High cholesterol is rampant in this country. About 100 million Americans have total cholesterol above 200, which is at the upper limits of the desirable or recommended range. This helps explain why heart attack is America's number one killer. In the famous Framingham Heart Study, 35 percent of heart attacks occurred in people who had total cholesterol between 150 and 200![14] These people likely never got any warning from their doctors that there was anything wrong. For optimal protection from heart attack, you should keep your total cholesterol below 150: No one in the Framingham study who maintained total cholesterol less than 150 died from coronary heart disease.[15] Our recommendations are to keep your total cholesterol below 150 and your low-density (LDL) cholesterol below 70, if you want near-total protection from heart attack. A PBD and physical activity have been shown to be effective in accomplishing these goals.[16] It has been our observation at LCA that the diet and physical activity of the 30-Day Diabetes Miracle program usually lowers cholesterol levels by 15 to 20 percent within the first 2 weeks. Many patients see more dramatic results.

Autoimmune disorders, such as rheumatoid arthritis, are also improved when our program is followed. Research shows a PBD can significantly improve those with rheumatoid arthritis.[17] If, like Dr. House's wife, Bonnie, you suffer the uniquely unpleasant pain associated with arthritis, you'll know that significant improvement will truly feel like a miracle. Other autoimmune conditions, such as lupus, multiple sclerosis, Crohn's disease, ulcerative colitis, and psoriasis can also be helped by discontinuing the standard American diet (SAD) and adopting a PBD, with much of the improvement coming from increasing omega-3 fatty acids in the diet.[18] Some experts recommend fish oil preparations as a source of the omega-3s. However, we recommend eating freshly ground flaxseed, walnuts, and hemp oil as better alternatives. There is also a plant-based version of dehydroepiandrosterone (DHA),[19] one of the key omega-3 fatty acids in fish oil, which is available for those contemplating taking fish oil (you can find information about it on our website, www.diabetesmiracle.org).

Osteoporosis is a debilitating condition that affects 10 million Americans and accounts for 1.5 million fractures per year.[20] The public has been lead to believe this disease is caused by a deficiency of calcium in the diet. It's safe to say that Americans suffer from very few conditions caused by dietary *deficiencies.* Our diseases are caused by our dietary *excesses,* and osteoporosis is no exception. Countries with the *lowest* calcium intakes have the lowest hip fracture rates, and countries with the highest calcium intakes have the highest rates.[21] This doesn't mean calcium is bad for your bones. The problem isn't how much calcium is consumed—rather, it is how much our bodies are losing in urine. The same countries that have high calcium intakes also have high amounts of animal protein in the diet.[22] Animal proteins make the body fluids more acidic, causing calcium to be removed from bone and eliminated by the kidneys. The result is osteoporosis. The 30-Day Diabetes Miracle program, consisting of a plant-based diet containing adequate calcium and no animal protein, as well as physical activity that includes strength training, will help prevent osteoporosis.

Because of the high fiber content of the plant-based diet, *constipation, hemorrhoids, varicose veins,* and even symptoms of *heartburn* can be expected to improve, too. After stopping dairy product consumption, many report fewer *allergies, sinus infections,* and other *upper respiratory ailments.*

EXPERIENCE
LIFESTYLE CENTER OF AMERICA
FOR YOURSELF

CAN I REALLY DO THIS PROGRAM AT HOME?

Yes, you can do this program at home! It's a matter of choice and commitment, and it can be done. But you might find that you need that extra "push," that extra incentive. If you're the kind of person who would prefer to transition among like-minded comrades, you might consider an 18-day stay at Lifestyle Center of America (LCA) or a 12-day session at LCA's resort program in Sedona, Arizona. The benefits of a residential program are many. While you're developing and solidifying new, healthful habits, you'll not have to face the temptations of the outside world. You will also be able to immerse yourself in the educational environment of lifestyle specialists and be able to experience firsthand an abundant variety of delicious plant-based foods.

Call a stopping-diabetes program specialist at 800-685-7310 or visit our website (www.diabetesmiracle.org) for more information on our residential programs. You can also join our online community, log your results, learn, and share your experiences with others involved in the miracle.

Notes

STOP DIABETES BEFORE IT STOPS YOU

1. Centers for Disease Control and Prevention [CDC], *National Diabetes Fact Sheet: General Information and National Estimates on Diabetes in the United States, 2005* (Atlanta, GA: Department of Health and Human Services, 2005).
2. N. R. Kleinfeld, "Bad Blood: Diabetes and Its Awful Toll Quietly Emerge As a Crisis," *New York Times*, January 9, 2006: A1, A18–A19.
3. National Center for Chronic Disease Prevention and Health Promotion, CDC, *Preventing Diabetes and Its Complications* (Atlanta, GA: Department of Health and Human Services, 2005). Available at www.cdc.gov/nccdphp/publications/factsheets/prevention/diabetes .htm. Accessed July 2007.
4. Still, most doctors have not changed the advice they give their heart patients and treat them as if coronary artery disease were incurable, nonreversible, and at best only managed—usually with drugs.
5. Cabrillo College [California] Stroke and Acquired Disability Center, "The Fundamental Concepts of Healing and Curing." Available at www.cabrillo.edu/academics/strokecenter/ side2/healing.html. Accessed July 2007.
6. National Institute of Diabetes and Digestive and Kidney Diseases, *General Information and National Estimates on Diabetes in the United States, 2005* [National Diabetes Statistics Fact Sheet] (Bethesda, MD: U.S. Department of Health and Human Services, National Institutes of Health, 2005).
7. Ibid.
8. Statistical analysis done on data from patients attending Lifestyle Center of America's 18-day program from March 2003 to December 2006. Data analysis was conducted by the Loma Linda University School of Public Health, Department of Epidemiology and Biostatistics. All values are statistically significant at $p. <.001$. Sample sizes range from 213 to 312.
9. Fructosamines are blood proteins that have glucose attached to them. They are an indicator of what your blood sugar levels have been over the previous 2 to 3 weeks.
10. Dennis Deaton, *The Ownership Spirit Handbook* (Mesa, AZ: Quma Learning, 2003).
11. World Health Organization, Health Systems: *Improving Performance* [World Health Report 2000] (Geneva: World Health Organization, June 21, 2000), p. 164. Available at www.who.int/whr/2000/en/whr00_en.pdf. Accessed July 2007.
12. B. Starfield, "Is U.S. Health Really the Best in the World?" *Journal of the American Medical Association* 284 (2000): 483–485.

13. Derrick Z. Jackson, "Diabetes and the Trash Food Industry" [Editorial], *Boston Globe*, January 11, 2006. Available at www.boston.com/yourlife/health/diseases/articles/2006/01/11/diabetes_and_the_trash_food_industry. Accessed July 2007.
14. Kleinfeld, "Bad Blood: Diabetes and Its Awful Toll Quietly Emerge as Crisis."

CHAPTER 1

1. N. R. Kleinfeld, "Bad Blood: Diabetes and Its Awful Toll Quietly Emerge as a Crisis," *New York Times*, January 9, 2006: A1, A18–A19.
2. Douglas Lisle and Alan Goldhamer, *The Pleasure Trap* (Summertown, TN: Healthy Living, 2003), pp. 41–50.
3. Alan Cowell, "Deadly Bird Flu Confirmed in British Turkeys," *New York Times*, February 4, 2007. Available at www.nytimes.com/2007/02/04/world/europe/04birdflu.html?ex=1185508800&en=ba2601e491f68268&ei=5070. Accessed July 2007.
4. Eric Schlosser, *Fast Food Nation* (New York: Harper Perennial, 2005), p. 4.
5. *Super Size Me*, directed by Morgan Spurlock (Roadside Attractions, Samuel Goldwyn Films, and Showtime Independent Films, 2004).
6. T. Colin Campbell, *The China Study* (Dallas: BenBella Books, 2004).
7. Ibid., p. 76.
8. Janet E. Fulton and Harold W. Kohl III, "The Epidemiology of Obesity, Physical Activity, Diet, and Type 2 Diabetes Mellitus," in *Lifestyle Medicine*, ed. James Rippe (Malden, MA: Blackwell Science), p. 870; and M. I. Harris, "Epidemiological Studies on the Pathogenesis of Non-Insulin-Dependent Diabetes Mellitus (NIDM)," *Clinical and Investigative Medicine* 18 (1995): 231–239.
9. Mike Huckabee, *Quit Digging Your Grave with a Knife and Fork* (New York: Center Street, 2005).
10. Campbell, *The China Study*.
11. Peter Cox, quoted in Howard Lyman, *Mad Cowboy: Plain Truth from the Cowboy Who Won't Eat Meat* (New York: Scribner, 1998), p. 45.
12. Migration and modernization have led many Asian and Pacific Islander Americans to abandon their traditional plant-based diets and choose more animal protein, animal fat, and refined (processed) carbohydrates. University of Michigan Heath System Mulitcultural Health Team, reviewers, "Diabetes in Asian Americans." Available at www.med.umich.edu/1libr/aha/umasamer01.htm. Accessed July 2007. See also Joslin Diabetes Center, "Diabetes Growing Rapidly in Asian Americans." Available at www.joslin.org/1083_2004.asp. Accessed July 2007.
13. E. Ravussin, M. E. Vlanecia, J. Esparza, et al., "Effects of a Traditional Lifestyle on Obesity in Pima Indians," *Diabetes Care* 17, no. 9 (1994): 1067–1074.
14. Ibid.
15. L. O. Schulz, P. H. Bennett, E. Ravussin, et al., "Effects of Traditional and Western Environments on Prevalence of Type 2 Diabetes in Pima Indians in Mexico and the U.S.," *Diabetes Care* 29, no. 8 (2006): 1866–1871; and D. E. Williams, W. C. Knowler, C. J. Smith, et al., "The Effect of Indian or Anglo Dietary Preference on the Incidence of Diabetes in Pima Indians," *Diabetes Care* 24, no. 5 (2001): 811–816.
16. Lyman, *Mad Cowboy*, p. 35.
17. John Robbins, *Diet for a New America* (Walpole, NH: Stillpoint Publishing, 1987), p. 277.
18. Dennis Deaton, *The Book on Mind Management*, 2nd ed. (Mesa, AZ: Quma Learning Systems, 2003), p. 180.
19. Alison Fleming, *Motivational Issues from a Psychobiological Perspective* (Toronto: University of Toronto, 2007).
20. E. Shiloah, S. Witz, Y. Abramovitch, et al., "Effect of Acute Psychotic Stress in Non-Diabetic Subjects on β-Cell Function and Insulin Sensitivity," *Diabetes Care* 26 (2003): 1262–1467.
21. M. Cosgrove, "Do Stressful Life Events Cause Type 1 Diabetes?" *Occupational Medicine* 54 (2004): 250–254.

22. Cited in Marilyn Elias, "The Fit May Produce Less of Harmful, Stress-Related Chemicals," *USA Today*, March 8, 2007: D9.

CHAPTER 2

1. Albert Einstein, "Albert Einstein Quotes." Available at www.heartquotes.net/einstein.html. Accessed July 2007.
2. Maya Angelou. Interview with the Academy of Achievement (January 22, 1999: High Point, NC). Available at www.achievement.org/autodoc/page/ang0int-1. Accessed July 2007.
3. Albert Einstein, "Albert Einstein Quotes." Available at http://thinkexist.com/quotation/learn_from_yesterday-live_for_today-hope_for/222120.html. Accessed July 2007.
4. Tim Arnott, *Dr. Arnott's 24 Realistic Ways to Improve Your Health* (Nampa, Idaho: Pacific Press, 2004), p. 19.
5. M. E. Seligman, "Explanatory Style and Cell-Mediated Immunity in Elderly Men and Women," *Health Psychology* 10, no. 4 (1991): 229–235. Italics added.
6. T. Maruta, "Optimists vs. Pessimists: Survival Rate among Medical Patients over a 30-Year Period," *Mayo Clinic Proceedings* 72, no. 2 (2000): 140–143.
7. Viktor Frankl, *Man's Search for Meaning*, 1st ed. (Boston: Beacon Press, 2006), p. 66.
8. Marilyn Elias, "A Laugh a Day May Help Keep Death Further Away." *USA Today*, March 12, 2007: 5D.
9. John 15:13.
10. Albert Schweitzer, "Albert Schweitzer Quotes." Available at www.brainyquote.com/quotes/authors/a/albert_schweitzer.html. Accessed July 2007.
11. Edmund Burke, "Authors: Edmund Burke." Available at www.quotedb.com/quotes/862. Accessed July 2007.
12. Thomas Jefferson, "Service Quotes to Inspire and Challenge." Available at www.wisdom quotes.com/cat_service.html. Accessed July 2007.
13. Dennis Deaton, *The Book on Mind Management*, 2nd ed. (Mesa, AZ: Quma Learning Systems, 2003), p. 128.
14. G. Gallup, *Religion in America: 1990* (Princeton, NJ: Princeton Religious Research Center, 1990).
15. D. A. Matthews, M. E. McCullough, and D. B. Larson, "Religious Commitment and Health Status," *Archives of Family Medicine* 7 (1998): 118–124.
16. H. G. Koenig, M. McCullough, and D. Larson, *Handbook of Religion and Health* (New York: Oxford University Press, 2000), pp. 7–14.
17. H. G. Koenig, "Religion, Spirituality, and Medicine: Application to Clinical Practice," *Journal of the American Medical Association* 284, no. 13 (2000): 1708.

CHAPTER 3

1. American Diabetes Association, "Diabetes: Heart Disease and Stroke." Available at www.diabetes.org/diabetes-heart-disease-stroke.jsp. Accessed July 2007.
2. W. B. Kannel and D. L. McGee, "Diabetes and Cardiovascular Disease. The Framingham Study," *Journal of the American Medical Association* 241, no. 19 (1979): 2035–2038.
3. S. P. Dhindsa, S. Prabhakar, M. Sethi, et al., "Frequent Occurrence of Hypogonadotropic Hypogonadism in Type 2 Diabetes," *Journal of Clinical Endocrinology and Metabolism* 89, no. 11 (2004): 5462–5468; and B. Goldfarb, "Low Testosterone Should Arouse Clinical Interest," *DOC News* 2, no. 12 (2005): 1.
4. A. K. Schroeder, S. Tauchert, O. Ortmann, et al., "Insulin Resistance in Patients with Polycystic Ovary Syndrome," *Annals of Medicine* 36, no. 6 (2004): 429–439; S. M. Carlsen, K. A. Salvesen, E. Vanky, et al., "Polycystic Ovarian Syndrome and Diabetes," *Tidsskrift for den Norske Laegeforening* 125, no. 19 (2005): 2619–2621; and J. Wider, "Male Hormones May Cause Menstrual Problems in Diabetic Women" [Press Release] (Society for Women's Health Research, August 21, 2003).

5. Jim Nuovo, "Type 2 Diabetes," in *Chronic Disease Management*, ed. Jim Nuovo (New York: Springer, 2007), p. 148.
6. Testing should be done especially if the following risk factors are present:
   - Family history of diabetes
   - Overweight: body mass index (BMI) (in kilograms per meter squared; kg/m2) greater than 25
   - Previous birth of baby weighing more than 9 pounds
   - American Indian, African American, Latino, South or East Asian, Pacific Island ethnicity
   - Own birth size greater than 9 pounds or smaller than 6 pounds
   - PCOS
   - Unexplained miscarriage or previous baby born with defects
   - Older than age 29
7. Between 10 and 15 percent of adults diagnosed with type-2 diabetes turn out to have something different, called type-1.5 diabetes, also called slow-onset type-1 diabetes or latent autoimmune diabetes in adults (LADA). At first, it looks and acts like type 2, even responding to some common type-2 oral medications. These patients look a little different from the average patient with type-2 diabetes, though. Their weight is usually normal, and their cholesterol and blood pressure are also usually within normal limits because they do not have the high insulin levels that cause such changes. Further testing, which may be ordered when the medications lose efficacy, often reveals little or no insulin resistance, which is why the oral medications used to decrease insulin resistance stop working. So the disease starts looking more like type-1 diabetes, in that it seems lifestyle choices (too much energy in, not enough energy out) are not the principle cause. And, like type 1, we see pancreatic beta-cell function dropping off, but at a much slower rate (3 to 7 years, as opposed to 3 to 6 months).

   We don't know exactly why this happens, though we have ideas. Several studies have uncovered antibodies in these patients that attack beta-cells in the pancreas (not unlike the presumptive culprit in type-1 diabetes), caught right in the middle of the destruction (hence the terms *slow-onset type-1 diabetes* and *latent autoimmune diabetes in adults*). The cause could be environmental toxins, and/or it might be a genetic disorder. Another intriguing possibility lies in prenatal conditions: Perhaps when such a patient was still in the womb, his or her mother took in too much energy without enough physical activity, which weakened the fetal pancreas, affecting its ability to function later in life.

   No matter what the cause of type-1.5 diabetes, individuals with the problem will probably need insulin with time. If they follow the principles of the 30-Day Diabetes Miracle program, their blood sugars will be easier to control and they may avoid the problems that come from getting too much insulin. This will help ensure that this patient's total insulin dosage per day is the same as that which is necessary for someone with uncomplicated type-1 diabetes or even someone without diabetes. (A normal adult produces 20 to 30 units per day from the pancreas.)

   Now, type-3 diabetes is really fascinating. In 2005, researchers at Brown University Medical School discovered what seems to be another, quite different, type of diabetes. This one, which they termed *type 3*, doesn't affect blood sugar, but does have to do with insulin. Only the insulin involved here doesn't come from the pancreas. Pretty stunning revelation. So where's it coming from? We've thought for years that there are some tissues in the body that don't need insulin to transport glucose energy into their cells. For example, the medical establishment has know for a long time that brain cells don't seem to require pancreatic insulin for energy metabolism. The Brown researchers discovered that, in fact, the brain does need insulin—but it makes its own! That means that brain cells produce insulin in tiny amounts, but enough to metabolize energy for normal brain functioning. It also means that brain cells have their own sensitivity and resistance to brain insulin. Now, the most interesting (and still unproven) theory is that when things go awry with brain insulin, the brain suffers because of poor energy metabolism. The Brown scientists believe they've found a link between brain insulin resistance and Alzheimer's disease. Most diabetes experts agree that there is some kind of link between diabetes and Alzheimer's disease. For example, people with type-2 diabetes have a two to three times greater risk of developing Alzheimer's disease. The researchers have also discovered deposits of a protein in the pancreases of many type-2 diabetes patients that correspond to similar protein deposits found in the brain tissue of people with Alzheimer's.

But more studies must be done to determine if there really is a type-3 diabetes, if a brain insulin–related central nervous system malfunction is at the root of the disease, or whether the effects of the more common forms of diabetes contribute to the death of memory cells, which is the basis for Alzheimer's disease. We believe there's enough evidence to posit that Alzheimer's, one way or the other, is caused by too much energy in and not enough energy out.

8. S. Tauriainen, K. Salminen, and H. Hyöty, "Can Enteroviruses Cause Type 1 Diabetes?" *Annals of the New York Academy of Science* vol. 1005, ed. C. B. Sanjeevi and G. S. Eisenbarth (New York: New York Academy of Sciences, 2003), pp. 13–22.

9. H. Malcova, Z. Sumnik, P. Drevinek, et al., "Absence of Breast-Feeding Is Associated with the Risk of Type 1 Diabetes: A Case-Control Study in a Population with Rapidly Increasing Incidence," *European Journal of Pediatrics* 165, no. 2 (2006): 114–119.

10. T. Colin Campbell and H. C. Gerstein, "Cow's Milk Exposure and Type 1 Diabetes Mellitus: A Critical Overview of the Clinical Literature," *Diabetes Care* 17 (1994): 13–19.

11. M. F. Holick, "Vitamin D: Importance in the Prevention of Cancers, Type 1 Diabetes, Heart Disease, and Osteoporosis," American Journal of Clinical Nutrition 79, no. 3 (2004): 362–371.

12. D. Hyppönen, E. Läärä, A. Reunanen, et al., "Intake of Vitamin D and Risk of Type 1 Diabetes: A Birth-Cohort Study," *Lancet* 358 (2001): 1500–1503.

13. Back then, medical school instructors told students a well-worn joke (truth); they said, "Fifty percent of what we teach you in medical school isn't true. We just don't know *which* 50 percent!"

14. Prenatal influences, a couch-potato youth culture, our reliance on automobiles, the cutting of school physical education programs, the promotion of junk foods in school, and other factors are all leading us down a diabetic path at an early age.

15. Julian Whitaker, *Reversing Diabetes* (New York: Warner Books, 2001), p. 42.

16. Nuovo, "Type 2 Diabetes," p. 145

17. These side effects appear to occur most often when Lyrica is taken in combination with the thiazolidinedione class of drugs, which include Actos (pioglitazone) and Avandia (rosiglitazone), according to Pfizer. Available at www.lyrica.com/content/main_safety_information.jsp; www.lyrica.com/content/dpn_common_questions.jsp; www.pfizer.com/pfizer/download/ppi_lyrica.pdf. All accessed July 2007.

18. E. G. Campbell, R. L. Gruen, J. Mountford, et al., "A National Survey of Physician-Industry Relationships," *New England Journal of Medicine* 356 (2007): 1742–1750.

19. American Diabetes Association, available at www.diabetes.org/diabetes-heart-disease-stroke.jsp. Accessed July 2007.

CHAPTER 4

1. Brenda Davis and Vasanto Melina, *Becoming Vegan: The Complete Guide to Adopting A Healthy Plant-Based Diet* (Summertown, TN: Book Publishing, 2000), p. 206.

2. Worldwatch Institute, *State of the World 2000*. Available at www.worldwatch.org. Accessed July 2007.

3. Davis and Melina, *Becoming Vegan*.

4. Julia Layton, "How Calories Work." Available at www.health.howstuffworks.com/calorie.htm. Accessed July 2007.

5. *Super Size Me*, directed by Morgan Spurlock (Roadside Attractions, Samuel Goldwyn Films, and Showtime Independent Films, 2004).

6. Bruce Horovitz, "Burger King of Cool? KK Wants to 'Stay on the Cutting Edge of Pop Culture,'" *USA Today*, February 7, 2007. Available at www.usatoday.com/money/industries/food/2007-02-06-burger-king-usat_x.htm. Accessed July 2007.

7. Allan Borushek, *The Calorie King: Calories, Fat, and Carbohydrate Counter* (Costa Mesa, CA: Family Health, 2006).

8. P. A. Cotton, A. F. Subar, J. E. Friday, and A. Cook, "Dietary Sources of Nutrients among US Adults, 1994 to 1996," *Journal of the American Dietetic Association* 104 (2004): 921–930.

9. J. Salmeron, F. B. Hu, J. E. Manson, et al., "Dietary Fat Intake and Risk of Type 2 Diabetes in Women," *American Journal of Clinical Nutrition* 73 (2001): 1019–1026.

10. U.S. Department of Agriculture and U.S. Department of Health and Human Services, *Nutrition and Your Health: Dietary Guidelines for Americans* [Home and Garden Bulletin 232], 5th ed. (Washington, DC: U.S. Government Printing Office, 2000). Other government data from the Economic Research Service of the U.S. Department of Agriculture estimates the daily intake of sugar in 2004 was 29.7 teaspoons; however, the authors used aggregate food supply data and assumed serving sizes based on the government's My Pyramid Plan, which skews the results downward.

11. Economic Research Service, U.S. Department of Agriculture, *Data Sets: Loss-Adjusted Food Availability*. Available at www.ers.usda.gov/Data/FoodConsumption/FoodGuideIndex.htm. Accessed July 2007. See also Stephen Haley, Economic Research Service, U.S. Department of Agriculture, *Sugar and Sweeteners Outlook* [SSS-248], February 5, 2007. Available at http://usda.mannlib.cornell.edu/usda/ers/SSS//2000s/2007/SSS-02-06-2007.pdf. Accessed July 2007.

12. J. F. Guthrie and J. F. Morton, "Food Sources of Added Sweeteners in the Diets of Americans, *Journal of the American Dietetic Association* 100 (2000): 152–154.

13. Fructose, pure floral honey, and some sugar alcohols such as sorbitol and xylitol as well as maltodextrin will raise your blood sugar more slowly and less steeply than pure glucose, but some diabetes experts caution against using these sweeteners at all if you're trying to avoid postprandial blood sugar elevation. This is important to note because both dextrose and maltodextrin, are the first ingredients in most sugar-free powdered sweeteners like Equal, Splenda, and Sweet'N Low. Grain Processing Corporation, a major manufacturer of maltodextrin, includes this statement on its website (www.grainprocessing.com) and in its promotional materials: "Diabetics should follow the advice of their physicians. . . . [M]altodextrin's glycemic index should be considered metabolically equivalent to glucose (dextrose)." Wow. That's interesting considering all those artificial sweeteners are specifically marketed to people with diabetes and most are approved by major diabetes organizations like the American Diabetes Association (ADA).

14. Sharon Fowler, "Abstract 1058-P," paper presentation at the 65th Annual Scientific Sessions of the American Diabetes Association, San Diego, CA, June 2005.

15. T. Colin Campbell, *The China Study* (Dallas: BenBella Books, 2004), p. 29.

16. Ibid.

17. Campbell, *The China Study*, pp. 30–31.

18. Edward Abramson, *Emotional Eating* (San Francisco: Jossey-Bass, 2001).

19. L. Christensen, "The Role of Caffeine and Sugar in Depression," *Nutrition Report* 9, no. 3 (1991): 17–23.

20. T. Wells, "World Food: People, Plants & Politics," *New Internationalist*, November 1991. Available at www.newint.org/issue225/keynote.htm. Accessed July 2007.

21. *Food Safety and Foodborne Illness*. Factsheet no. 237, published by the World Health Organization, revised January 2002.

22. Centers for Disease Control and Prevention, *Salmonella enteritidis: Frequently Asked Questions*. Available at www.cdc.gov/ncidod/dbmd/diseaseinfo/salment_g.htm#How%20Eggs%20Become%20Contaminated. Accessed July 2007.

23. Centers for Disease Control and Prevention, *Foodborne Illness: Frequently Asked Questions*. Available at www.cdc.gov/ncidod/dbmd/diseaseinfo/files/foodborne_illness_FAQ.pdf. Accessed July 2007.

24. "Dirty Birds: Even 'Premium' Chickens Harbor Dangerous Bacteria," *Consumer Reports*, January 2007: 20–23.

25. G. P. Gui, P. R. Thomas, M. L. Tizard, et al., "Two-Year Outcomes Analysis of Crohn's Disease Treated with Rifabutin and Macrolide Antibiotics," *Journal of Antimicrobial Chemotherapy* 39, no. 3 (1997): 393–400.

26. Partnership for Food Safety Education, *About Foodborne Illness*. Available at www.fight bac.org/content/view/14/21. Accessed July 2007.

27. G. C. Buehring, S. M. Philpott, and K. Y. Choi, "Humans Have Antibodies Reactive with Bovine Leukemia Virus," *AIDS Research and Humam Retroviruses* 19, no. 12 (2003): 1105–1113.

28. G. C. Buehring, "Evidence of Bovine Leukemia Virus in Human Mammary Epithelial Cells," *Seminars in Cell and Developmental Biology* 35 (1997): 27A; Abstract V-1001.

29. N. Franscini, A. E. Gedaily, U. Matthey, et al., "Prion Protein in Milk," *PLoS ONE* 1(1) (2006): 1–71.

30. N. Hellmich, "Health Spending Soars for Obesity," *USA Today*, June 27, 2005: A1.

CHAPTER 5

1. See Brian Wansink, *Mindless Eating* (New York: Bantam Dell, 2006); a fantastic book by a Cornell food scientist.

2. National Institute of Diabetes and Digestive and Kidney Diseases, *Diabetes Control and Complications Trial (DCCT)*. Available at http://diabetes.niddk.nih.gov/dm/pubs/control/ index.htm. Accessed July 2007. UK Prospective Diabetes Study (UKPDS) Group, "Intensive Blood-Glucose Control with Sulphonylureas or Insulin Compared with Conventional Treatment and Risk of Complications Patients with Type 2 Diabetes (UKPDS 33)," *Lancet* 352 (1998): 837–853.

3. National Institute of Diabetes and Digestive and Kidney Diseases, *Diabetes Control and Complications Trial (DCCT)*.

4. Wansink, *Mindless Eating*.

5. R. J. Barnard, M. R. Massey, S. Cherny, et al., "Long-Term Use of a High-Complex-Carbohydrate, High-Fiber, Low-Fat Diet and Exercise in the Treatment of NIDDM Patients," *Diabetes Care* 6, no. 3 (1983): 268–273.

6. T. Colin Campbell, *The China Study* (Dallas: BenBella Books, 2004), p. 29:
   > Major McKay, a prominent English physician in the early twentieth century, provided one of the more entertaining, but most unfortunate, moments in this history. Physician McCay was stationed in the English colony of India in 1912 in order to identify good fighting men in the Indian tribes. Among other things, he said that people who consumed less [animal] protein were of a "poor physique, and a cringing effeminate disposition is all that can be expected."

7. E. G. White, "Diet and Health," in *The Ministry of Healing* (Altamont, TN: Harvestime Books, 1999), p. 194.

8. A. Trichopoulou, "Adherence to a Mediterranean Diet and Survival in a Greek Population," *New England Journal of Medicine* 348 (2003): 2599–2608.

9. Gary E. Fraser, *Diet, Life Expectancy, and Chronic Disease: Studies of Seventh-Day Adventists and Other Vegetarians* (New York: Oxford University Press, 2003).

10. Note that the association between meat eating and diabetes was more apparent among men than women. See D. A. Snowdon and R. L. Phillips, "Does a Vegetarian Diet Reduce the Occurrence of Diabetes?" *American Journal of Public Health* 75, no. 5 (1985): 507–512.

11. Neal Nedley, *Proof Positive: How to Reliably Combat Disease and Achieve Optimal Health through Nutrition and Lifestyle*, 4th ed. (Ardmore, OK: Author, 1999), p. 181.

12. J. W. Anderson, B. M. Smith, and N. J. Gustafson, "Health Benefits and Practical Aspects of High-Fiber Diets," *American Journal of Clinical Nutrition* 5 (1994; Suppl.): 1242S–1247S.

13. J. C. Brand, B. J. Snow, G. P. Navhan, et al., "Plasma Glucose and Insulin Responses to Traditional Pima Indian Meals," *American Journal of Clinical Nutrition* 51, no. 3 (1990): 416–420.

14. Nedley, *Proof Positive*, p. 181.
15. *The Food Processor SQL* [computer program], by ESHA Research, Salem, OR. Nutrition analysis and fitness software.
16. R. S. Beaser, *Outsmarting Diabetes: A Dynamic Approach for Reducing the Effects of Insulin-Dependent Diabetes* (Minneapolis: Chronimed Publishing, 1994), p. 87.
17. Ibid.; Anderson, Smith, and Gustafson, "Health Benefits and Practical Aspects of High-Fiber Diets."
18. Nedley, *Proof Positive*, p. 180.
19. M. Chandalia, A. Garg, and D. Lutjohann, "Beneficial Effects of High Dietary Fiber Intake in Patients with Type 2 Diabetes Mellitus," *New England Journal of Medicine* 342 (2000): 1392–1398; and M. A. Pereira, D. R. Jacobs, J. J. Pins, et al., "Effect of Whole Grains on Insulin Sensitivity in Overweight Hyperinsulinemic Adults," *American Journal of Clinical Nutrition* 75, no. 5 (2002): 848–855.
20. E. Lanza, D. Y. Jones, G. Block, et al., "Dietary Fiber Intake in the U.S. Population," *American Journal of Clinical Nutrition* 46 (1987): 790–797.
21. J. Montonen, P. Knekt, A. A. Järvinen, et al., "Whole-Grain and Fiber Intake and the Incidence of Type 2 Diabetes," *American Journal of Clinical Nutrition* 77, no. 3 (2003): 622–629; and T. T. Fung, F. B. Hu, S. L. Pereira, et al., "Whole-Grain Intake and the Risk of Type 2 Diabetes: A Prospective Study in Men," *American Journal of Clinical Nutrition* 76, no. 3 (2002): 535–540.
22. U.S. Department of Agriculture, *National Nutrient Database for Standard Reference*. Available at www.nal.usda.gov/fnic/foodcomp/search. Accessed July 2007.
23. Two exceptions are brown rice and oats, both of which are whole grain, but often aren't labeled with the word *whole*.
24. Fraser, *Diet, Life Expectancy, and Chronic Disease*, p. 132.
25. M. S. Eberhardt, C. Ogden, M. Engelgau, et al., "Prevalence of Overweight and Obesity among Adults with Diagnosed Diabetes—United States, 1988–1994 and 1999–2002," *Morbidity and Mortality Weekly Report* 53, no. 45 (2004): 1066–1068.
26. The LCA diet has about 3 percent saturated fat, 0 trans-fat, and 17 to 22 percent good plant-based fats.
27. J. Salmerón, F. B. Hu, J. E. Manson, et al., "Dietary Fat Intake and Risk of Type 2 Diabetes in Women," *American Journal of Clinical Nutrition* 73 (2001): 1019–1026.
28. J. A. T. Pennington and Douglass J. Spungen, *Bowe's and Church's Food Values of Portions Commonly Used*, 18th ed. (Philadelphia: Lippincott Williams & Wilkins, 2005).
29. Too much fat in the blood is toxic to the β-cells that make insulin; it's called *lipotoxicity*. The most toxic of fats for β-cells is saturated fat. So lots of fat contributes to β-cell death, which, of course, leads to diabetes.
30. There was about a 57 percent insulin reduction with a low-fat diet versus a 1 percent reduction with a high-fat diet among a mixed group of patients with type-1 and type-2 diabetes. See I. M. Rabinowitch, "Effects of the High Carbohydrate-Low Calorie Diet upon Carbohydrate Tolerance in Diabetes Mellitus," [Abstract] *Canadian Medical Association Journal*, August 1935: 136–144. The original paper was presented at the Joint Meeting of the Ontario and Quebec Dietetic Associations, Ottawa, April 27, 1935.
31. John Goley, "What Causes Diabetes?" lecture presented January 2005, at Lifestyle Center of America. A study focused on 80 people recently diagnosed with diabetes. They were put on a low-fat diet in which 75 to 78 percent of calories came from carbs. At the end of 6 weeks, 62 percent of the subjects were off their insulin because their blood sugar levels were under control without it. The researchers followed the group for another 5 years. And here's what's incredibly exciting: At the end of those 5 years, 80 of the original group of patients with diabetes were functioning as people who did not have diabetes—without insulin. They had a loaded gun, but they had stopped pulling the trigger.
32. J. W. Anderson, R. H. Herman, and D. Zakim, "Effect of High Glucose and High Sucrose Diets on Glucose Tolerance of Normal Men," *American Journal of Clinical Nutrition* 26 (1973): 600–607.

33. C. Lara Castro and T. W. Garvey, "Diet, Insulin Resistance, and Obesity: Zoning In on Data for Atkins Dieters Living in South Beach," *Journal of Clinical Endocrinology and Metabolism* 89, no. 9 (2004): 4197–4205.

34. A. M. Rosenfalck, "A Low-Fat Diet Improves Peripheral Insulin Sensitivity in Patients with Type 1 Diabetes," *Diabetes Medicine* 23, no. 4 (2006): 384–392.

35. Soy protein is linked with a reduction in LDL cholesterol: People who regularly consume it, in the form of soy milk, tofu, and soybeans, have cholesterol levels 13 points lower than those who don't. And some of these foods, like garbanzo beans, have more beneficial effects on blood sugar than whole wheat foods. See P. Nestel, M. Cehun, and A. Chronopouls, "Effects of Long-Term Consumption and Single Meals of Chickpeas on Plasma Glucose, Insulin, and Triacylglycerol Concentrations," *American Journal of Clinical Nutrition* 79 (2004): 390–395.

36. B. H. Sung, T. L. Whitesett, W. R. Lovallo, et al., "Prolonged Increase in Blood Pressure by a Single Oral Does of Caffeine in Hypertensive Men," *American Journal of Hypertension* 7, no. 8 (1994): 755–758; and W. Lovallo, M. F. Wilson, A. S. Vincent, et al., "Blood Pressure Response to Caffeine Shows Incomplete Tolerance after Short-Term Regular Consumption," *American Journal of Hypertension* 43 (2004): 760–765.

37. R. W. Stout, "Blood Glucose and Atherosclerosis, Thrombosis, and Vascular Biology," *Journal of the American Heart Association* 1 (1981): 1:227–234.

38. U.S. Department of Health and Human Services, *The Surgeon General's Report on Nutrition and Health* [Public Health Service DHHS (PHS) Publication Number 88–50210] (Washington, DC: Government Printing Office, 1988), p. 658.

39. W. P. Castelli and K. Anderson, "A Population at Risk. Prevalence of High Cholesterol Levels in Hypertensive Patients in the Framingham Study," *American Journal of Medicine* 80, no. 2A (1986): 23–32.

40. Kenneth J. Carpenter, "A Short History of Nutritional Science: Part 4 (1945–1985)," *Journal of Nutrition* 133 (2003): 3331–3342.

41. Campbell, *The China Study*, p. 95.

42. Ibid.

43. J. D. Wright, J. Kennedy-Stephenson, C. Y. Wang, et al., "Trends in Intake of Energy and Macronutrients—United States, 1971–2000," *Morbidity and Mortality Weekly Report* 53, no. 4 (2004): 80–82.

44. Much of the current science and government recommendations on protein intake are based on the work of Dr. William Rose and his colleagues at the University of Illinois conducted in the 1940s and 1950s. By studying both rats and prisoners, Rose isolated the 20 amino acids that are the building blocks of proteins in humans. He found that eight of them, called *essential amino acids,* cannot be synthesized by the body and, therefore, must come from the diet. Without them, we would fall ill and eventually die. Rose reduced each of the essential amino acids from the prisoners' diet, one at a time, and when the prisoners started showing symptoms of protein deficiency, Rose doubled that highest measured minimum, just to be on the safe side. This became the recommended minimum daily amount. He ultimately determined that the total protein necessary for good health is 20 g per every 3,000 calories consumed. This translates to 2.6 percent of our calories coming from protein. This, by the way, is much, much less protein than the original German scientists believed was necessary.

45. T. Colin Campbell, "Muscling Out the Meat Myth." Available at www.vsdc.org/meat myth.html. Accessed July 2007.

46. Nedley, *Proof Positive*, p. 487.

47. Mark Messina and Virginia Messina, *The Simple Soybean and Your Health* (New York: Avery, 1994).

48. Pennington and Spungen, *Bowe's and Church's Food Values of Portions Commonly Used*, p. 153.

49. U.S. Department of Agriculture, *National Nutrient Database for Standard Reference.*

50. American Diabetes Association, "Complications of Diabetes in the United States." Available at www.diabetes.org/diabetes-statistics/complications.jsp. Accessed July 2007.

51. The Diabetes Control and Complications Trial Research Group, "The Effect of Intensive Treatment of Diabetes on the Development and Progression of Long-Term Complications in Insulin-Dependent Diabetes Mellitus," *New England Journal of Medicine* 329 (1993): 977–986.

52. J. W. Anderson, B. M. Johnstone, and M. E. Cook-Newell, "A Meta-Analysis of the Effects of Soy Protein Intake on Serum Lipids," *New England Journal of Medicine* 333, no. 5 (1995): 276–282.

53. E. L. Knight, M. J. Stampfer, S. E. Hankinson, et al., "The Impact of Protein Intake on Renal Function Decline in Women with Normal Renal Function or Mild Renal Insufficiency," *Annals of Internal Medicine* 138 (2003): 460–467; and J. Coresh, B. C. Astor, T. Greene, et al., "Prevalence of Chronic Kidney Disease and Decreased Kidney Function in the Adult US Population: Third National Health and Nutrition Examination Survey," *American Journal of Kidney Disease* 41 (2003): 1–12.

54. B. U. Ihle, G. J. Becker, J. A. Whitworth, et al., "The Effect of Protein Restriction on the Progression of Renal Insufficiency," *New England Journal of Medicine* 321, no. 26 (1989): 1773–1777.

55. Robert C. Atkins, *Dr. Atkins' New Diet Revolution* (New York: Avon Books, 2002), p. 100.

56. C. R. Sirtori, E. Agradi, F. Conti, et al., "Soybean-Protein Diet in the Treatment of Type-II Hyperlipoproteinaemia," *Lancet* 1, no. 8006 (1977): 275–277.

57. Actually, feedlot cattle are usually fed a mix that includes animal protein and even chicken litter (chicken droppings and chicken-house floor waste). This practice is legal in the United States as long as no protein is obtained from renderings of cows, deer, elk, sheep, or goats.

58. National Center for Health Statistics, *Deaths—Leading Causes.* Available at www.cdc.gov/nchs/fastats/lcod.htm. Accessed July 2007.

59. D. J. A. Jenkins, C. W. C. Kendal, A. Marchie, et al., "Type 2 Diabetes and the Vegetarian Diet," *American Journal of Clinical Nutrition* 78 (2003; Suppl.): 610S–616S.

60. Atkins, *Dr. Atkins' New Diet Revolution.*

61. Campbell, *The China Study,* p. 97.

62. If you're interested in the subject, you can see Katy McLaughlin and Ron Winslow, "Report Details Dr. Atkins's Health Problems: Diet Guru's Weight, Heart History Are Cited by Medical Examiner," *Wall Street Journal,* February 10, 2004; and Nancy Hellmich and Steve Sternberg, "Atkins Wasn't Obese, Hospital File Shows," *USA Today,* February 10, 2004. Available at www.usatoday.com/life/people/2004-02-10-atkins_x.htm. Accessed July 2007.

63. S. A. Bilsborough and T. C. Crowe, "Low-Carbohydrate Diets: What Are the Potential Short- and Long-Term Health Implications?" *Asia Pacific Journal of Clinical Nutrition* 12 (2003): 396–404; and A. Stevens, D. P. Robinson, J. Turpin, et al., "Sudden Cardiac Death of an Adolescent during Dieting," *Southern Medical Journal* 95, no. 9 (2002): 1047–1049.

64. Campbell, *The China Study,* p. 97.

65. Richard K. Bernstein, *Dr. Bernstein's Diabetes Solution,* (New York: Little, Brown, 2003), p. 120.

66. Ibid.

67. Campbell has visited LCA, eaten in our restaurant, and affirmed our dietary practices.

68. Bernstein, *Dr. Bernstein's Diabetes Solution,* p. 145.

69. Ibid.

70. James F. Balch, *The Super Anti-Oxidants: Why They Will Change the Face of Healthcare in the 21st Century* (New York: Evans, 1998), p. 8.

71. Nedley, *Proof Positive.*

72. Balch, *The Super Anti-Oxidants,* p. 9.

73. B. Halliwell, "Reactive Oxygen Species in Living Systems: Source, Biochemistry, and Role in Human Disease," *American Journal of Medicine* 91, no. 3C (1991): 14S–22S.

74. Jim Nuovo, "Type 2 Diabetes" in *Chronic Disease Management,* ed. Jim Nuovo (New York: Springer, 2007), p. 180.

75. D. Ziegler, "Oral Treatment with Alpha-Lipoic Acid Improves Symptomatic Diabetic Polyneuropathy," *Diabetes Care* 29 (2006): 2365–2370.

76. M. F. Melhem, P. A. Craven, and F. R. Derubertis, "Effects of Dietary Supplementation of Alpha-Lipoic Acid on Early Glomerular Injury in Diabetes Mellitus," *Journal of the American Society of Nephrology* 12 (2001): 124–133.

77. M. N. Diaz, B. Frei, J. A. Vita, and J. F. Keaney, "Antioxidants and Atherosclerotic Heart Disease," *New England Journal of Medicine* 337, no. 16 (1997): 408–416; D. W. Laight, M. J. Carrier, and E. E. Anggard, "Antioxidants, Diabetes and Endothelial Dysfunction," *Cardiovascular Research* 47 (2000): 457–464; and S. Bursell, A. C. Clermont, L. P. Aiello, et al., "High-Dose Vitamin E supplementation Normalizes Retinal Blood Flow and Creatinine Clearance in Patients with Type 1 Diabetes," *Diabetes Care* 22, no. 8 (1999): 1245–1251.

78. J. G. Eriksson, "The Effects of Coenzyme Q10 Administration on Metabolic Control in Patients with Type 2 Diabetes Mellitus," *Biofactors* 9, nos. 2–4 (1999): 315–318; J. Henriksen, C. B. Andersen, O. Hother-Nielsen, et al., "Impact of Ubiquinone (Coenzyme Q10) Treatment on Glycaemic Control, Insulin Requirement and Well-Being in Patients with Type 1 Diabetes Mellitus," *Diabetes Medicine* 16 (1999): 312–318; P. Langsjoen, A. Langsjoen, R. Willis, and K. Folkers, "Treatment of Essential Hypertension with Coenzyme Q10," *Molecular Aspects of Medicine* 15 (1994): S265–S272.

79. N. G. Congdon and K. P. West, "Nutrition and the Eye," *Current Opinion in Ophthalmology* 10 (1999): 484–473.

80. S. Hercberg, P. Galan, and P. Preziosi, "Antioxidant Vitamins and Cardiovascular Disease: Dr. Jekyll or Mr. Hyde?" *American Journal of Public Health* 89, no. 3 (1999): 289–291; and The Alpha-Tocopherol, Beta-Carotene Cancer Prevention Study Group, "The Effect of Vitamin E and Beta Carotene on Incidence of Lung Cancer and Other Cancers in Male Smokers," *New England Journal of Medicine* 330 (1994): 1029–1035.

81. A. M. de Burgos, M. Wartanowicz, and S. Ziemlanowski, "Blood Vitamin and Lipid Levels in Overweight and Obese Women," *European Journal of Clinical Nutrition* 46 (1992): 803–808; and B. Frei, "The Role of Vitamin C and Other Antioxidants in Atherogenesis and Vascular Dysfunction," *Proceedings of the Society of Experimental Biology and Medicine* 222, no. 3 (1999): 196–204.

82. H. Hemilia and R. M. Douglas, "Vitamin C and Acute Respiratory Infections," *International Journal of Tuberculosis and Lung Disease* 3, no. 9 (1999): 756–761.

83. A. B. Chausmer, "Zinc, Insulin and Diabetes." *Journal of the American College of Nutrition* 17, no. 2 (1998): 109–115.

84. James F. Balch and Phyllis A. Balch, *Prescription for Nutritional Healing*, 2nd ed. (Garden City Park, NY: Avery Publishing, 1997), pp. 45 and 230.

85. Virginia Messina and Mark Messina, *The Vegetarian Way: Total Health for You and Your Family* (New York: Three Rivers Press, 1996), p. 28.

86. Walter C. Willett, *Eat, Drink, and Be Healthy: The Harvard Medical School Guide to Healthy Eating* (New York: Free Press, 2001), p. 182.

87. Balch and Balch, *Prescription for Nutritional Healing*, p. 7.

88. Kristine Napier, *Eat Away Diabetes* (New York: Prentice Hall Press, 2002), p. 35.

89. Willett, *Eat, Drink, and Be Healthy*, p. 144.

90. Michelle Heimburger, "Caffeine Nation Marches On," *The Spark*, March 1, 2007. Available at http://dir.yahoo.com/thespark/7145/caffeine-nation-marches-on. Accessed July 2007.

91. Nedley, *Proof Positive*, pp. 499–500.

92. G. B. Keijzers, B. D. De Galan, C. J. Tack, et al., "Caffeine Can Decrease Insulin Sensitivity in Humans," *Diabetes Care* 25 (2002): 364–369; and A. Pizziol, V. Tikhonoff, C. D. Paleari, et al., "Effects of Caffeine on Glucose Tolerance: A Placebo-Controlled Study," *European Journal of Clinical Nutrition* 52 (1998): 846–849.

93. Stephen Cherniske, *Caffeine Blues: Wake Up to the Hidden Dangers of America's #1 Drug* (New York: Warner Books, 1998), pp. 199–200.

94. This would be a dose that would be lethal for 50 percent of individuals weighing 115 pounds. The dose amount would be higher for individuals weighing more. Information taken from the Material Safety Data Sheet for caffeine. Available at www.sciencelab.com/xMSDS-Caffeine-9927475. Accessed July 2007.

95. Marshall Brain, *How Caffeine Works*. Available at www.howstuffworks.com/caffeine4.htm. Accessed July 2007.

96. Which is why Excedrin makes headaches go away: It contains caffeine. The pain you experience around the same time the next day is called an *analgesic rebound headache*, and the makers of Excedrin count on it. Like caffeinated beverages, and hardcore narcotics, it's a self-perpetuating product. It can take a full week of serious discomfort before the symptoms abate.

97. L. A. Martini and R. J. Wood, "Vitamin D Status and the Metabolic Syndrome," *Nutrition Reviews* 4, no. 11 (2006): 479–486.

98. K. C. Chiu, A. Chu, V.L.W. Go, et al., "Hypovitaminosis D Is Associated with insulin Resistance in Beta Cell Dysfunction," *American Journal of Clinical Nutrition* 79 (2004): 820–825.

99. W. B. Grant and M. F. Holick, "Benefits and Requirements of Vitamin D for Optimal Health: A Review," *Alternative Medicine Review* 10, no. 3 (2005): 94–111.

100. B. W. Hollis, "Circulating 25-Hydroxyvitamin D Levels Indicative of Vitamin D Sufficiency: Implications for Establishing a New Effective Dietary Intake Recommendation for Vitamin D," *Journal of Nutrition* 135 (2005): 317–322; B. Dawson-Hughes, "Estimation of Optimal Serum Concentrations of 25-Hydroxyvitamin D for Multiple Health Outcomes," *American Journal of Clinical Nutrition* 84, no. 1 (2006): 18–28; and C. M. Weaver and J. C. Fleet, "Vitamin D Requirements: Current and Future," *American Journal of Clinical Nutrition* 80 (2004; Suppl.): 1735S–1739S.

101. Willett, *Eat, Drink, and Be Healthy*, p. 23.

102. A. S. Nicholson, M. Sklar, N. D. Barnard, et al., "Toward Improved Management of NIDDM: A Randomized, Controlled, Pilot Intervention Using a Low-Fat, Vegetarian Diet," *Preventive Medicine* 29, no. 3 (1999): 87–91.

103. N. D. Barnard, J. Cohen, D. J. Jenkins, et al., "A Low-Fat Vegan Diet Improves Glycemic Control and Cardiovascular Risk Factors in a Randomized Clinical Trial in Individuals with Type 2 Diabetes," *Diabetes Care* 29, no. 8 (2006): 1777–1783.

104. In an LCA study, hemoglobin A_{1c} (HgA_{1c}) was measured in 21 patients who ate a highly PBD. (HgA_{1c} values directly correlate with average blood sugar levels over the preceding 120 days prior to measuring the HgA_{1c}. Higher HgA_{1c} values indicate higher average blood sugar levels.) There was an 18.76 percent reduction in HgA_{1c}, from an average of 7.25 on entry to LCA to an average of 5.89 after 6 months (data were self-reported). In 16 patients who did not eat a highly PBD, there was only a 4.8 percent reduction in HgA_{1c}, from an average of 6.9 on entry to LCA to an average of 6.4 after 6 months (data were self-reported). These results were independent of other factors, including medicine intake.

105. M. Segasothy and P. A. Phillips, "Vegetarian Diet: Panacea for Modern Lifestyle Diseases?" [Commentary] *Quarterly Journal of Medicine* 92 (1999): 531–544.

106. T. Sherard, "Lifestyle Treatment of Type-2 Diabetes," paper presented to the Loma Linda University Preventive Medicine Department, October 2003.

CHAPTER 6

1. C. K. Roberts, D. Won, S. Pruthi, et al., "Effect of Diet and Exercise Intervention on Oxidative Stress, Inflammation, MMP-9 and Monocyte Chemotactic Activity in Men with Metabolic Syndrome Factors," *Journal of Applied Physiology* 100 (2005): 1657–1665.

2. Ibid.; and M. G. Crane and C. Sample, "Regression of Diabetic Neuropathy on Total Vegetarian (Vegan) Diet," *Journal of Nutrition and Medicine* 4 (1994): 431–439.

3. Virginia Messina, Reed Manels, and Mark Messina, *The Dietitian's Guide to Vegetarian Diets: Issues and Applications*, 2nd ed. (Sudbury, MA: Jones and Bartlett, 2004), p. 415; M. B. Schulze, S. Liu, E. B. Rimm, et al., "Glycemic Index, Glycemic Load, and Dietary Fiber Intake and Incidence of Type 2 Diabetes in Younger and Middle-Aged Women," *American Journal of Clinical Nutrition* 80 (2004): 348–356; and J. Brand-Miller, S. Hayne, P. Petocz, et al., "Low-Glycemic Index Diets in the Management of Diabetes: A Meta-Analysis of

Randomized Controlled Trials," *Diabetes Care* 26 (2003): 2261–2267.

4. It's the white rice, in case you're wondering.

5. Michael Pollan, *The Omnivore's Dilemma: A Natural History of Four Meals* (New York: Penguin Press, 2006).

6. Shauna S. Roberts, "Meat-Free Diets Pay Off," *Diabetes Forecast*, March 2007, p. 42. Also, N. D. Barnard, J. Cohen, D. Jenkins, et al., "A Low-Fat Vegan Diet Improves Glycemic Control and Cardiovascular Risk Factors in a Randomized Clinical Trial in Individuals with Type 2 Diabetes," *Diabetes Care* 29 (2006): 1777–1783.

7. R. Giacco, M. Parillo, A. A. Rivellese, et al., "Long-Term Dietary Treatment with Increased Amounts of Fiber-Rich Low-Glycemic Index Natural Foods Improves Blood Glucose Control and Reduces the Number of Hypoglycemic Events in Type 1 Diabetes Patients," *Diabetes Care* 23 (2000): 1461–1466.

8. S. J. Gillespie, K. D. Kulkarni, and A. E. Daly, "Using Carbohydrate Counting in Diabetes Clinical Practice," *Journal of the American Dietetic Association* 98, no. 8 (1998): 897–905.

9. Diabetes Control and Complications Trial Research Group, "Nutrition Interventions for Intensive Therapy in the Diabetes Control and Complications Trial," *Journal of the American Dietetic Association* 93 (1993): 768–772.

10. R. Laredo, "Carbohydrate Counting for Children and Adolescents," *Diabetes Spectrum* 13 (2000): 149–152.

11. S. Saffel-Shrier, "Carbohydrate Counting for Older Patients," *Diabetes Spectrum* 13 (2000): 158–162.

12. D. Reader, "Carbohydrate Counting for Pregnant Women," *Diabetes Spectrum* 13 (2000): 152–153.

13. M. A. Johnson, "Carbohydrate Counting for People with Type 2 Diabetes," *Diabetes Spectrum* 13 (2000): 156–158; Diabetes Control and Complications Trial Research Group, "Nutrition Interventions for Intensive Therapy in the Diabetes Control and Complications Trial"; and Diabetes Control and Complications Trial Research Group, "The Effect of Intensive Treatment of Diabetes on the Development and Progression of Long-Term Complications in Insulin-Dependent Diabetes Mellitus," *New England Journal of Medicine* 329 (1993): 977–986.

14. B. W. Paddock, "Carbohydrate Counting in Institutions," *Diabetes Spectrum* 13, no. 3 (2000): 149.

15. A. Albright, "Carbohydrate Counting for Athletes," *Diabetes Spectrum* 13 (2000): 154–156.

16. Richard Bernstein, *Dr. Bernstein's Diabetes Solution* (New York: Little, Brown, 2003), p. 177.

17. Diabetes Control and Complications Trial Research Group, "Nutrition Interventions for Intensive Therapy in the Diabetes Control and Complications Trial."

18. Z. T. Bloomgarden, "Diet and Diabetes," *Diabetes Care* 27, no. 11 (2004): 2755–2761.

19. N. M. McKeown, J. B. Meigs, S. Liu, et al., "Carbohydrate Nutrition, Insulin Resistance, and the Prevalence of the Metabolic Syndrome in the Framingham Offspring Cohort," *Diabetes Care* 27, no. 2 (2004): 538–546.

20. American Diabetes Association, "Postprandial Blood Glucose" [Consensus Statement], *Diabetes Care* 24 (2001): 775–778; P. Reichard, B. Y. Nilsson, and U. Rosenqvist, "The Effect of Long-Term Intensified Insulin Treatment on the Development of Microvascular Complications of Diabetes Mellitus," *New England Journal of Medicine* 329 (1993): 304–309; and UK Prospective Diabetes Study Group, "Intensive Blood-Glucose Control with Sulphonylureas or Insulin Compared with Conventional Treatment and Risk of Complications in Patients with Type 2 Diabetes (UKPDS 33)," *Lancet* 352 (1998): 837–853.

21. J. Brand-Miller, T. M. S. Wolever, S. Colagiuri, et al., *The New Glucose Revolution*, 3rd ed. (New York: Marlowe, 2007).

22. A. E. Brynes, J. L. Lee, R E. Brighton, et al., "A Low Glycemic Diet Significantly Improves the 24-h Blood Glucose Profile in People with Type-2 Diabetes, as Assessed Using the Continuous Glucose MiniMed Monitor," *Diabetes Care* 26, no. 2 (2003): 548–549. In short, a low-GI diet is related to better long-term blood sugar control through more insulin sen-

sitivity. See A. E. Buyken, M. Toeller, G. Heitkamp, et al., "Glycemic Index in the Diet of European Outpatients with Type 1 Diabetes: Relations to Glycated Hemoglobin and Serum Lipids," *American Journal of Clinical Nutrition* 73 (2001): 574–581. This study found that a lower dietary GI was related to lower long-term blood sugars (HgA$_{1c}$), *independent of fiber intake*. See also, T. Wu, E. Giovannucci, T. Pischon, et al., "Fructose, Glycemic Load, and Quantity and Quality of Carbohydrate in Relation to Plasma C-Peptide in US Women," *American Journal of Clinical Nutrition* 80 (2004): 1043–1049.

23. Jennie Brand-Miller and Kay Foster-Powell, *The New Glucose Revolution Shopper's Guide to GI Values 2007* (New York: Marlowe, 2007), p. 79.

24. Ibid.

25. Real people who don't have diabetes, that is, and who probably don't have insulin resistance. So the effects on your own blood sugar might differ—we've seen this happen.

26. J. C. Brand-Miller, "Glycemic Load and Chronic Disease," *Nutrition Reviews* 61 (2003): S49–S55.

27. D. S. Ludwig, J. A. Majzoub, A. Al-Zahrani, et al, "High Glycemic Index Foods, Overeating, and Obesity," *Pediatrics* 103, no. 3 (1999): 1–6.

28. While cornstarch, raw flour, and Thicken Up have not been officially GI tested yet, our experience at LCA is that when we substitute cornstarch or Thicken Up for flour—especially white flour—in our recipes, the patients we informally test tend to have lower postprandial blood sugar spikes.

29. J. McMillan-Price, P. Petrocz, F. Atkinson, et al., "Comparison of 4 Diets Varying Glycemic Load on Weight Loss and Cardiovascular Risk Reduction in Overweight and Obese Young Adults: A Randomized, Controlled Trial," *Archives of Internal Medicine* 166, no. 14 (2006): 1438–1439.

30. See L. M. Steffen, D. R. Jacobs, M. A. Murtaugh, et al., "Whole Grain Intake Is Associated with Lower Body Mass Index and Greater Insulin Sensitivity among Adolescents," *American Journal of Epidemiology* 158 (2003): 243–250. This study examined adolescents living in Minnesota.

CHAPTER 7

1. F. J. Service, L. D. Hall, R. E. Westland, et al., "Effects of Size, Time of Day, and Sequence of Meal Ingestion on Carbohydrate Tolerance in Normal Subjects," *Diabetologia* 25 (1983): 316–321; E. Van Cauter, E. T. Shapiro, H. Tillil, et al., "Circadian Modulation of Glucose and Insulin Responses to Meals: Relationship to Cortisol Rhythm," *American Journal of Physiology* 262 (1992): E467–E475; A. Verrillo, A. De Teresa, C. Martino, et al., "Differential Roles of Splanchnic and Peripheral Tissues in Determining Diurnal Fluctuation of Glucose Tolerance," *American Journal of Physiology* 257 (1989): E459–E465; and A. Lee, M. Ader, G. A. Bray, and R. N. Bergman, "Diurnal Variation in Glucose Tolerance. Cyclic Suppression of Insulin Action and Insulin Secretion in Normal Weight, but Not Obese Subjects," *Diabetes* 41, no. 6 (1992): 742–749.

2. J. O. Hill, H. Wyatt, S. Phelan, and R. Wing, "The National Weight Control Registry: Is It Useful in Helping Deal with Our Obesity Epidemic?" *Journal of Nutrition Education and Behavior* 37, no. 4 (2005): 206–210; R. R. Wing and S. Phelan, "Long-Term Weight Loss Maintenance," *American Journal of Clinical Nutrition* 82 (2005; Suppl.): 222S–225S; and H. R. Wyatt, G. K. Grunwald, C. L. Mosca, et al., "Long-Term Weight Loss and Breakfast in Subjects in the National Weight Control Registry," *Obesity Research* 10, no. 2 (2002): 78–82.

3. The National Weight Control Registry, a database of more than 4,000 individuals who have been successful at long-term weight loss maintenance, reports that 78 percent of registry members eat breakfast every day of the week. Eating breakfast was also one of the habits associated with better health status and even *prolonged life* in another famous study, this one from Alameda County, California. In this population, not eating breakfast regularly was associated with 1.5 times increased risk of death compared to those who ate breakfast reg-

ularly. The other habits included never smoking, drinking fewer than five alcoholic beverages at one sitting, sleeping 7 to 8 hours a night, getting physically active, maintaining ideal weight, and avoiding snacks. See R. M. Masheb and C. M. Grilo, "Eating Patterns and Breakfast Consumption in Obese Patients with Binge Eating Disorder," *Behavior Research and Therapy* 44, no. 11 (2006): 1545–1553; and G. A. Kaplan, T. E. Seeman, R. D. Cohen, et al., "Mortality among the Elderly in the Alameda County Study: Behavioral and Demographic Risk Factors," *American Journal of Public Health* 77, no. 3 (1987): 307–312. Most important meal of the day? How about most important meal of your *life*?

4. S. A. Morse, P. S. Ciechanowski, W. J. Katon, and I. B. Hirsch, "Isn't This Just Bedtime Snacking? The Potential Adverse Effects of Night-Eating Symptoms on Treatment Adherence and Outcomes in Patients with Diabetes," *Diabetes Care* 29, no. 8 (2006): 1800–1804.

5. Kaya Chong, one of our LCA nutritionists, puts it simply: Snacking is associated with obesity in part because it increases the number of times you have to "face food"; and if you tend to overeat, this is one way you wind up adding unnecessary calories to your diet, not to mention a heavier workload for your tired pancreas.

6. Morse et al., "Isn't this Just Bedtime Snacking?"

7. C. A. Schoenborn, "Health habits of US adults, 1985: The 'Alameda 7' revisited," *Public Health Report* 101, no. 6 (1986): 571–580.

8. M. G. De Verdier and M. P. Longnecker, "Eating Frequency—A Neglected Risk Factor for Colon Cancer?" *Cancer Causes and Control* 3, no. 1 (1992): 77; and M. A. Lane, J. Mattison, D. K. Ingram, and G. S. Roth, "Caloric Restriction and Aging in Primates: Relevance to Humans and Possible CR Mimetics," *Microscopy Research and Technique* 59, no. 4 (2002): 335–338.

9. Lane et al., "Caloric Restriction and Aging in Primates."

10. L. Fontana and S. Klein, "Aging, Adiposity, and Calorie Restriction," *Journal of the American Medical Association* 297, no. 9 (2007): 986–994.

11. J. B. Johnson, D. R. Laub, and S. John, "The Effect on Health of Alternate Day Calorie Restriction: Eating Less and More Than Needed on Alternate Days Prolongs Life," *Medical Hypotheses* 67, no. 2 (2006): 209–211; and G. S. Roth, D. K. Ingram, and M. A. Lane, "Caloric Restriction in Primates and Relevance to Humans," *Annals of the New York Academy of Science* 928 (2001): 305–315.

CHAPTER 8

1. H. Mayer, D. DeRose, Z. Charles-Marcel, et al., "A Comparison between Intermittent Versus Continuous Aerobic Training on Cardiorespiratory and Body Composition Responses in Sedentary Adults," *Medicine and Science in Sports and Exercise* 32, no. 5 (2000): S218; K. Mayer, L. Samek, M Schwaibold, et al., "Interval Training in Patients with Severe Chronic Heart Failure: Analysis and Recommendations for Exercise Procedures," *Medicine and Science in Sports and Exercise* 29, no. 3 (1997): 377–381; and P. Ekkekakis and S. Petruzzello, "The Affective Beneficence of Vigorous Exercise Revisited, *British Journal of Health Psychology* 7 (2002): 47–66.

2. A. M. Wolf, M. R. Conaway, J. Q. Crowther, et al., "Translating Lifestyle Intervention to Practice in Obese Patients with Type 2 Diabetes: Improving Control with Activity and Nutrition (ICAN) Study," *Diabetes Care* 27 (2004): 1570–1576.

3. S. C. S. Sushruta, *Vaidya Jadavaji Trikamji Acharia* (Bombay, India: Sagar, 1938) cited in Carol Mensing, *The Art and Science of Diabetes Self-Management Education: A Desk Reference for Healthcare Professionals* (Chicago: American Association of Diabetes Educators, 2006), p. 208.

4. R. H. Lawrence, "The Effects of Exercise on Insulin Action in Diabetes," *British Medical Journal* 1 (1926): 648–653.

5. J. Tuomilehto, J. Lindstrom, J. G. Eriksson, et al., "Prevention of Type 2 Diabetes Mellitus by Changes in Lifestyle among Subjects with Impaired Glucose Tolerance," *New England*

Journal of Medicine 344 (2001): 1343–1350; Diabetes Prevention Research Group, "Reduction in the Incidence of Type 2 Diabetes with Lifestyle Intervention or Metformin," *New England Journal of Medicine* 346, no. 6 (2002): 393–403; X. R. Pan, G. W. Li, Y. H. Hu, et al., "Effects of Diet and Exercise in Preventing NIDDM in People with Impaired Glucose Tolerance: The Da Quing IGT and Diabetes Study," *Diabetes Care* 20 (1997): 537–544; and Diabetes Prevention Program, "Reduction in the Incidence of Type 2 Diabetes with Lifestyle Intervention and Metformin," *New England Journal of Medicine* 346, no. 6 (2002): 393–403.

6. K. Mulcahy, M. Maryniuk, M. Peeples, et al., "Diabetes Self-Management Education Core Outcomes," *Diabetes Education* 29, no. 5 (2003): 768–803.

7. Adapted from American College of Sports Medicine, *Exercise Management for Persons with Chronic Diseases and Disabilities* (Champaign, IL: Human Kinetic, 1997).

8. K. F. Eriksson and F. Lindarde, "Prevention of Type II Diabetes Mellitus by Diet and Physical Exercise: The 6-Year Malmo Feasibility Study," *Diabetologia* 34 (1991): 891–898; G. W. Heath, R. H. Wilson, J. Smith, and B. E. Leonard, "Community-Based Exercise and Weight Control: Diabetes Risk Reduction and Glycemic Control in Zuni Indians," *American Journal of Clinical Nutrition* 53 (1991): S1642–S1646; and S. H. Schneider, A. K. Khachadurian, L. F. Amorosa, et al., "Ten-Year Experience with an Exercise-Based Outpatient Lifestyle Modification Program in the Treatment of Diabetes Mellitus," *Diabetes Care* 15 (1992; Suppl. 4): 1800–1810.

9. W. D. McArdle, F. I. Katch, and V. L. Katch, *Essentials of Exercise Physiology* (Philadelphia: Lippincott Williams & Wilkins, 2004).

10. J. F. P. Wojtaszewki, B. F. Hansen, J. Gade, et al., "Insulin Signaling and Insulin Sensitivity after Exercise in Human Skeletal Muscle," *Diabetes* 49 (2000): 325–331; K. Cusi, K. I. Maezono, A. Osman, et al., "Insulin Resistance differentially Affects the PI 3-Kinase and MAP Kinase-Mediated Signaling in Human Muscle," *Journal of Clinical Investigation* 88 (2000): 797–803; and J. P. Kirwan, L. F. del Aguila, J. M. Hernandes, et al., "Regular Exercise Enhances Insulin Activation of IRS-1-Associated PI3K in Human Skeletal Tissue," *Journal of Applied Physiology* 88 (2000): 797–803.

11. McArdle et al., *Essentials of Exercise Physiology.*

12. K. E. Powel, "Physical Activity and the Incidence of Coronary Heart Disease," *Annual Review of Public Health* 8 (1987): 253–287.

13. B. S. McEwen, "Protective and Damaging Effects of Stress Mediators," *New England Journal of Medicine* 338, no. 3 (1998): 171–179.

14. A. L. Dunn, M. H. Trivedi, J. B. Kampert, et al., "Exercise Treatment for Depression: Efficacy and Dose Response," *American Journal of Preventative Medicine* 28, no. 1 (2005): 140–141. Between 30 and 35 minutes of aerobics, three to five times a week, reduced moderate depressive symptoms by almost 50 percent. See M. H. Trivedi, T. L. Greer, B. D. Grannemann, et al., "Exercise as an Augmentation Strategy for Treatment of Major Depression," *Journal of Psychiatric Practice* 12, no. 4 (2006): 205–213.

15. From a study done at Leeds Metropolitan University in Britain, reported by Wayne Kalyn, "The Best News in Fitness," *Parade*, April 23, 2006. Available at www.parade.com/articles/editions/2006/edition_04-23-2006/zfitness_news. Accessed July 2007.

16. Debbie Fentress and Ed Coord, "Live Fit: A Family-Friendly Guide to Getting More Physical Activity," *Diabetes Forecast* 58, no. 3 (2005): 49–53, 56–65.

17. This one's weird, but true. People who work out moderately three to five times a week reduced their chances of getting gum disease by 40 percent. M. S. Al-Zahrani, E. A. Borawski, and N. F. Bissada, "Increased Physical Activity Reduces Prevalence of Periodontitis," *Journal of Dentistry* 23, no. 9 (2005): 703–710; and Nabil F. Bissada, quoted in Kalyn, "The Best News in Fitness."

18. Many studies have found that exercise improves mental function in seniors with dementia. Two studies that came out in 2004 alone showed that merely walking appeared to reduce the risk of dementia in both men and women in their 70s and older. R. D. Abbott, L. R. White, G. Webster-Ross, et al., "Walking and Dementia in Physically Capable Older Men,"

Journal of the American Medical Association 12, no. 292 (2004): 1447–1453; J. Weuve, J. H. Kang, J. E. Manson, et al., "Physical Activity, Including Walking, and Cognitive Function in Older Women," *Journal of the American Medical Association* 12, no. 292 (2004): 1454–1461; Dr. Eric Larson, quoted in Nicholas Bakalar, "Fitness Delays Onset of Dementia," *New York Times*, May 23, 2006, available at www.nytimes.com/2006/05/23/health/23agin.html, accessed September 2007; and Laura Dehaven Baker, "Exercise: Can It Help You Think?" *Diabetes Forecast* 59, no. 2 (2006): 69–71.

19. According to the National Cancer Institute, physical activity appears to cut the risk of developing colon cancer by 40 to 50 percent, breast cancer by up to 40 percent, endometrial (uterine) cancer by 30 to 40 percent, and prostate cancer by 10 to 30 percent. *National Cancer Institute Factsheet.* Available at www.cancer.gov/newscenter/pressreleases/physical activity. Accessed August 2007.

20. National Heart, Lung, and Blood Institute, National Institute of Diabetes and Digestive and Kidney Diseases, and the National Institutes of Health, *Clinical Guidelines on the Identification, Evaluation, and Treatment of Overweight and Obesity in Adults* (Washington, DC: U.S. Government Printing Office, 1998).

21. Adapted from American College of Sports Medicine, *Exercise Management for Persons with Chronic Diseases and Disabilities.* Some of these principles were adapted from Ed D. Boyer, John L. Boyer, and Fred W. Kasch, *Adult Fitness Principles and Practices* (Mountain View, CA: Mayfield Publishing, 1970).

22. About 80 percent of people with diabetes are overweight, and many are dealing with neuropathy (nerve pain or numbness) and lower extremity, kidney, heart, or eye problems.

23. American College of Sports Medicine, *ACSM's Guidelines for Exercise Testing and Prescription*, 6th ed. (Philadelphia: Lippincott Williams & Wilkins, 2000).

24. Some people with tightly controlled diabetes—and experience—can get physically active in the 80–90 blood sugar range without risking hypoglycemia (low blood sugar), but unless you know this is true for you, we don't recommend it.

25. Mensing, *The Art and Science of Diabetes Self-Management Education*, p. 208.

26. V. Koivisto and P. Felig, "Effects of Leg Exercise on Insulin Absorption in Diabetic Patients," *New England Journal of Medicine* 298 (1978): 79–83.

27. R. Peter, S. D. Luzio, G. Dunseath, et al., "Effects of Exercise on the Absorption of Insulin Glargine in Patients with Type 1 Diabetes," *Diabetes Care* 28 (2005): 560–565.

28. Mensing, *The Art and Science of Diabetes Self-Management Education*, p. 307.

29. Susan McQuillan and Edward Saltzman, *The Complete Idiot's Guide to Losing Weight* (New York: Alpha Books, 1998), p. 189.

30. Sheila A. Ward, "Diabetes, Exercise, and Foot Care: Minimizing Risks in Patients Who Have Neuropathy," *Physician and Sportsmedicine* 33, no. 8 (2005).

31. Even people with type-1 diabetes can see drastic decreases in their insulin level with a proper PBD and daily activity.

32. Bariatric or weight loss surgery is not without major risks. In a study of Medicare recipients who underwent bariatric surgery of various types, mortality rates 30 days after the procedure were 3.7 percent for men and 1.5 percent for women. Mortality rates at 1 year were 7.5 percent for men and 3.7 percent for women. See D. R. Flum, L. Salem, J.A.B. Elrod, et al., "Early Mortality among Medicare Beneficiaries Undergoing Bariatric Surgical Procedures," *Journal of the American Medical Association* 294 (2005): 1903–1908.

33. T. L. Trus, G. D. Pope, S. R. Finlayson, "National Trends in Utilization and Outcomes of Bariatric Surgery," *Surgical Endoscopy* 19 (2005): 616–620.

34. Nanci Hellmich, "Anti-Fat Pill Goes Over-the-Counter: No 'Magic Bullet,' Experts Caution," *USA Today*, February 8, 2007: 1A. What about the so-called superpill or polypill, which generated so much hubbub in the summer of 2003? Headlines across America and Europe promised that this pill, a combination of drugs and vitamins, could add years to your life. See Jacqui Thornton, "Take a Pill and Live 12 Years Longer," *The Sun* (UK), June 27, 2003, p. 8; and Jeremy Laurance, "For Only 60p a Day, the 'Magic Bullet' That Could Prevent Heart Attacks and Strokes," *The Independent* (UK), June 27, 2003, p. 3.

35. L. M. Steffen, D. R. Jacobs Jr., J. Stevens, et al., "Associations of Whole-Grain, Refined-Grain, and Fruit and Vegetable Consumption with the Risks of All-Cause Mortality and Incident of Coronary Artery Disease and Ischemic Stroke: The Atherosclerosis Risk in Communities (ARIC) Study," *American Journal of Clinical Nutrition* 78 (2003): 383–390.

36. O. H. Franco, C. de Laet, A. Peeters, et al., "Effects of Physical Activity on Life Expectancy with Cardiovascular Disease," *Archives of Internal Medicine* 165 (2005): 2355–2360.

37. L. DiPietro, D. F. Williamson, C. J. Caspersen, et al., "The Descriptive Epidemiology of Selected Physical Activities and Body Weight among Adults Trying to Lose Weight: The Behavioral Risk Factor Surveillance System Survey, 1989," *International Journal of Obesity and Related Metabolic Disorders* 17, no. 2 (1993): 69–76.

38. Department of Human Biology, University of Limburg, Maastricht, Netherlands, "Digestion, Absorption and Exercise," *Sports Medicine* 15, no. 4 (1993): 242–257.

39. Wendy McLaughlin, ed., *American College of Sports Medicine (ASCM) Fitness Book,* 3rd ed. (Champaign, IL: Human Kinetics, 2003).

40. Adapted from Bob Anderson, *Stretching,* 20th anniversary rev. ed. (Bolinas, CA: Shelter, 2000), p. 11.

41. Vern Cherewatenko and P. Berry, *The Stress Cure* (New York: Collins, 2004); and K. E. Innes, C. Bourguignon, and A. G. Taylor, "Risk Indices Associated with the Insulin Resistance Syndrome, Cardiovascular Disease, and Possible Protection with Yoga: A Systematic Review," *Journal of the American Board of Family Practice* 18 (2005): 491–519.

42. "When the muscles of the neck and upper back become taut, blood flow from the heart to the head is impeded. As a result, thought, judgment, and decision-making are adversely affected. In turn, constrictions in the neck hamper optimum flow of the secretions from the brain back to the body." Dennis Deaton, *The Book on Mind Management,* 2nd ed. (Mesa, AZ: Quma Learning Systems, 2003), p. 196.

43. Bob Anderson, *Stretching* (Bolinas, CA: Shelter, 2006), p. 12.

44. Reported in Michael O'Shea, "Better Fitness," *Parade,* February 19, 2006. On the study's 16-week program, the guys didn't change their diet—but don't get any ideas!

45. K. A. Wiley and M. A. Fiatarone-Singhm, "Battling Insulin Resistance in Elderly Obese People with Type 2 Diabetes: Bring on the Heavy Weights," *Diabetes Care* 26 (2003): 1580–1588.

46. I Astrant, P. O. Astrand, E. Christensen, and R. Hedman, "Intermittent Muscular Work," *Acta Physiologica Scandinavic* 48 (1960): 448; Mayer et al., "A Comparison between Intermittent Versus Continuous Aerobic Training on Cardiorespiratory and Body Composition Responses in Sedentary Adults"; H. Mayer, D. DeRose, Z. Charles-Marcel, et al., "Hemodynamic and Metabolic Effects of Intermittent Versus Continuous Aerobic Training," *Medicine and Science in Sports and Exercise* 33, no. 5 (2001): S19; and T. M. McLellan and J. S. Skinner, "Blood Lactate Removal during Active Recovery Related to the Aerobic Threshold," *International Journal of Sports Medicine* 3 (1982): 224.

47. J. D. Branch, R. R. Pate, and S. P. Bourque, "Moderate Intensity Exercise Training Improves Cardiorespiratory Fitness in Women," *Journal of Women's Health and Gender-Based Medicine* 9 (2000): 65–73; I. M. Lee and R. S. Paffenbarger, "Associations of Light, Moderate and Vigorous Intensity Physical Activity with Longevity—The Harvard Alumni Study," *American Journal Epidemiology* 151 (2000): 293–299. J. Manson, F. Hu, J. Rich-Edwards, et al., "A Prospective Study of Walking as Compared with Vigorous Exercise in the Prevention of Coronary Heart Disease in Women," *New England Journal of Medicine* 341 (1999): 650–658; J. A. Romijn, E. F. Coyle, L. S., Sidossis, et al., "Regulation of Endogenous Fat and Carbohydrate Metabolism in Relation to Exercise Intensity and Duration," *American Journal of Physiology* 265 (1993): E380–E391; and A. Tremblay, J. A. Semoneau, and C. Bouchard, "Impact of Exercise Intensity on Body Fatness and Skeletal Muscle Metabolism," *Metabolism* 43 (1994): 814–818.

48. Astrant et al., "Intermittent Muscular Work."

49. Mayer et al., "A Comparison between Intermittent Versus Continuous Aerobic Training on Cardiorespiratory and Body Composition Responses in Sedentary Adults."

50. E. E. Hall, P. Ekkekakis, and S. J. Petruzzello, "The Affective Beneficence of Vigorous Exercise Revisited," *British Journal of Health Psychology* 7 (2002): 47–66.

51. P. M. Dubbert, "Exercise in Behavioral Medicine," *Journal of Consulting and Clinical Psychology* 60, no. 4 (1992): 613–618.

52. A. C. King, W. J. Rejeski, and D. M. Buchner, "Physical Activity Interventions Targeting Older Adults," *American Journal of Preventative Medicine* 15, no. 4 (1998): 316–333.

53. Statistical analysis done on data from patients attending the LCA 18-day program from March 2003 to December 2006. All values are statistically significant ($p < .001$).

54. P. O. Astrand and K. Rodahl, *Textbook of Work Physiology: Physiological Bases of Exercise*, 3rd ed. (New York, McGraw-Hill, 1986).

55. Ibid.

56. D. Costill, "Physiology of Marathon Running," *Journal of the American Medical Association* 221 (1972): 1024–1029; and J. Davi, P. Vodak, and J. Wilmore, "Anaerobic Threshold and Maximal Aerobic Power for Three Modes of Exercise," *Journal of Applied Physiology* 41 (1976), 544–550.

57. L. Gauvin and W. Rejeski, "The Exercise-Induced Feeling Inventory: Development and Initial Validity," *Journal of Sport and Exercise Psychology* 15 (1993): 403–423.

58. G. Borg, "Pyschophysical Bases of Perceived Exertion," *Medicine and Science in Sports and Exercise* 14 (1982): 377–381

59. D. J. Macfarlane, L. H. Taylor, and T. F. Cuddihy, "Very Short Intermittent vs. Continuous Bouts of Activity in Sedentary Adults," *Preventative Medicine* 43, no. 4 (2006): 332–336.

60. James A. Levine, "Nonexercise Activity Thermogenesis (NEAT): Environment and Biology," *American Journal of Physiology, Endocrinology, and Metabolism* 286 (2004): E675–E685.

61. R. Andersen, C. Crespo, S. Bartlett, et al., "Relationship of Physical Activity and Television Watching with Body Weight and Level of Fatness among Children: Results from the Third National Health and Nutrition Survey," *Journal of the American Medical Association* 279 (1998): 28–32.

62. Heinz Drexel, presentation to the American Heart Association 2004 Scientific Assembly, New Orleans, November 10, 2004) Abstract 3826.

63. Kristen Gerencher, "Burning Calories on the Job," *MarketWatch*, February 23, 2006. Available at www.marketwatch.com/news/story/coming-soon-desk-near-you/story.aspx?guid=%7B76AF581E-6C89-456E-86DC-59699C6B5FE0%7D. Accessed July 2007.

CHAPTER 9

1. M. de Groot, B. Pinkerman, J. Wagner, et al., "Depression Treatment and Satisfaction in a Multicultural Sample of Type 1 and Type 2 Diabetes Patients," *Diabetes Care* 29 (2006): 549–553.

2. Anthony Robbins, *Unlimited Power* (New York: Fireside, 1986), p. 4

3. M. R. Cobain and J. P. Foreyt, "Designing 'Lifestyle Interventions' with the Brain in Mind," *Neurobiology of Aging* 62S (2005): S85–S87.

4. Douglas Lisle and Alan Goldhamer, *The Pleasure Trap* (Summertown, TN: Healthy Living Publications, 2003), pp. 9–13.

5. Terry Burnham and Jay Phelan, *Mean Genes* (Cambridge, MA: Perseus, 2000), p. 60.

6. Lisle and Goldhamer, *The Pleasure Trap*, p. 158.

7. Ibid.

8. Did you know that it's fat that gives us the biggest brain buzz? Fat has the most calories per serving, so our brains and genes are wired to find it the most pleasurable. In the old days, more calories equaled more chance of survival. Burnham and Phelan, *Mean Genes*, p. 53.

9. Dan Baker and Cameron Stauth, *What Happy People Know* (New York: St. Martin's Griffin, 2004), p. 228.

10. S. Melamed, A. Shirom, S. Toker, and I. Shapira, "Burnout and Risk for Type 2 Diabetes: A Prospective Study of Apparently Healthy Employed Persons," *Psychosomatic Medicine* 68, no. 6 (2006): 863–869.

11. F. E. Van der Does, J. N. De Neeling, F. J. Snoek, et al., "Symptoma and Well-Being in Relation to Glycemic Control in Type II Diabetes," *Diabetes Care* 19, no. 3 (1996): 204–210. The team discovered that subjects with higher hemoglobin A_{1c} (HgA_{1c}) levels (showing higher average blood sugar levels over a 3-month period) were more likely to be in a bad mood and less likely to be in a state of general well-being compared to those with lower long-term blood sugar levels.

12. Marcia Hughes, *Life's 2% Solution: Simple Steps to Achieve Happiness and Balance* (Boston: Nicholas Brealey, 2006), p. 205

13. R. S. Surwit and M. S. Schneider, "Role of Stress in the Etiology and Treatment of Diabetes Mellitus," *Psychosomatic Medicine* 55, no. 4 (1993): 380–393.

14. T. Chandola, E. Brunner, and M. Marmot, "Chronic Stress at Work and the Metabolic Syndrome: Prospective Study," *British Medical Journal* 332 (2006): 521–525.

15. J. E. Williams, C. C. Paton, I. C. Siegler, et al., "Anger Proneness Predicts Coronary Heart Disease Risk," *Circulation* 101 (2000): 2034.

16. Matthew Kelly, *The Rhythm of Life: Living Every Day with Passion and Purpose* (New York: Fireside, 2005), p. 218.

17. R. S. Surwit, M. A. Tilburg, N. Zucker, et al., "Stress Management Improves Long-Term Glycemic Control in Type 2 Diabetes," *Diabetes Care* 25, no. 1 (2002): 30–34. Measurement was HgA_{1c}.

18. A. Attari, M. Sartippour, M. Amini, and S. Haghighi, "Effect of Stress Management Training on Glycemic Control in Patients with Type 1 Diabetes," *Diabetes Research and Clinical Practice* 73, no. 1 (2006): 23–28. Measurement was HgA_{1c}.

19. Earl Nightingale, "Earl Nightingale Quotes." Available at www.brainyquote.com/quotes/authors/e/earl_nightingale.html. Accessed July 2007.

20. Hughes, *Life's 2% Solution*, p. 205.

21. Kate Ruder, "Lousy Mood: A Link to Blood Glucose," *Diabetes Forecast*, November 2006, p. 22.

22. F. Talbot and A. Nouwen, "A Review of the Relationship between Depression and Diabetes in Adults: Is There a Link?" *Diabetes Care* 23, no. 10 (2000): 1556–1562; and L. C. Brown, S. R. Majumdar, and S. C. Newman, "Type 2 Diabetes Does Not Increase Risk of Depression," *Canadian Medical Association Journal* 175, no. 1 (2006): 42–46.

23. P. Lustman and R. Clouse, "Section III: Practical Considerations in the Management of Depression in Diabetes," *Diabetes Spectrum* 17 (2004): 160–166.

24. J. L. Jackson, K. DeZee, and E. Berbano, "Can Treating Depression Improve Disease Outcomes?" [Editorial], *Annals of Internal Medicine* 140, no. 12 (2004): 1054–1056.

25. P. J. Lustman, R. J. Anderson, K. E. Freedland, et al., "Depression and Poor Glycemic Control: A Meta-Analytical Review of the Literature," *Diabetes Care* 23 (2000): 934–942.

26. M. de Groot, R. Anderson, K. E. Freedland, et al., "Association of Depression and Diabetes Complications: A Meta-Analysis," *Psychosomatic Medicine* 63 (2001): 619–630.

27. D. L. Musselman, E. Betan, H. Larsen, et al., "Relationship of Depression to Diabetes Types 1 and 2: Epidemiology, Biology, and Treatment," *Biological Psychiatry* 54 (2003): 317–329.

28. R. J. Anderson, P. J. Lustman, R. E. Clouse, et al, "Prevalence of Depression in Adults with Diabetes: A Systematic Review," *Diabetes* 49 (2000; Suppl. 1): A64.

29. C. Fortes, S. Farchi, F. Forastiere, et al., "Depressive Symptoms Lead to Impaired Cellular Immune Response," *Psychotherapy and Psychosomatics* 72 (2003): 253–260.

30. B. W. Pennix, S. B. Krichevsky, K. Yaffe, et al., "Inflammatory Markers and Depressed Mood in Older Persons: Results from the Health, Aging and Body Composition Study," *Biological Psychiatry* 54 (2003); 566–572.

31. R. Ramasubbu, "Insulin Resistance: A Metabolic Link between Depressive Disorder and Atherosclerotic Vascular Diseases," *Medical Hypotheses* 59 (2002): 537–551.

32. D. J. Wexler, "Low Risk of Depression in Diabetes? Would That It Were So," *Canadian Medical Association Journal* 175, no. 1 (2006): 47.

33. Baker and Stauth, *What Happy People Know*, pp. 224, 228.

34. Aileen Ludington and Hans Diehl, *Health Power: Health by Choice Not Chance* (Hagerstown, MD: Review and Herald, 2000), p. 220.

35. National Institute of Mental Health, *Depression and Diabetes* [NIH Publication No. 02–5003] (Bethesda, MD: National Institutes of Health, U.S. Department of Health and Human Services, 2002).
36. Again, if you're experiencing chronic depression or thoughts of death or suicide, you should *contact a mental health professional immediately.* You needn't suffer this way!
37. National Institute of Mental Health, *Depression and Diabetes.*
38. P. J. Lustman, L. S. Griffith, K. E. Freedland, et al., "Cognitive Behavior Therapy for Depression in Type 2 Diabetes Mellitus: A Randomized, Controlled Trial," *Annals of Internal Medicine* 129, no. 8 (1998): 613–621.
39. Norman Vincent Peale, *The Power of Positive Thinking* (New York: Ballantine Books, 1996).
40. Ludington and Diehl, *Health Power,* pp. 216–217.
41. Dennis Deaton, *The Ownership Spirit Handbook* (Mesa, AZ: Quma Learning Systems, 2003), p. 14.
42. Lynn Clark, *SOS Help for Emotions: Managing Anxiety, Anger & Depression*, 2nd ed. (Bowling Green, KY: SOS Programs & Parents Press, 2005), pp. 21–27.
43. Edward Abramson, *Emotional Eating: What You Need to Know before Starting Another Diet* (San Francisco: Jossey-Bass, 2001), p. 69.
44. Albert Ellis and Windy Dryden, *The Practice of Rational Emotive Behavior Therapy*, 2nd ed. (New York: Springer, 1997), p. 204.
45. Ellis, *Reason and Emotion in Psychotherapy.*
46. REBT therapists call this one *awfulizing*, or, less artfully, *catastrophizing.*
47. Albert Ellis, *Techniques for Disputing Irrational Beliefs (DIBS)*, rev. ed. (New York: Institute for Rational-Emotive Therapy, 1994).
48. Viktor Frankl, *Man's Search for Meaning* (New York: Washington Square Press, 1985), comes to mind. Hope in the Holocaust? It's possible. It's what saved Frankl, even after he saw his family slaughtered.
49. David D. Burns, *The Feeling Good Handbook*, rev. ed. (New York: Plume, 1999), pp. 8–10.
50. Earl Nightingale, "Earl Nightingale Quotes." Available at www.brainyquote.com/quotes/authors/e/earl_nightingale.html. Accessed July 2007.
51. I. S. Rallidis, "Dietary Alpha-Linolenic Acid Decreases C-Reactive Protein, Serum Amyloid A, and Interleukin-6 in Dyslipidaemic Patients," *Atherosclerosis* 167, no. 2 (2003): 237–242; D. Lanzmann-Petithory, "Alpha-Linolenic Acid and Cardiovascular Diseases," *Journal of Nutritional, Health, and Aging* 5, no. 3 (2001): 179–183; B. Davis, *Essential Fatty Acids in Vegetarian Nutrition.* Available at www.vegetarian-nutrition.info/vn/essential_fatty_acids.htm. Accessed July 2007. D. R. Illingworth, "The Influence of Dietary N-2 Fatty Acids on Plasma Lipids and Lipoproteins, *Annuals of the New York Academy of Science* 676 (1993): 70–82. A. P. Simopoulos, "Essential Fatty Acids in Health and Chronic Disease," *American Journal of Clinical Nutrition* 70 (1999; Suppl.): 560S–569S; and M. De Lorgeril, "Mediterranean Alpha-Linolenic Acid-Rich Diet in Secondary Prevention of Coronary Heart Disease," *Lancet* 343, no. 8911 (1994): 1454–1459.
52. S. E. Hyman and M. V. Rudorfer, "Depressive and Bipolar Mood Disorders," in *Scientific American Medicine*, Vol. 3, ed. D. C. Dale and D. D. Federman (New York: Healtheon/WebMD, 2000), p. 13.II:1.
53. F. M.Gloth, W. Alam, B. Hollis, "Vitamin D vs. Broad Spectrum Phototherapy in the Treatment of Seasonal Affective Disorder," *Journal of Health, Nutrition, and Aging* 3, no. 1 (1999): 5–7.
54. G. W. Lambert, C. Reid, D. M. Kaye, "Effect of Sunlight and Season on Serotonin Turnover in the Brain," *Lancet* 360, no. 9348 (2002): 1840–1842.
55. E. Hypponen and C. Power, "Vitamin D Status and Glucose Homeostasis in the 1958 British Birth Cohort: The Role of Obesity," *Diabetes Care* 29, no. 10 (2006): 2244–2246.
56. M. L. Perlis, L. J. Smith, J. M. Lyness, et al., "Insomnia as a Risk Factor for Onset of Depression in the Elderly," *Behavioral Sleep Medicine* 4, no. 2 (2006): 104–113; and D. Riemann and U. Voderholzer, "Primary Insomnia: A Risk Factor to Develop Depression?" *Journal of Affective Disorders* 76, nos. 1–3 (2003): 255–259.

57. Tim Arnott, *Dr. Arnott's 24 Realistic Ways to Improve Your Health* (Nampa, ID: Pacific Press, 2004).

58. Ibid.

59. K. Spiegel, "Impact of Sleep Debt on Metabolic and Endocrine Function," *Lancet* 354, no. 9188 (1999): 1435–1439.

60. G. Lac, "Elevated Salivary Cortisol Levels as a Result of Sleep Deprivation in a Shift Worker," *Occupational Medicine* 53, no. 2 (2003): 143–145; and R. Rosamond, "Stress Induced Disturbances of the HPA Axis: A Pathway to Type 2 Diabetes," *Medical Science Monitor* 9, no. 2 (2003): 35–39.

61. Adapted from Neal Nedley, *Proof Positive: How to Reliably Combat Disease and Achieve Optimal Health through Nutrition and Lifestyle*, 4th ed. (Ardmore, OK: Author, 1999), p. 397.

62. Richard Wolf, "States Consider Tobacco Tax Hikes," *USA Today*, February 27, 2007. Available at www.usatoday.com/news/nation/2007-02-27-tobacco-tax_x.htm. Accessed July 2007.

63. B. Eliasson, "Cigarette Smoking and Diabetes," *Progress in Cardiovascular Diseases* 45, no. 5 (2003): 405–413.

64. P. Nilsson, S. Gudbjornsdottir, and J. Cederholm, "Diabetes and Tobacco—A Double Health Hazard," *Lakartidningen* 99, no. 20 (2002): 2281–2282, 2285.

65. Eliasson, "Cigarette Smoking and Diabetes."

66. D. Magis, I. Geronooz, and A. J. Scheen, "Smoking, Insulin Resistance, and Type 2 Diabetes," *Revue Médicale de Liège* 57, no. 9 (2002): 575–581; and Nilsson et al. "Diabetes and Tobacco."

67. G. Reaven and P. Tsao, "Insulin Resistance and Compensatory Hyperinsulinemia: The Key Player Between Cigarette Smoking and Cardiovascular Disease?" *Journal of the American College of Cardiology* 41, no. 6 (2003): 1044–1047.

68. There was no increase for patients with type-2 diabetes. P. McCulloch, S. Less, R. Higgins, et al., "Effect of Smoking on Hemoglobin A1c and Body Mass Index in Patients with Type 2 Diabetes Mellitus," *Journal of Investigative Medicine* 50, no. 4 (2002): 284–287.

69. Magis et al., "Smoking, Insulin Resistance, and Type 2 Diabetes."

70. C. Filozokc, M. C. Fernandez Pinilla, and A. Fernandez-Cruz, "Smoking Cessation and Weight Gain," *Obesity* 5, no. 2 (2004): 95–103.

71. Smoking cessation alone won't prevent or cure diabetes, which has several risk factors. See J. Tuomilehto, "Primary Prevention of Type 2 Diabetes: Lifestyle Intervention Works and Saves Money, but What Should Be Done with Smokers?" *Annals of Internal Medicine* 142, no. 5 (2005): 381–383.

72. Lisle and Goldhamer, *The Pleasure Trap*, p. 172.

73. S. M. Montgomery and A. Ekbom, "Smoking during Pregnancy and Diabetes Mellitus in a British Longitudinal Birth Cohort," *British Medical Journal* 324, no. 7328 (2002): 26–27.

74. M. Weitzman, S. Cook, P. Auinger, et al., "Tobacco Smoke Exposure Is Associated with the Metabolic Syndrome in Adolescents," *Circulation* 112 (2005): 862–869.

75. H. G. Koenig, "Religion, Spirituality, and Medicine: Application to Clinical Practice," *Journal of the American Medical Association* 284 (2000): 1708.

76. H. G. Koenig, M. McCullough, and D. Larson, *Handbook of Religion and Health* (New York: Oxford University Press, 2000), pp. 7–14.

77. Albert Ellis, *How to Stubbornly Refuse to Make Yourself Miserable about Anything, Yes Anything!* (New York: Lyle Stuart, 1988), p. 144.

78. Dennis Deaton, *The Book on Mind Management*, 2nd. ed. (Mesa, AZ: Quma Learning Systems, 2003), p. 147.

79. Maxwell Maltz, *Psycho-Cybernetics* (New York: Pocket Books, 1969), pp. 95–96.

80. U.S. Bureau of the Census, *Statistical Abstract of the United States 1998* (Washington, DC: U.S. Bureau of the Census, 1998).

81. D. P. O'Neill and E. K. Kenny, "Spirituality and Chronic Illness." *Image* 30, no. 3 (1998): 275–280.

82. T. P. Daaleman, A. Kuckelman Cobb, and B. B. Frey, "Spirituality and Well-Being: An Exploratory Study of the Patient Perspective," *Social Science & Medicine* 53, no. 11 (2001): 1503–1511.

83. K. M. C. Cline and K. F. Ferraro, "Does Religion Increase the Prevalence and Incidence of Obesity in Adulthood?" *Journal for the Scientific Study of Religion* 45, no. 2 (2006): 269–281; and K. F. Ferarro, "Firm Believers? Religion, Body Weight, and Well-Being," *Review of Religious Research* 39 (1998): 224–244.

84. To wit, a 1998 study by researchers at Purdue University looked at 2,500 people's weight and religion. Religious activity can promote obesity. Weight is highest in states where religious affiliation is highest. Of all the religious groups surveyed, Southern Baptists were heaviest, followed by Fundamentalist and Pietistic Protestants. Catholics were in the middle, and the lowest average body weight was found among Jews and other non-Christians. "Consolation and comfort from religion and from eating," the lead researcher wrote, "may be a couple of the few pleasures accessible." It is interesting that this study also found that modern religion did not inhibit gluttony or obesity. In fact, higher religious practice is more common among overweight people. See Cline and Ferraro, "Does Religion Increase the Prevalence and Incidence of Obesity in Adulthood"; and Ferarro, "Firm Believers? Religion, Body Weight, and Well-Being."

85. P. S. Mueller, D. J. Plevak, and T. A. Rummans, "Religious Involvement, Spirituality, and Medicine: Implications for Clinical Practice," *Mayo Clinic Proceedings* 76 (2001): 1225–1235.

86. Koenig, "Religion, Spirituality, and Medicine."

87. Psalms 46:10.

88. Proverbs 17:22.

89. Maltz, *Psycho-Cybernetics*, p. 96.

90. John 3:2.

91. Jeremiah 30:17.

92. James 5:15.

93. Carl Jung, *Modern Man in Search of a Soul*, trans. Cary Baynes (London: Routledge & Kegan Paul, 1933).

94. Kelly, *The Rhythm of Life*, p. 203

95. A. J. Palmer, S. Rose, W. G. Valentine, et al., "Intensive Lifestyle Changes or Metformin in Patients with Impaired Glucose Tolerance: Modeling the Long-Term Health Economic Implications of the Diabetes Prevention Program in Australia, France, Germany, Switzerland, and the United Kingdom," *Clinical Therapeutics* 26 (2004): 304–321.

96. If we live long enough, life is going to become stormy for all of us. Acceptance, again, is the first step to coping with life's storms. If we believe that there should be no storms in life, there should be no aberrant blood sugar levels, there should be no consequences for our diets and lifestyle, then when a storm comes, we will be totally unprepared for it. If, on the other hand, we accept uncertainly as a part of life, we will still experience healthy and appropriate emotions like sadness and disappointment, but we won't be destroyed by unexpected events.

97. Lisle and Goldhamer, *The Pleasure Trap*, pp. 163–172.

CHAPTER 10

1. Douglas Wood, *Paddle Whispers* (Duluth, MN: Pfeifer-Hamilton, 1993), p. 49.

2. M. Namdar, P. Koepfli, R. Gratwohl, et al., "Caffeine Decreases Exercise-Induced Myocardial Flow Reserve," *Journal of the American College of Cardiology* 47 (2006): 405–410.

APPENDICES

1. K. M. Narayan, "'Polypill' for Cardiovascular Disease Prevention," *Clinical Diabetes* 22 (2004): 157–158.

2. American Heart Association, *Know the Facts, Get the Stats 2007* [Pamphlet] (American Heart Association, 2007).

3. D. Ornish, S. E. Brown, L. W. Scherwitz, et al., "Can Lifestyle Changes Reverse Coronary Artery Disease? The Lifestyle Heart Trial," *Lancet* 336 (1990): 129–133.

4. D. B. Esselstyn Jr., "Updating a 12-Year Experience with Arrest and Reversal Therapy for Coronary Heart Disease: An Overdue Requiem for Palliative Cardiology," *American Journal of Cardiology* 84 (1999): 339–341.

5. American Cancer Society, *Cancer Facts and Figures* (Atlanta: American Cancer Society, 2007).

6. A. Tavani and C. La Vecchia, "Fruit and Vegetable Consumption and Cancer Risk in a Mediterranean Population," *American Journal of Clinical Nutrition* 61, no. 6 (1995; Suppl.): 1374S–1377S; E. Riboli and T. Norat, "Epidemiologic Evidence of the Protective Effect of Fruit and Vegetables on Cancer Risk," *American Journal of Clinical Nutrition* 78, no. 3 (2003: Suppl.): 559S–569S; and J. L. Slavin, "Mechanisms for the Impact of Whole Grain Foods on Cancer Risk," *Journal of the American College of Nutrition* 19, no. 3 (2000; Suppl.): 300S–307S.

7. D. A. Snowden, "Animal Product Consumption and Mortality because of all Causes Combined: Coronary Heart Disease, Stroke, Diabetes, and Cancer in Seventh-Day Adventists," *American Journal of Clinical Nutrition* 48 (1988): 739–748; and L. Chatenoud, C. La Vecchia, S. Francechi, et al., "Refined-Cereal Intake and Risk of Selected Cancers in Italy," *American Journal of Clinical Nutrition* 70 (1999): 1107–1110.

8. C. M. Freidenreich and M. R. Orenstein, "Physical Activity and Cancer Prevention: Etiologic Evidence and Biologic Mechanisms," *Journal of Nutrition* 132 (2002): 3456S–3464S.

9. American Heart Association, *Know the Facts, Get the Stats 2007*.

10. Ibid.

11. M. W. Gillman, L. A. Cupples, D. Gagnon, et al., "Protective Effect of Fruits and Vegetables on Development of Stroke in Men," *Journal of the American Medical Association* 273 (1995): 1113–1117; and K. J. Joshipura, "The Effect of Fruit and Vegetable Intake on Risk for Coronary Artery Disease," *Annuals of Internal Medicine* 134 (2001): 1106–1114.

12. A. V. Chobanian, G. Bakris, H. Black, et al., "The Seventh Report of the Joint National Committee on Prevention, Detection, Evaluation, and Treatment of High Blood Pressure," *Hypertension,* 42 (2003): 1206–1252.

13. Ibid.

14. W. P. Castelli, J. T. Doyle, T. Gordon, et al., "HDL Cholesterol and Other Lipids in Coronary Heart Disease: The Cooperative Lipoprotein Phenotyping Study," *Circulation* 55 (1977): 767–772.

15. Ibid; and C. B. Esselstyn Jr., "In Cholesterol Lowering, Moderation Kills," *Cleveland Clinic Journal of Medicine* 67, no. 8 (2000): 560–564.

16. J. McDougall, K. Litzau, E. Haver, et al., "Rapid Reduction of Serum Cholesterol and Blood Pressure by a Twelve-Day, Very Low Fat, Strictly Vegetarian Diet," *Journal of the American College of Nutrition* 14, no. 5 (1995): 491–496.

17. J. Kjeldsen-Kragh, "Rheumatoid Arthritis Treated with Vegetarian Diet," *American Journal of Clinical Nutrition* 70 (1999): 594S–600S.

18. A. P. Simopoulos, "Omega-3 Fatty Acids in Inflammation and Autoimmune Diseases," *Journal of the American College of Nutrition* 21, no. 6 (2002): 495–505.

19. Omega-Zen 3, available at www.veganessentials.com. Accessed July 2007.

20. National Osteoporosis Foundation, *Annual Report, 2003* (Washington, DC: National Osteoporosis Foundation, 2003).

21. B. Abelow, "Cross-Cultural Association between Dietary Animal Protein and Hip Fracture: A Hypothesis," *Calcified Tissue International* 50 (1992): 14–18.

22. L. A. Frassetto, "Worldwide Incidence of Hip Fracture in Elderly Women: Relation to Consumption of Animal and Vegetable Foods," *Journals of Gerontology: Series A, Biological Sciences and Medical Sciences* 55, no. 10 (2000): M585–M592.

Acknowledgments

THE THREE OF us are greatly indebted to the fine staff of Lifestyle Center of America (LCA), past and present, for their invaluable assistance while we put this book together. In particular, we wish to acknowledge: Sid Lloyd, Kevin Brown, Dr. Diana Fleming, Amy Hanus, Linda Kennedy, Linda Brinegar, Lonnie Carbaugh, Dan Braun, Al Trace, Ricky Seiler, Jim Pinder, Kaya Chong, J. P. Wegmuller, Holly Graves, George Krajewski, Michelle Jones, Harold Mayer, Larry Imes, Dr. Iris Paul, Dr. Myron Mills, Dr. George Guthie, Dr. Tim Arnott, Dr. David De Rose, and Dr. John Goley. Thanks to our photographic models, Dr. Teresa Sherard, Bonnie House, and Rico Flores; our photographer, Dave Smith; and our designer, David Hemmer. We also thank Dr. Floyd Petersen of the Loma Linda University School of Public Health, Department of Epidemiology and Biostatistics, for his enthusiastic assistance in reviewing our research data; and Megan H. Schrader, MS, dietetic intern, at the Oklahoma State University, Stillwater, Department of Nutritional Sciences, for her able research assistance. But mostly, this book would not have been completed without the tireless efforts of executive assistant Rosie Gagel (*vielen, vielen Dank!*). We're also grateful for the faith, discipline, and literary élan of our agent, Celeste Fine, at Folio Literary Management, who somehow pulled off a major book auction (now if only she would give up coffee and cigarettes!). Finally, we honor our priceless publisher at Perigee, John Duff, who believed in our miracle. Celeste and John, we thank you for taking LCA "off the hill!"

FRANKLIN HOUSE

TO MY WIFE, Bonnie, who has stood by me for 50 years, discovered with me the joys "of eating to live" in contrast to "living to eat," and in the process transitioned from an excellent meat cook to a gourmet plant-based cook.

To our three boys—Rick, Ray, and Rollin—who, as they grew up, put up with our lifestyle wanderings and who have adopted most of them as adults.

To our dog, Conji, a 10-year-old Basenji who twice daily demands a long, fast-paced walk. Conji gets most of the credit for our faithfulness to a decision made years ago to stay active.

To my patients in Killeen, Copperas Cove, Alpine, and Marfa, Texas, who shared with me their lives and sorrows and through whom I learned the difference between curing and healing. They drove my passion to learn and teach lifestyle choices for healing those who suffer with diabetes.

To everybody affiliated with Lifestyle Center of America, who welcomed me into their healing sanctuary and allowed me to lead, follow, and learn.

To Ian Blake Newman, without whose courage, passion, and ability this book would never have been written.

To the alumni of LCA, who repeatedly assure us that we are doing a good, life-changing thing.

STUART SEALE

TO MY MOTHER and father, who always encouraged and supported me in my efforts and dreams.

To my children, who inspired me to be introspective about my health and who were the motivating force I needed to make changes in my own lifestyle.

To my former patients and friends in my Springfield, Missouri, private practice. It was difficult to leave them when I joined LCA, and I am indebted to them for understanding my need for a career-path change. They will forever be my friends.

To Jane Henson, my receptionist, office manager, and right hand for more than 20 years in Springfield. Jane was supportive of my career move, even though it meant a change of career for her also.

To Sandra Bagge, my assistant and lifestyle coach in my current Sedona practice. Sandra gave valuable advice while helping me put my thoughts into words for this book, and she continues to inspire me daily.

To Sid Lloyd, and coauthors Franklin and Ian, who invited me to join this fantastic project, thus giving me the opportunity to change more lives than I ever imagined possible.

IAN BLAKE NEWMAN

FOR HIS DOGGED faith and support for the past 10 years and for his great good humor and luminous patience during my manifold illnesses and recoveries, I am indebted to my partner, David Hemmer.

For inspiring through his vibrancy and strength my commitment to help his generation prevent debilitating chronic diseases, I thank Kyle Werthmann.

For their generosity and grace beyond measure, I thank my parents, Maris and Steve Newman, who taught me how to hustle and gave me all I needed to transform any challenge—even cancer and type-1 diabetes—into an opportunity.

For granting me a much-needed sabbatical to complete this book, I thank the SUNY Rockland Community College administration and board of trustees.

And for their trust, which means more to me than I can say, I thank my own personal doctors without borders, Franklin House and Stuart Seale—healers, helpers, scholars, friends.

Index

Dr. Franklin House received his M.D. in 1962 from Loma Linda University. The founder of a multispecialty clinic, community hospital, and a long-term care company in Texas, Dr. House went on to hone his philosophy and skills in lifestyle medicine in the North Pacific island chain of Micronesia. He came to Lifestyle Center of America in 2000, first as its president, and now as chairman of the board.

●

Dr. Stuart A. Seale, a board-certified family physician who has been in private practice since 1983, served as lifestyle educator, medical clinic director, and staff physician at Lifestyle Center of America in Sulphur, Oklahoma. He currently resides in Sedona, Arizona, where he provides medical supervision and health education for patients who attend the LCA Diabetes Wellness Program, and for the WELL Experience, an advanced wellness workshop.

●

Ian Blake Newman is the author and editor of *Managing the College Newsroom*, which is used by more than seven hundred colleges and universities across the country. A contributor to numerous publications, he has twice been nominated for the Pushcart Prize. Newman first came to LCA in 2005 as a type-1 diabetes patient in search of a miracle. He found it.

Experience Lifestyle Center of America for Yourself

If you liked the advice in The 30-Day Diabetes Miracle and want to experience the added benefits of attending one of our residential programs, call a Stopping Diabetes Program specialist at **800.685.7310** or visit **www.diabetesmiracle.org** for more details.

FREE Special Offer

I would like to learn how to avoid the pitfalls of the most common diabetes treatments. Please mail me the booklet, *The Nine Costly Mistakes People with Diabetes Make... and How to Avoid Them!*

This offer is good while supplies last.

Mail requests to:
Lifestyle Center of America
Free Booklet
Rt. 1, Box 4001
Sulphur OK 73086

E-mail requests to:
freebooklet@lifestylecenter.org

Please provide name, full mailing address & phone number

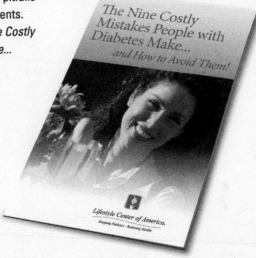

Lifestyle Center of America®

Stopping Diabetes - Restoring Health